Clinical Forensic Me

Clinical Forensic Medicine

3rd edition

Edited by

W.D.S. McLay

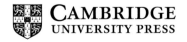

CAMBRIDGE
UNIVERSITY PRESS

CAMBRIDGE UNIVERSITY PRESS
Cambridge, New York, Melbourne, Madrid, Cape Town, Singapore,
São Paulo, Delhi

Cambridge University Press
The Edinburgh Building, Cambridge CB2 8RU, UK

Published in the United States of America by Cambridge University Press,
New York

www.cambridge.org
Information on this title: www.cambridge.org/9780521705684

First edition 1990
Second edition 1996 © GMM
Third edition 2009

Printed in the United Kingdom at the University Press, Cambridge

A catalogue record for this publication is available from the British Library

Library of Congress Cataloging-in-Publication Data

Clinical forensic medicine / edited by W.D.S. McLay. – 3rd ed.
    p. ; cm.
    Includes bibliographical references and index.
    ISBN 978-0-521-70568-4 (paperback)
1. Medical jurisprudence. I. McLay, W. D. S. (W. David S.) II. Title.
    [DNLM: 1. Forensic Medicine–Great Britain. W 700 C6415 2009]
    RA1051.C57 2009
    614'.1–dc22

                                           2008044169

ISBN 978-0-521-70568-4 paperback

Contents

Contributors

Anthony Busuttil OBE MOM KHS MD FRCPath FRCPE FRCPG FRCSE FFFLM DMJ [Path]
Regius Professor of Forensic Medicine Emeritus
University of Edinburgh, UK
Medical Director of Forensic Medical Examiner Service
NHS Lothian

Cathy Cobley LLB LLM [Wales]
Senior Lecturer in Law
Cardiff Law School
Cardiff, UK

Jack Crane MBBCh FRCPath FFPathRCPI DMJ [Clin et Path]
Professor of Forensic Medicine
at The Queen's University of Belfast, UK
State Pathologist for Northern Ireland

Peter Dean MBBS BDS [Hons] LLM FFFLM DRCOG DFFP
HM Coroner for Suffolk and South East Essex
Principal Forensic Medical Examiner
Metropolitan Police
London, UK

Victoria Evans LLM FFFLM MRCGP DMJ DFFP
Senior Consultant Forensic Physician
Greater Manchester Police
Manchester, UK

C. George M. Fernie LLB MBChB MPhil FFFLM FRCGP DFM
Medico-Legal Adviser
The Medical and Dental Defence Union of Scotland
Glasgow, UK

Peter J. Franklin MBBS LLM MA FFFLM DMJ
Senior Police Surgeon for Staffordshire Police
Honorary Lecturer in Clinical Forensic Medicine
Keele University, UK

Jeanne Herring MBBS BSc FFFLM DMJ [Clin]
Principal Forensic Medical Examiner
Metropolitan Police Service
Examiner to Worshipful Society of Apothecaries
for DMJ
Chief Examiner Faculty of Forensic and
Legal Medicine
Royal College of Physicians
London, UK

Judith A. Hinchliffe BDS DipFOd Hon FFFLM
Independent Forensic Dentist
UK and New Zealand

Ian Hogg
Chief Inspector
Scottish Police Services Authority Forensic
Services
Glasgow, UK

**The late Michael A. Knight MBE MBBS LLM FFFLM
MRCGP DMJ [Clin] DOccMed**
Former Force Medical Advisor
Suffolk Constabulary
Ipswich, UK

W.D.S. McLay OBE MBChB LLB FRCS FFFLM
Formerly Chief Medical Officer
Strathclyde Police and
Honorary Clinical Senior
Lecturer in Forensic Medicine
University of Glasgow, UK

Julie Mennell BSc PhD FFSSoc FInstMC FRSA PGCTLHE
Dean
School of Applied Sciences
Northumbria University
Newcastle, UK

Felicity Nicholson BSc MBBS FRCPath
Forensic Medical Examiner
Metropolitan Police
London, UK

**Guy A. Norfolk MBChB LLM FRCP FFFLM
MRCGP DMJ**
President
Faculty of Forensic and Legal Medicine
Royal College of Physicians
London, UK

**W.T.M. Ransom MSc FRCS MFFLM MRCGP
DRCOG DMJ**
Barrister-at-Law
Principal Forensic Medical Examiner
Metropolitan Police
London, UK

Gavin Reid MBChB BMSc [Hons] MRCPsych
Consultant Forensic Psychiatrist
Glasgow, UK

**Deborah J. Rogers MBBS FFFLM MRCGP MMJ DCH
DRCOG DFFP DMJ**
Forensic Physician
UK

Ian C. Shaw BSc
School of Applied Sciences
Northumbria University
Newcastle, UK

**Margaret M. Stark LLM MBBS FFFLM FACBS DGM
DMJ DAB**
Academic Dean
Faculty of Forensic and Legal Medicine
Royal College of Physicians
London, UK

Crispian Strachan CBE OStJ QPM DL MA
Formerly Chief Constable
Northumbria Police, UK

Robert Sunderland MD MBChB FRCP FRCPCH MFFLM
Consultant Paediatrician
Birmingham Children's Hospital
Birmingham, UK

Ian F. Wall MBChB [Hons] FFFLM FRCGP DMJ DOccMed
David Jenkins Professor of Forensic and Legal
Medicine
Faculty of Forensic and Legal Medicine
Royal College of Physicians
London, UK
Honorary Senior Lecturer in Forensic Medicine
and Bioethics
University of Central Lancashire
Preston, UK

Catherine White MBChB FFFLM MRCGP DMJ DRCOG DCH DFFP
Clinical Director
St. Mary's Sexual Assault Referral Centre
Manchester, UK

Michael Wilks MBBS FFFLM
Senior Forensic Physician
Metropolitan Police
London, UK

Preface

This third edition of *Clinical Forensic Medicine* has been regrettably slow in gestation. Each year, it seemed, impending major legislation affecting the work of the forensic clinician made delay necessary or justifiable, until delay became a habit.

More important than legislation has been the long-awaited establishment of the Faculty of Forensic and Legal Medicine at the Royal College of Physicians of London, under the presidency of Guy Norfolk, one of our authors. Another author, Ian Wall, is the first to occupy the chair set up in memory of the late David Jenkins, a stalwart of the Association of Police Surgeons. Other friends and colleagues are no longer with us, most poignantly the writer of Chapter 4, Michael Knight, who, with characteristic self-discipline, delivered a polished manuscript on time, and still found it possible to discuss other contributions before he died.

Thanks are, of course, due to all the authors. Several of these, and other colleagues who were not contributors, have given me advice on contentious matters (Vicky Evans, George Fernie, Judy Hinchliffe, Alistair Irvine, Archie McConnell, Jason Payne-James, Mac Ransom). I have not always taken that advice, so the responsibility for error lies with me.

During discussions with Cambridge University Press editors Nick Dunton and Laura Wood about format, the suggestion of a dedicated website emerged. Some material, mainly large figures and colour illustrations, will be posted there; this will help to keep down the cost of production and allow for periodic updating.

Lastly, putting authors' contributions in order has been the work of months, requiring great spousal tolerance.

Legal systems: a world view

W.T.M. Ransom

The English legal system is based on the *common law*. Consistency and predictability are assured by prior decisions of the courts on similar matters establishing judicial *precedent*. The continuing role of the courts is to apply and develop the common law. Statute law is created by Parliament and takes precedence over common law, Parliament being the supreme legal authority of the United Kingdom. This supremacy has been affected by the UK's membership of the European Union (EU), with European Law taking precedence over British Acts of Parliament (although it is still thought possible by many that Parliament could reassert its supremacy if it should so choose).

The alternative legal tradition in most of Europe is derived originally from the legal system of Ancient Rome, also known as *Civil Law* (the latter not to be confused with English 'civil law' which refers to non-criminal legal matters – see below). Over the centuries the code developed as a body of international law, the *ius commune* and was later codified in many countries as their own national expression of law. In contrast to common law precedent, consistency is achieved by judicial application and interpretation of the code, rather than prior case law decisions.

The United Kingdom exported the English legal system to its colonies, including the United States, and the countries of the Commonwealth. Most retained it after independence. By similar colonial expansion many countries of Europe established Roman law as the predominant legal system. Other nations, including Turkey and Japan, adopted Roman law as the basis of their legal systems. A few countries have systems exhibiting a mixture of common and Roman law elements.

A third international legal system is based on religious law, mainly the Sharia Law, derived from the Islamic faith, which exhibits many differences from Western systems, such as a prohibition on exacting interest. It is the basis of law in countries such as Saudi Arabia and Iran.

Wales shares the same common law tradition as England. Scotland had developed its own more Roman law-based tradition and continues with this system today (see Chapter 2). The modern law in Northern Ireland is also based on the common law, a consequence of the Plantation in the seventeenth century, followed by the Union of Great Britain and Ireland in 1801. After Partition in 1922, Northern Ireland retained the common law system.

Civil and criminal law

Most legal systems are divided into civil and criminal jurisdictions. Civil law regulates the conduct of persons (which can include 'corporate' persons such as companies) toward one another. Criminal law regulates conduct sufficiently unacceptable to

Clinical Forensic Medicine, third edition ed. W.D.S. McLay. Published by Cambridge University Press. © Cambridge University Press 2009.

society in general as to warrant the enforcement of penalties by the state. The law, procedural rules and courts which hear cases differ between civil and criminal jurisdictions in the United Kingdom.

Sources of law

The main sources of law in England and Wales are Parliament, the EU, and case law adjudicated by the courts.

Parliament

Statute law is enacted by Parliament. All Acts of Parliament must be passed by both Houses and receive Royal Assent. Statute law takes precedence over all other law. In addition to statute law (or *primary* legislation), Parliament passes a huge volume of *secondary* legislation, including Statutory Instruments and Bye-laws. The authority for these laws is derived from statute law. Such a mechanism enables the passage of many measures impracticable to enact fully as statutes.

Approved *Codes of Practice* issued by government departments comprise a special category. Such guidance has a quasi-legal status. Although not law, it can be admitted in court as evidence of recognized good practice; to disregard it could very rarely be justified. The most important examples for forensic physicians (FPs) are the Codes of Practice governing certain key areas of police procedure issued by the Home Office under the Police and Criminal Evidence Act 1984 (PACE), of which the most important is Code C governing the detention, treatment and questioning of suspects in police custody.

Legislation is also passed by representative bodies in the other UK nations. Since devolution in 1998 Scotland has its own Parliament whose responsibilities include criminal justice. Wales has a National Assembly capable of passing secondary legislation. Northern Ireland has recently seen devolved government restored, with an Executive and Legislative Assembly.

European Union (EU)

The United Kingdom acceded to the EU in 1973. Since then EU legislation has had growing effects on domestic law. The EU is governed by a Council of Ministers, has an elected Parliament, and is administered by a Commission from which all European legislation originates. *Regulations* automatically become the law in member states. *Directives* require member states to legislate to achieve the directive's intent.

The EU has traditionally not had much influence on the UK criminal justice system but this may change in future. A recent change has been the introduction of the European Arrest Warrant (Extradition Act 2003). An arrest warrant can be issued by a court in one member state, leading to the arrest of a suspect in another, and speedy extradition.

The European Court of Justice (ECJ) sits in Luxembourg. It should not be confused with the European Court of Human Rights (ECHR) in Strasbourg, which adjudicates on the European Convention on Human Rights. The ECJ is the final authority on European Law throughout member states, and its decisions take precedence over national law. Where UK law is found to be in conflict with European Law, the former must be changed. The UK courts may refuse to enforce a conflicting national law (*R* v. *Secretary of State for Transport ex parte Factortame* [1990] 2 AC 85).

Case law and the courts

The role of the courts is to determine the facts of a matter, and then apply the law in judgment. This involves application of both legislation and prior case law. Good legislative drafting should reduce the need for arguments about interpretation. Court judgments much more commonly involve case law.

Consistency results from judicial *precedent*, applying the legal principle of *stare decisis* ('let the decision stand'). This means that courts are bound to act in accordance with prior rulings in other courts when faced with similar facts. Judgments are published in the Law Reports. All will contain

Hierarchy of the Courts

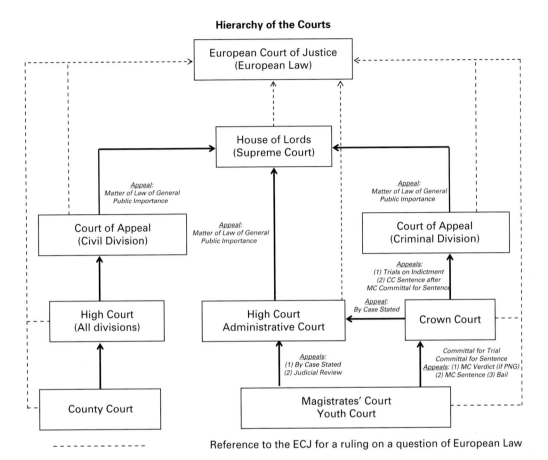

Fig. 1.1 Hierarchy of the courts. MC, magistrates' court; CC, Crown Court; PNG, Pleaded Not Guilty.

a kernel of legal reasoning known as the *ratio deci-dendi* (the 'reason for deciding'), which explains the legal principles applied. This is the part of the judgment creating the *binding* precedent. The remainder of the judgment is termed *obiter dicta* ('things said by the way'). This may influence other courts, so being persuasive, but is not binding. Identifying the *ratio* of a case is an important legal skill. For precedent to work in practice, a hierarchy of the courts allows more difficult matters to be appealed at a higher level. The court system differs for civil and criminal cases.

Traditionally the Judicial Committee of the House of Lords (HOL), comprising the most senior judges (the 'Law Lords'), formed the highest court in the United Kingdom (see Fig. 1.1). This arrangement has been criticized as diminishing the constitutional separation of the judiciary and the legislature. As a result of reforms enacted in the Constitutional Reform Act 2005, the HOL will soon be renamed the Supreme Court of the UK, and will become completely separate from Parliament. For similar reasons, the judicial role of the Lord Chancellor has now been abolished and replaced with that of a Minister for Constitutional Affairs, more recently subsumed into the new Ministry of Justice.

The HOL binds all the courts beneath it. No other court binds it (other than the ECJ on matters of European Law) and it can depart from its own previous decisions. The next highest court, the Court of Appeal, is bound by the HOL, but also by its own prior decisions, and again binds all courts beneath it (with the exception of criminal appeals, where the Court of Appeal has the power to disregard precedent when it is deemed to be in the overall interests of justice).

Below the Court of Appeal, the Divisional Courts and High Court are bound by the courts above them, create precedent for those below and are in general also bound by their own prior decisions. The magistrates' and county courts are bound by precedents set in higher courts, but do not create precedent, and are not bound by other decisions of similar 'lower' courts. The Crown Court binds magistrates' courts and is bound by the higher courts, but not by itself.

In 1997, following concern about miscarriages of justice, the Government established an independent body, the Criminal Cases Review Commission, to investigate such possible cases in England, Wales and Northern Ireland. A similar body exists in Scotland. Anyone can apply for a case to be considered, although stringent criteria apply to avoid frivolous applications. The Commission assesses allegations of injustice and whether convictions or sentences should be referred to the Court of Appeal. The Court of Appeal may also direct the Commission to investigate appeal cases.

Matters of European Law can be referred to the ECJ, and ECJ rulings bind all courts including the HOL. Such referrals are not appeals, but requests for guidance on application of European Law. The ECJ also adjudicates on disputes involving member states, and the Institutions of the EU.

Civil cases are generally heard first at the county court. However, if complex, or involving large sums of money, they may be heard first at the High Court, to which county court cases may also be appealed.

In civil cases in general appeals are made to the next level of judge up in the court hierarchy. A county court appeal lies from a district judge to a circuit judge (who may also sit in the county court) and thence to a High Court judge. Appeals from a High Court judge are heard by the Civil Division of the Court of Appeal, and thence in turn by the HOL.

Roughly 95% of criminal cases are heard in the magistrates' courts. Many are minor matters such as speeding or parking, and can be dealt with by the accused pleading guilty by post (s12 Magistrates Court Act 1980). Summary trial usually takes place before a panel of three lay persons appointed as magistrates, assisted by a legally qualified court clerk. In some larger courts, a salaried district judge replaces the panel.

After a first appearance in a magistrates' court, more serious 'indictable' offences will be sent for Crown Court trial. Transfers to Crown Court are now made by a simple 'allocation' procedure. (Sch. 3 Criminal Justice Act 2003 (CJA 2003)). Both the verdict and sentence of a magistrates' court may also be appealed to Crown Court. The prosecution also have limited rights of appeal. Appeals from Crown Court are heard by the Administrative Court, part of the Queen's Bench Division of the High Court. The sole ground for appeal is now that the conviction is 'unsafe' (s2 Criminal Appeal Act 1995). From the High Court cases may be appealed to the Criminal Division of the Court of Appeal, and from there in turn again to the HOL.

The youth court is effectively a specialized form of magistrates' court, in which procedure has been amended to make the court less intimidating for juveniles (who are classed as those under 18). It is one result of a widespread change in managing youth offenders since passage of the 1998 Crime and Disorder Act. New police powers were created to issue warnings and reprimands, and new sentences, including reparation and parenting orders were introduced. Juveniles have no power to elect Crown Court trial, and all matters except homicide can be tried before the youth court. Public access to youth court trials is not permitted and reporting strictly controlled.

The ECHR adjudicates on disputes involving issues of human rights as in the European Convention. Forty-five member states are signatories to the Convention, and half have incorporated the Convention into their national law, as Britain did with the 1998 Human Rights Act (HRA). This Act has enabled UK nationals to seek redress in the UK national courts for infringement of Convention rights. An appeal to the ECHR is only possible if domestic redress is exhausted. Detailed discussion of the Convention and HRA 1998 are outside the scope of this chapter but they have had far-reaching effects on UK law.

Criminal law and procedure

Investigation of crime

The criminal justice process begins with the suspicion that an offence has been committed. Upon receiving a report of an alleged offence the police, whose role is to uphold the law, will consider an investigation, dependent on the nature of the report, the gravity of the matter, and the resources available. The police are not the only body with power to investigate suspected crime, and other agencies may also do so, for example HM Revenue and Customs (HMRC) and Trading Standards.

Arrest

The Police and Criminal Evidence Act 1984, and the provisions of the PACE Codes of Practice, apply to all criminal investigations, ensuring a balance between the rights of suspects and the conduct of enquiries. Once individuals become 'suspects' they should be cautioned, before further questioning. The Police and Criminal Evidence Act 1984 powers of arrest have been substantially amended by s110 Serious Organised Crime and Police Act 2005 (SOCAPA) making all offences arrestable. Lawful arrest (without warrant) now requires the arresting officer to have formed an (objective) reasonable suspicion of guilt, a genuine (subjective) belief of probable guilt, and to believe that arrest is necessary. The necessity criteria are set out in PACE Code G para 2.4 to 2.9 and include such things as the need to prevent the person causing injury to himself or others, or damage to property, and the protection of children.

The Police and Criminal Evidence Act 1984 as revised also contains a new section 24A dealing with powers of arrest by persons other than a constable (so-called 'citizen's arrest'). These are of especial importance to the growing number of Police Community Support Officers (PCSOs) as well as workers in the security industry. Section 24A arrest powers apply only to indictable offences and it must also be impracticable for a constable to make the arrest, which must also be necessary, for example to prevent the suspect making off before a constable can assume responsibility for him/her.

Magistrates may also issue arrest warrants, usually when suspects fail to attend court, commonly called 'bench warrants'. If the magistrates are prepared to allow bail after arrest, they endorse the back of the warrant with the necessary conditions, and the warrant is then 'backed for bail'. Crown Court judges have similar powers.

A person must be told the reason for arrest as soon as practicable, after which they must be either bailed or taken to a police station suitable for detention purposes. Procedures at the police station, and the FP's role therein, are dealt with elsewhere in this book.

Decision to prosecute

The Crown Prosecution Service (CPS) is the body responsible for prosecuting criminal cases investigated by the police. When a decision is made whether to charge a person with an offence the CPS is responsible for this decision (s28 CJA 2003) in all but minor offences, and is now routinely consulted by the police before proceeding. The CPS decision is guided by the Code for Crown Prosecutors, which provides a test for decisions on prosecuting. There must be sufficient evidence to provide a realistic prospect of conviction (on the balance of probabilities), and the public interest must lie in favour of prosecution.

Adversarial trial process

In English law the trial process is an adversarial one, which tests the competing claims of the parties, rather than 'searching for the truth'. Each party presents their case, with the evidence to support it, and may seek to discredit the other party's case. The role of the judge is to ensure proper conduct between the parties. By contrast, the trial process in many civil (Roman) law systems is an inquisitorial one, characterized by a search for facts. In both systems, the court is normally the vehicle for determining the conclusion or verdict, and also the appropriate remedy or sentence.

Offence categories and mode of trial

Criminal cases follow a path through the courts determined by which of three categories they fall into. *Summary* offences are heard in the magistrates' court, including relatively minor matters such as obstructing police, and in the absence of a guilty plea will be listed for summary trial. Offences *triable only on indictment* (TOI) are immediately sent to the Crown Court for trial before a jury, and include the most serious offences, such as murder and rape. Several preparatory hearings frequently occur before the actual trial date.

In the third category of offences, *triable either way*, a further hearing will be held in the magistrates' court to determine where the trial will take place (Mode of Trial Determination – MOTD), depending on the seriousness of the offence, and the magistrates' sentencing powers in the event of a conviction. National guidelines from the Sentencing Guidelines Council help magistrates reach consistent decisions.

At the MOTD hearing the accused is offered the opportunity to enter a plea. If the plea is Guilty, the magistrates' court moves straight either to sentence (or to committal to Crown Court for sentence if the

magistrates consider their powers inadequate). If the plea entered is Not Guilty, the MOTD hearing proceeds. If the court decides that summary trial is appropriate, the accused can accept this, or elect for Crown Court trial instead. The effect of this procedure is that both court and accused must agree for summary trial to take place.

From the perspective of the accused, the main considerations will be that conviction rates in the magistrates' court are much higher (some studies suggest 70% or more) than in the Crown Court before a jury (somewhat less than 50%). However, if convicted, the sentencing options available at the Crown Court are much more stringent, including longer terms of imprisonment and heavy fines. A careful exercise in balancing the possible outcomes and sentences is necessary, with legal advice essential to making the best choice.

Criminal procedure reforms

Significant recent changes have taken place in the management of all criminal cases with the introduction of the Criminal Procedure Rules 2005 to govern all aspects of handling cases. An accompanying Consolidated Criminal Practice Direction consolidates all previous such directions. The system has introduced a stated overriding objective that criminal cases be dealt with justly, with active case management by judges and magistrates to speed up the court process. Plea and Case Management (PACM) hearings have been introduced to enable more efficient case management.

Juries

The main difference between trials in the Crown and magistrates' court is in the role of the jury. Magistrates and judges both serve as *tribunal of law* in their courts, applying the law to the facts laid before them in evidence. Magistrates also serve as the *tribunal of fact*, reaching conclusions on the facts and thus the verdict. However, the tribunal of fact in the Crown Court is the jury, which alone determines the verdict, and may acquit even when it appears the facts must lead to a conviction. This is a central part of the system of protection afforded to the accused. Some civil cases may also be heard by a jury (see below).

Recent reforms mean that, with very few exceptions such as the mentally ill, almost all adults on the electoral roll are eligible for jury service. Selection is at random and made by computer. In certain sensitive cases, those selected may be vetted by guidelines issued by the Attorney General. The jury must not discuss the case with other people and their deliberations must remain secret (Contempt of Court Act 1981). A unanimous verdict is always sought first, but if this cannot be reached after a reasonable interval, a majority verdict of not less than ten to two is permitted. This may be reduced to nine to one if jurors have been discharged in the course of the trial. Up to three jurors may be discharged during a trial (requiring a unanimous verdict of the remaining nine) before the jury must be dismissed and a retrial ordered (s16 Juries Act 1974).

Magistrates' court trial

In the magistrates' court the charges are put to the accused and the plea is taken. The prosecution may then make an opening speech giving an overview of the case. Usually this is confined to a brief account of the alleged facts of the offence(s), or foregone altogether. The prosecution then calls its witnesses, who take the oath (or affirm), and are then questioned by the prosecution; this is *examination in chief*, and the witness gives his *evidence in chief*.

After each witness is heard the defence can then question or *cross-examine* them. Finally the prosecution can make a brief further *re-examination*. Written statements agreed by both parties are read into the record.

At the end of the prosecution case the defence may make a submission of 'no case to answer', if insufficient evidence has been advanced to prove one of the essential facts for conviction or the evidence given has been discredited. If a no case submission is not made, or fails, the defence will then

present their case, by calling witnesses as did the prosecution. The accused must be called first if giving evidence. The defence must ensure that they 'put their case' to the court, that is adduce evidence to support all aspects of that case. Any facts advanced by the prosecution that the defence does not dispute are deemed accepted. The defence usually does not make an opening speech, saving their submissions for a closing speech, and thus having the last word.

The magistrates then retire to reach a verdict. If a guilty verdict is announced, unless then committed to the Crown Court for sentence, the case is usually adjourned. Typically this is for three or four weeks to obtain pre-sentence reports, before sentence is passed.

Crown Court trial

In the Crown Court the charge is put and plea taken (the *arraignment*) at a PACM hearing. At the start of the trial a jury is empanelled by selection of 12 jurors from a larger pool who enter court. Those selected, unless challenged, are then sworn. The indictment is then read to the jury and they are advised of the not guilty plea.

It may be asserted that the accused is unfit to plead, which has a specific meaning in law, namely that the accused is incapable of understanding the proceedings, and thus cannot advance a defence, follow the evidence, or instruct counsel (*R* v. *Podola* [1960] 1 QB 325). Under the Criminal Procedure (Insanity) Act 1964 (as later amended), the judge must hear evidence and determine the issue. If then found unfit to plead, the court proceeds to trial and the jury has to establish whether the accused committed the criminal act (*actus reus*) of the offence. If so, an order for detention in a secure hospital will normally be made.

Unlike the magistrates' court, the prosecution always make an opening speech giving the jury an overview of the case. Prosecution witnesses are then examined and cross-examined as in the magistrates' court. At the conclusion of the prosecution case, the defence may make a 'no case' or 'half-time' submission on similar grounds to the magistrates' court.

The defence may object to part of the prosecution evidence. Where possible such questions are resolved in preliminary hearings, but if they occur during a trial a hearing may be held to determine the matter in the absence of the jury, commonly called a *voir dire* (a trial within a trial). The position differs in the magistrates' court, where the bench are also the tribunal of fact, and the guiding principle is to ensure the fairness of the proceedings. Once a decision on admissibility is made, witnesses may require warning and written statements may require editing to exclude matters not admissible.

In complex cases the defence may start their evidence with a speech outlining their case, but if no witnesses to fact other than the accused (and any character witnesses) are to be called, the right to a defence opening speech is lost. The defence witnesses are then examined and cross-examined. As in the magistrates' court, the accused must be called first if giving evidence. Where multiple defendants are being tried, their defence cases are heard in the order in which their names appear on the indictment. A closing speech is sometimes made by the prosecution and always by the defence. The judge then sums up the case by instructing the jury on their role, on the applicable law and by summarizing the evidence. The jury then retire to consider their verdict.

Sentencing

Following conviction, sentence is passed. Magistrates and judges work within clear guidelines issued by the Sentencing Guidelines Council on their sentencing powers, such as the relevant aggravating and mitigating factors which should be considered and the credit to be given for an early guilty plea. Any significant departure from these is likely to form grounds for an appeal. The sentences available include fines, custody, community sentences and costs orders. Compensation orders may be awarded to victims.

Civil procedure

Civil law comprises actions brought by claimants against defendants in the county court or the High Court, which may lead to the award of remedies, such as damages and/or costs. Since 1999 the structure of civil justice has been radically reformed with the introduction of the Civil Procedure Rules, and an overriding objective to ensure that the courts deal with cases *justly*, ensure efficiency and save costs. These changes were the forerunner of the Criminal Procedure Rules, which have similar objectives. The rules provide a uniform framework for both county and High Court actions, which used to be subject to different rules and procedures.

The most common civil actions are for recovery of debt, recovery of land and personal injury. However, those most likely to involve FPs are actions against the police for assault, unlawful arrest, false imprisonment and malicious prosecution (the latter two classes of action are normally tried before a jury). In addition there is the risk of a medical negligence action directly involving the FP.

Such actions may be commenced several years (sometimes decades) after the events giving rise to them. Thus it is essential that the FP keep detailed notes on all the cases he sees and retains these for many years (effectively for life). Of particular importance are the notes kept on the injury or lack of injury resulting from the application of handcuffs, strikes by asps and batons, and the use of control and restraint agents such as CS spray and the Taser (Thomas A. Swift's electronic rifle). Where such methods have been employed it is unwise to rely on saying the absence of notes indicates normality, which can be made to sound a very weak assertion in court.

Claimant solicitors make an initial assessment of the possible claim, including potential costs. If the claimant proceeds, the solicitor arranges detailed investigation of the claim and assembly of relevant evidence, including witness statements. In certain types of case, including medical negligence, this process has been streamlined through the introduction of *pre-action protocols* enabling efficiency in the exchange of information and the use of experts.

The action commences with issue of a Claim Form (formerly a *writ*) served on the defendant, followed by details (the *particulars*) of the claim. The defendant must then acknowledge receipt of this and/or file a defence, or risk judgment being awarded against him/her in default. If either the original case or the defence is weak, either party may seek, or the court itself may enter, a summary judgment to bring proceedings to a close and minimize costs. Alternative Dispute Resolution by arbitration, mediation, or conciliation may also be suggested.

If the action proceeds it is then allocated to one of three tracks according to its value and complexity: the small claims track in the county court deals with sums less than £5000; fast track cases are usually allocated to the county court and deal with sums of between £5000 and £15000; multi-track cases of more than £15000 value may be allocated to the High Court.

Evidence is then disclosed by the parties, and the court may give directions for further such disclosure, including that of expert evidence. A trial date is eventually fixed. At the hearing the judge, who will have read the papers, will sometimes forego an opening address, otherwise the claimant's advocate makes an opening speech. Witness statements are in a standard form containing a signed statement of truth. These will usually simply be tendered as evidence in chief, and the witnesses then called are submitted to immediate cross-examination. After closing speeches judgment is given either immediately or after an adjournment. The judge may then award damages, make other remedial orders and award costs.

Case preparation and the law

For a criminal conviction, three things must normally be established, namely a criminal act (*actus reus*), an accompanying mindset (the *mens rea* – guilty mind) and the absence of an accepted defence. A prosecution lawyer confronted with criminal case papers will first determine what offences have been charged, and then examine the law to determine what are the above *elements* making up the offence(s). All the elements must be proved for a conviction to be established, and each has its own legal background. Alongside this there must be no recognized defence, of which there are a number of established legal categories, each with its own legal framework.

Once the offence(s) and the law are clarified, the next step will be to review the evidence to establish what are asserted to be the facts of the matter, and in particular those which are disputed. Applying the law to the facts will enable a prosecution lawyer to determine what facts must be proved to enable a conviction, and then to assess the strength of the evidence available to prove those facts. Those that must be proved and are disputed are the *facts in issue* of the case. A defence lawyer will perform the same exercise but with a view to disproving some of the facts in issue such that at least one element of the offence is not established, or a defence is proved.

A similar process underlies civil actions. For example, in a negligence action, success with a claim requires proof of four components; the existence of a duty of care, a breach of that duty, damage or harm and a causal link between breach and the damage.

The law of evidence

In an apocryphal legal tale, an English judge is said to have become impatient when witness after witness produced conflicting accounts before him. 'Am I never to hear the truth?' he finally asked a barrister. 'No my Lord, merely the evidence', replied counsel.

Evidence is information by which facts tend to be proved or disproved, by persuading a court of the probability of the facts asserted. Evidence can be of several forms, such as witness evidence, documentary evidence and real evidence (objects like clothing or specimens). Circumstantial evidence suggests the truth of a fact by inference rather than by direct observation.

Evidence must be both relevant and admissible. Evidence is relevant if it logically helps to prove or disprove some fact at issue in the case (*R* v. *Sang* [1980] AC 402). It is admissible if it is related either directly or circumstantially to the facts at issue, and (in general) has been properly obtained. The *weight* of evidence is how much probative effect it has.

For many years the English approach to evidence has tended to be exclusionary in nature, to provide safeguards against unfairness, particularly in criminal prosecutions. For example there were stringent restrictions on admissibility of evidence of the defendant's previous convictions. Such restrictions were aimed at preventing both undue prejudice against the accused, and reducing the risk of concocted or improperly obtained evidence.

In recent years the trend has been less protective, especially in the civil courts where most cases are heard before a judge rather than a jury. This change in approach has now also extended to large areas of criminal evidence. The Criminal Justice and Public Order Act 1994 (CJPOA) made the accused's right to silence subject to possible adverse inferences. The CJA 2003 has now allowed much wider admissibility of both hearsay and bad character criminal evidence, subject to certain restrictions.

Witness evidence

Witnesses are *competent* if they can be allowed to give evidence. They are *compellable* if they can be made to do so by law. In general everyone is considered both competent and compellable. Criminal defendants are competent but not compellable in their own defence, or that of co-defendants.

In civil actions spouses are competent and compellable. In criminal cases the defendant's spouse is competent and compellable as a defence witness. For the prosecution, he/she is competent but becomes compellable only in certain categories of offence that involve domestic violence or sexual abuse. He/she cannot be compelled in any case where he/she is a co-defendant.

Children (those under 18 – s105 Children Act 1989) (ChA) in civil cases are competent to give evidence on oath if they understand the nature of the oath and the duty it embodies (*R* v. *Hayes* [1977] 2 All ER 288). If not, they can give evidence unsworn if they understand their duty to be truthful, and have sufficient understanding to be heard (s98 ChA 1989). In criminal cases persons of all ages are competent unless they do not understand questions put to them and cannot give answers that can be understood (s53 Youth Justice and Criminal Evidence Act 1999) (YJCEA). Children under 14 give criminal evidence unsworn. Over the age of 14, they are presumed able to give evidence sworn (if disputed this is determined by a test similar to the Hayes test for civil cases – s55 YJCEA 1999).

The competence tests for mentally subnormal persons as criminal witnesses are similar to those for children. In civil cases, however, if a person does not satisfy the Hayes test there is no provision for them to give evidence unsworn, and they are deemed incompetent to testify.

Testimony in court

The aim of examination in chief is to elicit a witness's contribution to the story of the case. The technique permitted is *direct* questioning – using questions which do not suggest the response sought. An alternative form of impermissible questioning is the *leading* question – one suggesting a particular response. To speed the process a few simple leading questions will often be asked at the start of examination in chief, provided the other party agrees, where these relate to what may be uncontested matters such as simple names and dates.

The aim of cross-examination is to amend or undermine the prosecution's case and the technique permitted now includes leading questions. A final and usually very brief re-examination may follow to further clarify any matters raised in cross-examination, and leading questions are again not allowed. The same rules apply in reverse when the defence presents its case. It can only ask direct questions, and the prosecution can cross-examine with leading ones. Special rules apply to some forms of cross-examination. There are rules to prevent cross-examination of complainants in sexual offence cases on their past sexual experience, unless special exceptions apply (ss41–3 YJCEA 1999).

Notes and memory refreshment

In view of the time likely to have elapsed between relevant events and trial, witnesses are permitted to refresh their memory in the witness box by reference to notes made contemporaneously with the events in question. Contemporaneity is not literal, but means the document was made when the evidence is still fresh in the mind of the maker (*R* v. *Richardson* [1971] 2 QB 484).

The original notes should be used, which are then available for inspection in court. If counsel decides to cross-examine the witness on matters in the notes document beyond those used for memory refreshment, the document may be seized and made an exhibit, relevant to the witness's credibility (*Senat* v. *Senat* [1965] P 172). This might occur, for example, where the notes show alterations that raise suspicions that the contents do not accurately reflect the original matters recorded. For this reason, deletions made at the time contemporaneous notes are created should not obscure the original content, but merely make clear the amendment. Any subsequent amendments made later to such notes should always be signed and dated, and the reason should also be either self-evident or clearly recorded.

A witness may also refresh his/her memory by rereading any statement he/she made, before going before the court. If the witness does this, he/she should ensure counsel are told, so they can advise their opponent. Such a documentary statement will not normally be made contemporaneously and therefore may not normally be used in the witness box.

Vulnerable witnesses

Sections 16–33 YJCEA 1999 allow the use of special measures to assist vulnerable witnesses, such as the very young, and those at risk of intimidation. In some cases examination in chief can be given by video recording, and cross-examination performed by live video link. Witnesses present in court may be screened from the accused and the public. Gowns and wigs may be removed and the public excluded. The defendant conducting his/her own case is not permitted to cross-examine sexual offence complainants and some child witnesses (ss34–9 YJCEA 1999). In some cases other witnesses may be permitted to give evidence via live link, though not the defendant (s51 CJA 2003).

Burden and standard of proof

The burden of proof is the *obligation* to prove a fact in issue. The burden generally rests with the party bringing the case ('he who asserts must prove' – *Wakelin* v. *LSWR* (1886) 12 App Cas 41 HL). It is also known as the *legal* or *persuasive* burden. In criminal cases the prosecution bear this. The accused is innocent until proved guilty, and the prosecution must prove the case against him/her (*Woolmington* v. *DPP* [1935] AC 462 HL).

The standard of proof is the probative effect required to persuade the court and measures the quality of the evidence. In criminal cases the prosecution must prove their case 'beyond reasonable doubt' (another term for this level of proof is commonly used in judicial directions, that the jury must be 'satisfied so that they are sure' (*R* v. *Kritz* [1950] 1 KB 82 CCA)).

In civil cases the standard is the 'balance of probabilities'; the tribunal of fact must conclude the facts asserted are more probable than not to accept them (*Miller* v. *Ministry of Pensions* [1947] 2 All ER 372). However, this standard may vary in some civil cases, with the requirement of a degree of probability commensurate with the occasion (*Hornal* v. *Neuberger Products* [1957] 1 QB 247). This *sliding scale* version of the balance of probabilities has now replaced 'beyond reasonable doubt' as the standard of proof required in professional misconduct hearings at the General Medical Council.

A different burden is the *evidential* burden. This is the obligation to adduce *sufficient* evidence to justify admissibility of a fact by a court. The prosecution bears this burden and failure to fulfil it may lead to a 'no case' submission. It also lies upon the defence when seeking to plead a formal defence, such as duress or self-defence. Once the defence fulfils this burden, on the balance of probabilities, the prosecution then assumes the legal burden of disproving that defence beyond reasonable doubt.

The only exceptions to this for the defence are where insanity is pleaded as a defence, or some statutory exceptions (as for instance under s2 Homicide Act 1957 on a charge of murder where the accused bears the legal burden of proving a defence of diminished responsibility). In such exceptional cases, the standard of proof required of the defence remains the balance of probabilities.

Presumptions, admissions, notice and corroboration

Some facts do not require proof in legal proceedings. Presumptions arise when admission or proof of a *basic* fact means another may be presumed proved and may be of fact or of law. Those of fact express normal logic, for example that people are thought to intend the natural consequences of their actions.

Presumptions of law may be rebuttable or irrebuttable. An irrebuttable presumption is that children under the age of 10 years (in Scotland, 8 years) cannot be guilty of committing a criminal offence (s50 Children and Young Persons Act 1933). Once the age of the child is established the presumption cannot be challenged. A rebuttable presumption is that a child conceived during wedlock is the child of the woman's husband.

Formal admissions of facts made by any party in accordance with either Rule 14 Civil Procedure Rules or s10 CJA 1967 are accepted as conclusive. Facts may be judicially 'noticed' when they are such common knowledge for proof to be unnecessary, and may also be established by judicial enquiry, for example the diplomatic status of a foreign national (*Engelke* v. *Mussmann* [1928] AC 433 HL).

Corroboration is the confirmation of the reliability of one item of evidence by another. It used to be necessary for judges to warn juries about the risks of conviction upon the uncorroborated evidence of certain witnesses, such as children and sexual offence complainants. This requirement was abolished by s34 CJA 1988 and s32 CJPOA 1994. Corroboration warnings are now optional. Corroboration is only required when imposed by statute, as in cases of speeding where a person cannot be convicted by the evidence of a single witness (s89 Road Traffic Regulation Act 1984).

Hearsay evidence

Hearsay in criminal proceedings is defined as 'a statement not made in oral evidence in court, that is relied on as evidence of matter stated in it' (s212(2) CJA 2003). In civil proceedings the definition is similar (s1(2) Civil Evidence Act 1995)(CEA).

A functional example: suppose A wishes to give evidence stating that B told him/her (A) that he/she (B) saw C commit the crime. If A's words are allowed as evidence that C committed the crime, this would be hearsay. Where possible B should be called to give evidence in court that he/she saw C commit the crime.

The main objection to a hearsay statement is it cannot be challenged in cross-examination. Other objections to hearsay include the increased risk of concocted evidence, which may be higher still with multiple (second-, third- or fourth-hand) hearsay. Article 6(3)(d) of the European Convention on Human Rights reinforces the right to examine witnesses as part of a fair hearing. Breaches of Article 6(3)(d) may occur if hearsay evidence is admitted as the sole criminal evidence for a conviction, or where the defence has no opportunity to contradict or discredit it adequately (*Trivedi* v. *UK* [1997] EHRLR 521).

On the other hand, evidence of almost conclusive reliability may be hearsay. A number of exceptions to the exclusionary rule evolved at common law or were legislated. Common law exceptions have included statements in public records, such as birth and death certificates, expert works of reference, confessions, expert opinion and dying declarations (this last category now abolished by the CJA 2003). Despite this the rules remained complex, confusing and increasingly outmoded.

As a result, the rule was first restricted and then abolished in civil proceedings (s1(1) CEA 1995). In criminal proceedings the law has been radically reformed and widened by the CJA 2003; the common law rule has been removed and hearsay evidence will now be admissible provided certain safeguards are met. Hearsay made by persons is admissible as criminal evidence if it is admissible by statute (including s118 CJA 2003 which preserves some of the old common law exceptions), by agreement of the parties, or in the interests of justice. Section 116 largely replaces the old s23 CJA 1988 provisions where witnesses are unavailable through death, illness, residence abroad and intimidation. Section 117 replaces the s24 CJA 1988 provisions for business document admissibility.

Statement includes 'any representation of fact or opinion made by a person by whatever means' (s115(2) CJA 2003) and so now includes documents and sketches (unlike the old common law position which did not (*R* v. *Cook* [1987] QB 417). Word-processed statements are representations, so are also included. The definition does not encompass statements produced by machine as a result of human information input; admissibility of these requires the input information be proved accurate (s129 CJA 2003). This operates alongside a common law rebuttable presumption that the machine in question will have been operating properly (as for example was established for breath testing machines in *Castle* v. *Cross* [1985] 1 All ER 87 DC).

Machine-produced statements automatically recorded without human input are not hearsay, but real evidence. A document is 'anything in which information of any description is recorded' (s134(1)

CJA 2003); thus a tape or video of a person describing a crime they had committed would be a document, but real evidence, and not hearsay. The old s69 PACE which treated computer evidence as a special case was repealed by s60 YJCEA 1999.

A strict insistence that all witnesses be present in court to give oral evidence would cause a great deal of inconvenience. Section 9 CJA 1967 allows documentary hearsay in the form of witness statements, signed by their maker, and containing a declaration of truth, to be admitted when both parties to litigation consent. (See also page 46.)

Confessions

A confession is any statement, made to any person, which may be in words or actions and which is wholly or partly adverse to the person who made it (s82(1) PACE 1984). Significant tensions arise when considering the issues governing admissibility of confessional evidence. If unrestricted, such admissibility would undoubtedly aid the efficient disposal of cases. However, it would also create a serious risk of unwarranted and oppressive conduct at the hands of the police.

Confessional evidence was traditionally admissible at common law, as an exception to the rule against hearsay, on the basis that a person is unlikely to bear false witness against him- or herself. This principle, however, failed to recognize the risk of suggestion or coercion of the psychologically vulnerable being employed to obtain a false confession.

It is a fundamental principle of most civilized jurisdictions that any confession should be made freely, and with full knowledge of legal rights. It is on this principle that the statutory regulations in PACE are predicated, particularly with reference to the exclusion of confessional evidence under s76, s78 and s82, and the care of detainees under the attached Codes of Practice.

The admissibility of confessions is now governed by s76(1) PACE. This makes confessions admissible in criminal trials but subject, in particular, to s76(2). Section 76(2) provides that if anyone (usually the defence) suggests to the court that a confession to be admitted by the prosecution was obtained by oppression of its maker, or by anything else at the time which made it unreliable, it should not be admitted unless the prosecution prove (beyond reasonable doubt) that the confession was not obtained this way (the truth of the confession is irrelevant (*R* v. *Crampton* [1991] Crim LR 277 CA).

Oppression, under s76(2)(a), is defined in s76(8) PACE (in words similar to those of Article 3 of the ECHR) as including torture, violence or degrading behaviour. Other definitions have included unreasonable, burdensome, cruel and unjust treatment of subjects by those in authority. Alongside such objective concepts of the meaning of oppression, the court will also consider subjective influences such as the character and experience of the suspect (*R* v. *Seelig* (1992) 94 Cr App Rep 17 CA); for example, the effect of detention on a suspect will undoubtedly differ between first-time offenders and professional criminals.

Unreliability as grounds for exclusion under s76 (2)(b) must have resulted from something said or done (or omitted) in the overall circumstances applying, and includes consideration of the characteristics of the accused (such as age). The wording means that something external to the accused must have influenced him/her (e.g. police impropriety), and not merely something internal. Accordingly confessions made and later retracted by individuals who then claim they were suffering from drug withdrawal, and had confessed in order to get out of police detention quickly to deal with withdrawal, will not necessarily be regarded by the courts as unreliable. Such stresses have been held to be a factor internal to the accused (*R* v. *Goldenberg* (1988) 88 Cr App Rep 285 CA).

However, a confession may be excluded under s76(2)(b) if the detainee has been given medication (an external factor) which is held to have adversely affected his/her mind at interview as in *R* v. *Sat-Bhambra* ([1988] Crim LR 453) where the detainee was given Valium by a doctor prior to interview. In similar situations, where medication is necessary, and there is a realistic possibility of possible adverse effects on fitness to interview, the

appropriate course is reassessment of the detainee after the medication has taken effect, and prior to interview. Such confessions may also be excluded under discretionary powers in ss78 and 82 PACE. Confessional evidence may in exceptional circumstances be excluded even when there is no suspicion of police impropriety, as where the accused's mental state or physical condition is disordered.

Admissibility is assessed in a *voir dire*, in the absence of the jury, and if the confession is excluded the jury are never told of it. Even if the prosecution is able to discharge the burden of proof for admissibility under s76, the judge still has a discretion to exclude such evidence under the statutory provisions s78 PACE, where the test is whether allowing admission of the confession would have an adverse effect on the fairness of the proceedings. Less commonly, exclusion may be ordered under s82(3) PACE which preserves the pre-PACE common law power of the court to exclude evidence. Both ss78 and 82 PACE have an application beyond confessions and can be invoked to exclude any relevant evidence.

The issue of confessional evidence has become increasingly important in clinical forensic medicine. An increased awareness of the psychology of confessions has resulted in requests by the police for FPs to assess detainees' fitness to be interviewed. Any true confession made at interview may be later regretted and retracted, with the accused arguing that he/she was labouring under a physical or mental handicap at the time of the admissions.

Conversely, false confessions made by innocent individuals labouring under psychological or psychiatric disability have lead to more than one celebrated case of a miscarriage of justice. This issue is particularly acute in England and Wales where a person may be convicted on the evidence of his/her own confession alone, and in the absence of any other incriminating evidence (*R* v. *Mallinson* [1977] Crim LR 161). In consequence, the medical assessment is most likely to be challenged in court where the confession is the only evidence against the accused. In Scotland and the USA, in contrast, independent corroborative evidence is always required in order to warrant a conviction. The reader is referred further to Gisli Gudjonsson's *The Psychology of Interrogations, Confessions and Testimony* [1] and *R* v. *Ward* [1993] 619, 96 Cr App Rep 1 CA.

Character evidence and past convictions

Good character essentially means 'no previous convictions' (usually equivalent also to 'only spent' or 'very minor' convictions). The admission of good character evidence is governed by common law, and may be relevant both to the accused's credibility (whether he/she is believable) and his/her propensity (his/her tendency to commit an offence of the kind charged).

Before passage of the CJA 2003 the law largely prevented admission of evidence of the accused's bad character, including his previous convictions. Exceptions at common law allowed discretionary admission of so-called 'similar fact' cases in restricted circumstances. Some statutory exceptions existed under the provisions of s1(3) CEA 1898. Evidence of previous misconduct by another witness was admissible if relevant to his credibility.

The CJA 2003 abolished the old common law rules, and repealed s1(3) CEA 1898. The new Act defined bad character (in s98) as 'evidence of, or of a disposition towards, misconduct' other than that related to the facts of the case, but including any in relation to its investigation or prosecution. Misconduct is defined broadly in s112(1) CJA 2003 as 'commission of an offence or any other reprehensible behaviour'. It includes both previous convictions, acquittals, and charges not pursued.

A new inclusionary framework was enacted, with admission of the accused's bad character possible without leave through a number of 'gateways' though notice of the intent to use this evidence must be given. The seven gateways in s101 CJA 2003 include the agreement of the parties, relevance to the accused's propensity to be untruthful or to commit offences, and attacks made on the character of other persons. A residual

discretion to exclude is created, alongside that under s78 PACE.

For all other witnesses, bad character evidence can now only be given either by agreement of the parties, or by leave of the court (when it must be either important explanatory evidence in the context of the allegations, or have a substantial probative value).

The right of silence

Traditionally at common law no guilt could be inferred from an accused's silence. This was part of the privilege against self-incrimination, which is an element of the right to a fair trial guaranteed under Article 6(1) of the European Convention (*Murray* v. *UK* 1996 22 EHRR 29). However there were longstanding concerns that experienced criminals were exploiting the right to silence to obtain unjust acquittals. This pressure led to the passage of the CJPOA 1994 which made it possible for a court to draw adverse inferences from the accused's silence, thereby discouraging both deliberate silence as a tool to evade questioning, and the refusal to testify. The inference that may be drawn is that the defence was fabricated after the initial investigation. Remaining silent on legal advice may not protect the accused as the reasons for the advice will need exploration. The judge retains an exclusionary discretion under s34 CJPOA for example, where there is a breach of PACE or the Codes of Practice.

Adverse inference can also be drawn under s62 (10) PACE from a suspect's refusal to consent to provide intimate samples.

Similar provisions have been in operation in Northern Ireland since the Criminal Evidence (NI) Order 1988.

Opinion and expert evidence

Ordinary witnesses in court confine themselves to giving evidence to which they were eye witnesses (that is of fact), and not what they believe (that is opinion). Otherwise they risk usurping the role of the court by inviting it to accept their opinion, rather than forming its own. Nevertheless in many cases, the court must reach judgments involving complex matters beyond the experience of those present. Expert witnesses assist the court by giving opinion evidence on such matters, which typically involves the use of knowledge acquired by extensive experience or training.

When instructed, experts should request a clear outline of the issues on which their expertise is sought, and be sure that they are suitably qualified for the task. They have an overriding duty to the court to provide unbiased opinion evidence, and should never become an advocate for the party instructing them. Unlike ordinary witnesses to fact, experts can sit in court prior to giving evidence to hear other witnesses' evidence of fact. Inadequate performance by an expert may damage the proper conduct and outcome of a trial, and may lead to criticism by the judge, or worse the referral of the expert to a relevant professional body, such as the GMC (*Meadow* v. *General Medical Council* [2006] EWCA Civ 1390).

Experts should also be aware of the legal framework in which they work, and of the content of the Civil Procedure Rules Rule 35 and the Code of Guidance on Expert Evidence. Those in the criminal courts should also be familiar with Rule 33 of the new Criminal Procedure Rules.

Sudden infant death syndrome

One area of special recent concern has been the use of expert medical evidence in homicide cases which may instead have been due to sudden infant death syndrome (SIDS). The Court of Appeal in *R* v. *Cannings* ([2004] 1 All ER 725 CA) stated that in cases of multiple sudden infant deaths in the same family, the exclusion of known natural causes of death does not establish that death resulted from harm, but rather that its cause remains unknown. The court also said that, in investigations of such multiple deaths, where there is disagreement between experts, and some hold that natural causes cannot be excluded, a prosecution for murder

should not be started without support from adequately weighty additional extraneous (non-expert) evidence.

It should be noted that the same caution about commencing proceedings should not apply to civil care proceedings (*Re U (a child) (serious injury: standard of proof)*; *Re B (a child) (serious injury: standard of proof)* [2004] EWCA Civ 567, [2004] 2 FCR 257 CA)), however some considerations from *R* v. *Cannings* were applicable, such as the fact that recurrence is not in itself probative, and caution should be exercised in the use of medical expert evidence.

Privilege and public immunity

Privilege is the right to refuse to testify or withhold evidence. It has three modern expressions in English Law.

The privilege against self-incrimination is a long-standing common law right, whose rationale is to discourage mistreatment of suspects, and improperly obtained confessions. It applies to witnesses at common law in criminal proceedings, but does not apply to the accused who decides to give evidence. It allows a person to refuse to answer any question that would tend to expose the person to proceedings. If improperly disregarded this may breach Article 6 of the European Convention (*Saunders* v. *UK* (1996) 23 EHRR 313).

Privileged statements made 'without prejudice' apply between opposing parties in a civil dispute. They protect disclosures made in potential settlement negotiations, which would otherwise be at serious risk of being damagingly admitted in subsequent hearings. A party can therefore make statements 'without prejudice' to future hearings if agreement is not eventually reached.

Legal professional privilege is a common law right but also embodied in s10 PACE. It applies to communications between client (or his/her agent) and legal adviser for the purpose of legal advice (*legal advice privilege*). A variant form also applies to communications between either client or adviser and any third party where the dominant purpose is for litigation (*litigation privilege*), whether criminal or civil. However litigation privilege is only protected if the dominant purpose of the communication is prospective or actual use in litigation. The privilege does not protect communications to facilitate crime.

Third party expert reports remain privileged if unused (if used they will be disclosed and thus no longer privileged), with the exception of cases involving child welfare (where the paramount interests of the child require disclosure of all reports, including unfavourable ones). The privilege continues after conclusion of any proceedings. For doctors who provide expert reports for use in proceedings, this does not affect the separate issue of the obligations of professional confidentiality.

Public interest immunity applies to documents (usually but not always emanating from government), which may be excluded from admission as evidence by the courts.

This is either on grounds that their disclosure would be damaging to the public interest (usually national security or diplomatic matters), or that this would hinder 'proper function of the public service'. The court makes the decision (*Conway* v. *Rimmer* [1968] AC 910). In public prosecutions the names of informers, and those who assist police surveillance teams by allowing use of their premises, can be protected by the same means (*Marks* v. *Beyfus* (1890) 25 QBD 494).

REFERENCE

1. Gudjonsson GH. *The Psychology of Interrogations, Confessions and Testimony: A Handbook*. Chichester, John Wiley, 2002. ISBN-10 0470844612; ISBN-13 978-0470844618.

2

Scottish legal system

C. George M. Fernie

History

The Treaty of Union of 1707 provided for the retention of a separate system of law in Scotland, particularly where this concerned private rights. The extent to which the Roman-Dutch element in Scots law has persisted since, despite the loss of legislative understanding at Westminster, is a tribute to the strength of a system based on principle rather than on precedent, which inspires Anglo-Saxon common law. Not only is Roman law influence still felt, it remains entirely competent to appeal to the ancient institutional writers' statements of valid law when apparent gaps are identified during a case. When a civil litigant appeals to the House of Lords as the highest civil appeal court (no such appeal is competent in criminal cases) the case is heard on the basis of Scots law. Since 1876 there has been at least one Law Lord from the Scottish Bench. This appeal function will be transferred to the proposed UK Supreme Court when the Constitutional Reform Act 2005 comes into effect.

Corroboration has long been a supremely important principle but, in civil cases, facts can now be provided by evidence from a single source. Hearsay evidence is competent, though not desirable (Civil Evidence (Scotland) Act 1988). In the criminal sphere, with a few statutory exceptions, an accused may not be convicted on the testimony of a single witness, but corroboration is not required if the accused can be shown to have 'special knowledge' of a crime, that is to say, cannot have known details unless they themselves perpetrated the crime. Another well-known peculiarity of criminal evidence is that of mutual corroboration, now usually referred to as the *Moorov* (1930 JC 68) doctrine. Here a series of crimes, which could not be proved individually, may mutually corroborate one another, as in a series of individual sexual assaults against separate women – in other words, a course of conduct. The case of *HMA* v. *Khaliq* (1984 SLT 137) where the accused was convicted of selling glue-sniffing kits to children, often in exchange for stolen goods, is an example of the flexibility of the system. The defence argued that such a crime was unknown to the law of Scotland. The Court ruled that the act was a species of real injury and said that the law would always respond to new manifestations of criminality.

Criminal jurisdiction

Lay Justices of the Peace, sitting in the district court, deal with very minor common law and statutory offences, where a legal assessor advises them on the law. In Glasgow, many cases in the district court are heard by stipendiary magistrates, whose powers in summary cases are the same as a sheriff sitting alone. Sheriffs, most of whom are advocates,

Clinical Forensic Medicine, third edition ed. W. D. S. McLay. Published by Cambridge University Press. © Cambridge University Press 2009.

are professional judges who hear both civil and criminal cases. Criminal cases are heard in the sheriff court either summarily or by a jury of 15 (solemn procedure) when the accused (known as the 'panel') is charged on indictment. Minor exceptions apart, prosecution is a public duty under the control of the Lord Advocate, and the accused has very little choice of forum, nor does he/she pay costs if convicted. Some statutory authorities, for example the factory inspectorate, may institute prosecutions, but these are very unusual.

The Carol X case (*X* v. *Sweeney* 1982 JC 70) is a rare instance of private prosecution. The Crown declined to proceed with a case where several youths were accused of rape on the basis of advice that the complainer's suicidal tendency might be exacerbated by the strain of a trial. She was later able to show that she had recovered, and was successful in an application to the High Court for a Bill of Criminal Letters, permitting her to mount a private prosecution leading to conviction. The Lord Advocate had disqualified himself from prosecuting, having acted publicly on the previous advice, but afforded Miss X the whole facilities of the Crown Office once the Court had allowed her bill. It is thought that, without such aid, bringing a private prosecution would be all but impossible. Legal aid is not available in such proceedings.

Trials for particularly serious crimes, including the 'pleas of the Crown' – such as murder, rape, treason – must be heard on indictment in the High Court. The High Court sits in Edinburgh, but the judges regularly go on circuit to other cities and towns as necessary. All serious cases in the locality, and certainly those where the penalty is likely to be greater than may be imposed by a sheriff (five years for some cases heard on indictment, although he/she may remit a convicted accused to the High Court for sentence if he/she considers his/her own powers insufficient), are included in a calendar to be tried before an appropriate sitting of the High Court. The jury's verdict is by simple majority. A *not proven* verdict has the effect of acquitting the accused; from time to time campaigns are mounted against the continuation of this verdict on the

ground that it establishes neither guilt nor innocence, but the concept has found favour with a previous Lord Chief Justice of England on the basis that no-one is ever tried on no evidence – the only question for the Court is therefore whether the case is proved or not. The Criminal Procedure (Amendment) (Scotland) Act 2004 has amended the strict time limits intended to safeguard an imprisoned accused: committal to prison must be followed by the service of an indictment within 80 days, a preliminary hearing must be held within 110 days (40 days in the case of summary trials) and the trial itself must begin no later than 140 days. From time to time procedural mistakes are made, and the accused must be liberated. The Crown may show cause why the period should be extended, but the Court will look critically at any such application.

Since 1993 solicitors who have passed further examinations to satisfy the Court have rights of audience in the Supreme Courts, where they are known as solicitor-advocates. They are recognizable in court by the lack of a wig. Sheriffs and High Court judges are addressed as 'My Lord' or 'My Lady' and magistrates as 'Your Honour'.

Appeal from any court of first instance is to the High Court of Justiciary, in its capacity as Court of Criminal Appeal. Appeals are always heard in Edinburgh, the bench being composed of three judges, which may be increased to five or seven in particularly important or contentious cases. The right of appeal has existed only since 1926, partly due to the influence of Sir Arthur Conan Doyle, who took a great interest in the case of *Oscar Slater* (1928 JC 94) who was convicted of murder, but later exonerated by the new court. The House of Lords has no jurisdiction, but the new Supreme Court (Constitutional Reform Act 2005) may alter the criminal appeal process.

Procurator fiscal (see also Chapter 18)

The Crown Office and Procurator Fiscal Service (COPFS) is responsible for the prosecution of crime in Scotland, the investigation of sudden or suspicious deaths and the investigation of complaints against the police. The strategic aim of this organization is to serve the public interest, prosecuting cases independently, fairly and effectively.

The fiscal is a qualified lawyer and a member of the civil service. They have a large measure of independence within their own sheriff court district. Their office is situated within or near the sheriff court. The number of deputes, who perform much of the routine business, will depend upon the volume of work. The duties of fiscals include the investigation of criminal complaints brought to them, usually by the police. They scrutinize reports and statements; they may instruct officers on further lines of enquiry; they ensure that expert opinion beyond the resources of the police force is obtained; they may interview (precognosce) witnesses, or have them seen on their behalf by clerks. Such a witness's statement to a fiscal is not given upon oath; inconsistencies between what he/she has said during precognition and what he/she subsequently says in court may not be referred to. Police statements may be put to officers if they say something different in evidence (a 'prior inconsistent statement'). During their investigations, the fiscals have power to bring witnesses thought to be prevaricating before a sheriff, when answers must be given under oath or affirmation.

He/she deals directly with *summary cases* by serving a *complaint* on the accused who may plead guilty or stand trial, usually at a later date. About two weeks before the trial, the accused appears at a *Preliminary Hearing* to confirm his/her plea and to check on how well prepared is the defence. At this stage, a plea bargain may be struck between the accused's agent and the fiscal. The prosecution is led by one of the depute fiscals.

The Crown Office

Statements, reports and the written views of the fiscal form the *precognition* on which decisions about prosecution are made. In certain, mainly serious, cases the precognition is sent to the Crown Office in Edinburgh for consideration by one of the advocates depute who, if the case merits trial in the High Court, has the responsibility of leading for the Crown. Some types of case are invariably considered personally by the Lord Advocate or the Solicitor General (both of whom are government ministers although the Lord Advocate no longer sits in Cabinet) and either may lead in particularly difficult cases, or where considerations of the public interest are especially important. When proceedings are to be taken on indictment, this document is served in the name of the Lord Advocate (the case is called '*HMA* v. *So-and-so*') and narrates the circumstances giving rise to the charge. It is unnecessary to name the crime alleged, although in suitable cases, the narration will include the phrase, 'and did murder him/her'. During a trial in the High Court, the fiscal acts as solicitor to Crown Counsel.

Cases may be sent back to the fiscal for further enquiry, the papers may be marked 'no proceedings' or the fiscal may be instructed him/herself to prosecute (on indictment if the matter is serious enough, or by way of summary complaint before a sheriff sitting alone). The fiscal has authority in more minor cases not to take proceedings; this power has allowed the development of diversionary schemes where, as a matter of public policy, it has been decided that measures other than prosecution could be more effective. Since the end of 1996, for certain statutory offences, the fiscal has had extended powers to offer payment of a 'fiscal fine' to an accused instead of going to the expense of pre-trial procedure. The fiscal may also issue a warning or offer the chance of referral for specialist support or treatment. These alternatives to prosecution mean the accused doesn't get a formal criminal record, members of the public are spared the inconvenience of attending as witnesses, and courts are freed up to spend time dealing with more serious cases.

Solemn cases

More serious matters are set out in a *petition* to the sheriff who grants a warrant for the detention of the accused, for his/her *judicial examination*, the summoning of witnesses and so forth. The judicial examination before a sheriff gives the accused an opportunity to make a declaration about the allegations; the prosecutor examines the accused with a view to eliciting denial, admission, explanation or justification and questions him about any alleged confession. The accused need not answer, but their silence may be commented on at their trial, unless they are silent on the advice of their solicitor (agent). The solicitor, too, may question the accused. Following this examination, the accused must be granted bail, unless accused of treason or murder, or there are objections from the Crown.

Their next appearance in court is at a *preliminary hearing* in the High Court or a *first diet* in the sheriff court, unless they are applying for bail after incarceration. These appearances allow the Court to assess progress in preparing the case and the setting of a trial diet. If the accused is committed to prison at the judicial examination, the indictment narrating the alleged events together with a list of witnesses and productions (that is to say documents and material evidence such as weapons or stained garments) must be served with 80 days, to allow them or their solicitor adequate time to prepare their defence. Failure to serve the indictment timeously gives the accused the right to liberty forthwith. This requirement puts immense pressure on the police, forensic scientists and the fiscal, as does that other limitation on the time – six hours – during which an arrested person may be detained by the police (s14 Criminal Procedure (Scotland) Act 1995) before a charge is brought or the prisoner released. In preparing a defence, the solicitor is entitled to precognosce all the prosecution witnesses. This right is a main argument against the wholesale disclosure of unused evidence which so exercises the English courts.

At a solemn trial the Crown, in the person of an advocate depute (in the High Court) or the procurator fiscal (in the sheriff court) leads evidence first, calling witnesses in turn, with no preliminary statement. Witnesses are cited in advance, and will generally receive at least 48 hours notice. Medical and other expert witnesses should take care to ascertain exactly when to attend (the courts being generally aware of the other calls on the witnesses' time), and try to come to a suitable arrangement. Having said that, the duty to answer a citation is an over riding one; the witness must keep closely in touch with court staff. Failure to comply when lawfully cited results in even medical witnesses being held in contempt of court, with sanctions of varying severity being possible.

When a witness seeking to be excused because of illness consults a doctor, the certificate must be issued 'on soul and conscience' or it is ineffective; even then, the certifying doctor may be called without notice to give oral evidence, or the fiscal may seek another opinion: it is essential, therefore, to give the matter deep thought before certifying. The same consideration applies when an accused attempts to postpone or evade appearance on medical grounds.

The oath is administered to a witness by the judge, both standing, and the witness remains standing in the witness box throughout his/her evidence in chief, cross- and re-examination. In most cases doctors will have given documentary evidence in the form of a certificate or a report. They speak to these, not solely from memory, and may (with the permission of the Court) refer to notes made at the time of any examination. The judge may intervene to clarify points; it is not his/her function to ask questions on matters not raised by prosecution or defence. It endangers the evidence for the party calling the doctors if the doctors do not follow their court oath and try to answer questions they have not been asked. The witnesses should therefore not readily volunteer views. If they believe that the thrust of their evidence has been distorted by the manner in which questions have been put to them they should say so to the judge, who may offer a further opportunity to give evidence. No doctor should usurp the Court's function by deciding for him/herself which information the Court should hear. Occasionally, either prosecution or defence will seek the Court's leave to have an expert witness sit in Court to assess the evidence of lay witnesses to the facts; he/she is not permitted to remain while an adversarial expert is testifying unless the parties' counsel agree to the contrary.

Criminal procedure

The Criminal Procedure (Scotland) Act 1995 (CPSA 95) introduced major changes to the ways in which crimes are investigated and evidence gathered in Scotland. These changes are radical: doctors must be aware that their rights and duties in ordinary practice or acting under the auspices of the police have altered significantly. Any words or sounds heard, writings made before, during and/or after a medical examination (including, for instance, jottings made in a diary or at home, letters to primary care physicians or hospitals) may now be used in evidence in any criminal trial in ways never before envisaged. Moreover, types of examination of the body previously thought of as solely a doctor's prerogative can now be conducted by police officers in conditions which they dictate.

In Part II of the CPSA 1995, under Police functions, s18 gives police officers of the rank of inspector or above powers to take, using reasonable force, *internal* samples, by means of swabbing, of saliva or 'other material'. They can also cut hair (except pubic hair), toe- and fingernails, take samples from underneath such nails and swab the body externally for blood or 'other bodily fluid'. Section 19 gives the police in the course of investigation or within one month of conviction, general powers to take samples of the type mentioned in s18 for the purpose of comparison with other samples. Section 20 allows the comparison, and thereby paved the way for the creation of a national DNA database (see Chapter 16). All of this can be done without the presence or participation of a doctor. These powers are not subject to any direct permission or review, so a doctor could now find his/her objections or refusals to take such samples overridden by the police.

It follows that it is entirely possible for a police doctor to have been excluded from seeing a suspect at a crucial stage of investigation, but be asked to attend at a different stage. At that stage the suspect may be in an entirely different physical or mental state. This possibility, when taken together with the important exceptions to the 'hearsay' and 'prior statement' rules introduced by ss259, 260 and 261 CPSA 95, means that doctors must take the utmost care both for themselves and the suspect in observing and reporting the state of the suspect and anything the doctor may hear. These new exceptions only apply when the maker of the statement is dead, outwith the United Kingdom, missing or cannot reasonably be brought to Court or the Court allows him/her not to give evidence, say under the rule against self-incrimination.

So long as there is evidence that a statement was made and is contained in 'any document' or its making is in the 'direct personal knowledge' of a witness giving evidence (such as a doctor) that 'document' can be admissible evidence. Thus, as well as any formal note or report, any jottings may be admissible. Doctors may find the defence or prosecution or both seeking an order of the Court to search a surgery or home or both for any 'document' retained by the doctor and held to be admissible. Further, although the rule against double-hearsay is preserved, it is quite possible in a serious case that anyone living or working with the doctor who may have seen the 'document' could be called on to give evidence about its contents, when it was made and so on. It is important to note that the 'document' would be admissible just as much as the testimony of its author. But the situation could easily arise where the author did not give evidence, leaving the 'document' to stand alone. That situation could readily have civil consequences for doctors if the 'document' is founded upon but the accused is eventually found to have been wrongly convicted.

The standard of proof for those seeking to persuade a Court that, without such a 'document', a miscarriage of justice may ensue is the civil standard of the balance of probabilities. Judges are therefore likely to be slow to refuse such motions.

Civil jurisdiction

At common law, sheriffs retain the power to try a very wide range of civil causes arising within their district. Divorce, when uncontested, may be heard. Solicitors and advocates may appear before a sheriff, but only advocates and solicitor-advocates in the Supreme Court. There, actions are pursued before a *Lord Ordinary* in the *Outer House* of the *Court of Session*. Appeals by pursuer or defender, whether from a decision of a sheriff (usually) or a Court of Session judge (always) are to the *Inner House,* which has two Divisions, the First and Second. These, chaired respectively by the Lord President and the Lord Justice Clerk, are thought to have equal authority. Further appeal may, at times, lie to the House of Lords. Most of these judges, the Senators of the College of Justice, sit in both criminal and civil courts. As head of the Criminal Appeal Court, the Lord President sits *qua* Lord Justice General of Scotland.

Child protection procedures in Scotland

The Social Work (Scotland) Act 1968 brought radical changes to working with children and incorporated these into the Children (Scotland) Act 1995. Gone were juvenile courts: children who were themselves delinquent became subject to procedures no less applicable to children in need. Central to the new system is the Reporter to the Children's Panel.

The reporter

Formerly appointed by the local authority, reporters now form part of a national service (Local Government etc. (Scotland) Act 1994; Children (Scotland) Act 1995) headed by the Principal Reporter. The reporters' functions are part administrative, part investigative, part quasi-judicial. They act as the central clearing agency, considering reports from the police, social workers and teachers, indeed anyone with an interest in the welfare of a child, including the child him/herself. To paraphrase the Social Work Act, anyone with a reasonable cause to believe that a child needs compulsory measures of care may give information to the reporter.

When considering reports on a child they must satisfy themselves that they have grounds to refer the child to the children's hearing (see below) and that they could substantiate these grounds before a sheriff. They must also satisfy themselves that the child concerned is in need of compulsory measures of supervision (whether remaining at home, with foster parents or in an institution) as set out in s52 of the Children (Scotland) Act. The section lists examples, some from other Acts, of conditions giving rise to the need for compulsory supervision; these include moral danger or criminal association, lack of parental control or care, commission of offences, misuse of drugs or alcohol. Supervision means protection, guidance, treatment or control of the child.

If they cannot be satisfied on these two counts, they must either take no further action or refer the case to the local authority with a view to their making arrangements for advice, guidance and assistance. It must be emphasized that the reporter's view is not swayed by supposed criminality on the child's part: the sole criterion is the need of that child.

When conduct would have constituted an offence had the perpetrator been older, the police will report the case to the reporter rather than to the fiscal, unless the offence is a serious one or adults are accused of the same matter. In general, however, a child under 16 does not appear in court as an accused with the exception of serious offences such as murder, assault, putting a life in danger or certain road traffic offences which can lead to disqualification from driving.

A child who has been abused is seen to be vulnerable. Both fiscal and reporter, then, have distinct functions, the former as prosecutor, the latter as protector, but they will consult together, bearing always in mind the best interests of the victim.

Children's hearings

(publications and research are available at www.childrens-hearings.co.uk)

These, set up under the term of the Social Work (Scotland) Act 1968, replaced former juvenile courts. Serious criminal cases involving minors are still heard by a sheriff or even the High Court, particularly when there is an adult co-accused. Children attend hearings with their parents. Although the facts alleged may constitute an offence, hearings form part of the civil law structure, and the child is not an accused. He or his parents may dispute the facts, whereupon the hearing is adjourned until the sheriff has heard evidence led by the reporter, and reached a conclusion, not on guilt or innocence, but on the truth or otherwise of the facts.

The main interest of hearings to police surgeons is in relation to child abuse, when doctors may appear to give evidence at such a 'proof' before a sheriff (see below).

In each local authority area lay people constituting a Panel receive training to fit them to take part in a hearing, most often as one of three, the sexes always being mixed. Efforts are made, too, to ensure that Panel members come from varied social backgrounds but, as in other largely voluntary fields, the older and more leisured may be available to participate to a greater degree.

Hearings are conducted in private, the child being accompanied by parents, unless there is a good reason (an obvious cause of absence exists when one parent is accused of abusing the child and has been remanded in custody). Proceedings involving children may not be disclosed in newspapers or elsewhere. The reporter intimates to the hearing the grounds on which he/she is referring the child. If these grounds are not accepted by the child and his/her parent the hearing must be adjourned forthwith (see below).

If the hearing proceeds, the aim is to secure the co-operation of the whole family for the better care of the child. Where a hearing concludes that compulsory measures of care are indicated, the options are supervision at home or removal from the home. When the Social Work (Scotland) Act first came into force high hopes were entertained, but the reality is that too few places are available whether in local authority or voluntary social work premises. There has been an expansion of fostering on a short-term basis.

Proof hearings

To reduce the seeming intimidation of proceedings, parents and children are not legally represented at a children's hearing (although legal representation at central government expense has been available since 2002 in certain circumstances, for example where the panel thinks a recommendation for secure accommodation is likely), nor need the reporter and his deputes be legally qualified. Disputed grounds of referral are taken before a sheriff whose duty it is to decide whether the grounds are established. At this stage, legal representation is allowed (the child in care being represented by the reporter) and medical witnesses will often find themselves closely questioned if the case turns on evidence of, for example, sexual abuse. Because the sheriff is exercising civil powers, the standard of proof is not the 'beyond reasonable doubt' familiar in the criminal courts, but the lesser 'balance of probabilities'.

For the sake of children who appear at such a proof, formality is reduced to a minimum. The sheriff sits on the bench, but police officers do not wear uniform if they have to give evidence, nor are gowns and wigs to be seen. Evidence is given on oath or affirmation, as in any other court.

When he/she has heard all the evidence, the sheriff determines only the adequacy of the reporter's grounds of referral. If he/she considers them inadequate, the referral is discharged. If he/she is satisfied, the initiative returns to the children's hearing. The Court of Session has, on occasion, used its power to order what was, in effect, a further proof to be heard. Section 85 of the Children (Scotland) Act now allows the sheriff to review the proceedings (if the grounds were held adequate) in the light of new evidence that could not have been available at the original proof.

Place of safety

Police officers have powers under s61(5) of the Children (Scotland) Act 1995 to remove any child in need of emergency care to a place of safety (such as a police station or hospital). Social workers require the authorization of a justice before whom they must appear (s61(2)). Authorization may require any person to produce the child (s61(3)). A place of safety authorization should be exhibited to clinical staff if the child is to be kept in hospital, and has equal effect when the child is transferred to other premises, for example to a specialist unit. The staff of the place of safety must know the terms and consequences of the authorization as well as the action they ought to take in the face of any attempt to remove the child.

A justice's authorization is granted only when it is not practicable to seek a child protection order (s57) from a sheriff and depends upon the same grounds, namely neglect or significant harm, actual or potential to the child. In general, the order ceases when adequate arrangements have been made by the reporter, the children's hearing and the local authority for the care and protection of the child.

The order may allow the transfer of parental rights to the applicant (the local authority or other person). The order may overcome refusal of parents to permit operation or blood transfusion, or confer authority on a doctor to examine the child for evidence of sexual abuse. The question of consent for such an examination is a difficult one but the Act (s90) does not prejudice a child's capacity under s2(4) of the Age of Legal Capacity (Scotland) Act 1991 to consent to (or refuse consent to) surgical, medical or dental procedures or treatment. For forensic physicians, the importance is that consent to examine must be obtained from the child 'with capacity' (certainly of 12 years or older) despite any warrant to examine given under ss66, 69 and 70 of the Children (Scotland) Act.

A parent has the responsibility, as defined by s1 of the Children (Scotland) Act, to safeguard and promote the child's health, development and welfare; 'direction' is provided up to the age of 16, and 'guidance' up to 18. Mothers always possessed the rights necessary to perform these responsibilities as did the father if married to the mother at or after the time of conception. However, with the Family Law (Scotland) Act 2006 coming into force joint registration of a child by unmarried parents now confers automatic parental rights and responsibilities (PRRs) to both the mother and the father of the child, albeit this change is not retrospective.

Parental rights and responsibilities may be transferred by court order to the local authority (s11).

Case conferences

Personnel from the various agencies – these include social workers, teachers, clinical psychologist, hospital staff, police, primary case physician, health visitor, forensic physician – have an opportunity to pool knowledge, to discuss future management and, most significantly, to place a child on the 'at risk' register. Presence at the conference should be limited to those with a personal professional interest, for they can easily become unwieldy. Police officers may find themselves in a difficult position if any criminal record of parents is to be discussed, or some other investigation cannot be revealed. Parents may be invited to attend part, or even all, of the proceedings, but this must inevitably inhibit the exchange of views. They must, of course, be advised of the outcome. Primary care physicians often complain that the conference is arranged for a time when they are at a busy surgery, but a good deal of flexibility ought to be practised, and those who cannot attend should not hesitate to send a written report. The chair is usually taken by a senior social work administrator, and confidential minutes are kept but case conference reports would normally be accessible by a valid subject access request under the Data Protection Act 1998 although the usual exceptions apply.

Case discussions are held at the early stages of an investigation, to allow the agencies to decide upon a common approach, to agree to set procedures and to arrange for medical examinations. Follow-up conferences are held as required, for example, whenever a decision of major significance in the management of the child is proposed by one of the agencies. These are attended by a narrower spectrum of personnel. Only such a conference may decide to remove a child's name from the register.

Child Protection Register

The register is designed to assist the agencies having childcare responsibilities by listing those children who have been the subject of abuse or neglect, or are thought to be at risk of such abuse. The register should help in diagnosis and is a source of statistical data. It is maintained by social work departments, and may be consulted by staff of the relevant agencies, at any hour of the day or night.

3

The Police in the United Kingdom

Crispian Strachan

The duties and structure of the police service

In England and Wales there is no statutory definition of the duties and purposes of policing. It is commonly accepted that the Police should:

- prevent crime and disorder, extremism and terrorism;
- maintain law and order, and protect people and property against crime and emergencies (both natural and man-made);
- detect criminals of all kinds and play a part in the criminal justice system, guided and directed by the Crown Prosecution Service;
- provide road policing services; and
- by long tradition, serve any one who needs their help.

This last aspect in particular comes from the British tradition that the police service is to serve the public, not to control it on behalf of the Government, but that tradition is being diluted by the exigencies of the fight against terrorism. The style in which these duties should be performed is in the Statement of Common Purpose and Values published by the Association of Chief Police Officers (ACPO) in 1992: 'The purpose of the police service is to uphold the law fairly and firmly; to prevent crime; to pursue and bring to justice those who break the law; to keep the Queen's Peace; to protect, help and reassure the community; and to be seen to do all this with integrity, common sense and sound judgment. We must be compassionate, courteous and patient, acting without fear or favour or prejudice to the rights of others. We need to be professional, calm and restrained in the face of violence and apply only that force which is necessary to accomplish our lawful duty. We must strive to reduce the fears of the public and, so far as we can, to reflect their priorities in the action we take. We must respond to well-founded criticism with a willingness to change.' These sentiments are all the more true as the pressures of diversity and human rights have applied to the work of the police service in recent years.

The accomplishment of these duties is achieved within a tripartite arrangement. The Home Secretary has a wide and growing range of powers to make regulations affecting the pay and conditions of service of all police officers (but not police staff); to control the expenditure on each force, including the provision of a grant of 51% of each force's annual budget; to require performance information and achievement by police forces; and to provide or arrange for central police services such as some training, scientific support and Her Majesty's Inspectorate of Constabulary. Despite all this, the Home Secretary has no operational control of the police and no accountability for police conduct.

Police authorities for all forces in England and Wales (apart from the City of London Police) are a composite body of 17 people: nine local councillors,

Clinical Forensic Medicine, third edition ed. W. D. S. McLay. Published by Cambridge University Press. © Cambridge University Press 2009.

three local magistrates and five independent members (local volunteers). The Metropolitan Police Authority is larger, having 23 members because of the size of London. Each police authority sets objectives for its force (taking account of objectives already given by the Home Secretary) and sets out three-year and one-year plans, after consultation with residents and businesses in the force area. The authority holds the finance and assets of the force and sets the budget each year, including the relatively small element which comes from the council tax precept. The Metropolitan Police Authority receives a determination of its budget from the Mayor of London. The chief constable, deputy and assistant chief constables (commissioner and commander ranks in London) are selected and appointed on fixed-term appointments by the authority. However, the authority has no operational control of the police and no accountability for police conduct. For the City of London Police, the Common Council of the City is the police authority and exercises similar duties and powers.

The Chief Constable of each force is solely responsible for the operational direction and control of his/her force. This reflects the position of every police officer as a constable holding office under the Crown (not an employee) and possessing original legal powers and duties. The Senior Management Team of each force will include a deputy chief constable, one or more assistant chief constables, and usually senior support staff in specialist roles, regarded as assistant chief officers. Superintendent ranks, inspectors, sergeants and constables provide policing services to communities, through geographical police areas often known as 'basic command units'.

There are 43 geographical forces within England and Wales, each of which has its own budget, resources, management structure and police support staff, who are employed by the police authority. Each force has almost total responsibility for policing services within its area, unlike the systems of European countries or America, with Federal, state and local forces.

The Welsh Assembly Government holds a central budget for policing in Wales.

In Scotland, the policing duties and structure reflect the long-standing differences in the legal system and the administration of criminal law. A specific set of police duties is set out in the Police (Scotland) Act, 1967, whereby it is the duty of a police constable:

to guard, watch and patrol so as:

to prevent crime;

to preserve order; and

to protect life and property;

to investigate and detect crime; and

to enforce traffic legislation.

The Ministers of the Scottish Executive (Scottish Government) have central duties and powers similar to the Home Secretary, but matters of national security, terrorism, firearms and drugs are reserved to the UK Government. Common (central) police services include the Scottish Police College, the Scottish Criminal Record Office, the Scottish Crime and Drug Enforcement Agency and the Scottish Forensic Science Service. Crime scene examination, fingerprints and forensic science are all directed by the Scottish Police Services Authority.

The Joint Police Board for each force exercises the same functions as does a police authority, above, but in Scotland these Boards are comprised entirely of local councillors.

Each Chief Constable of a Scottish force is in the same position as in England and Wales, above.

The Police Service of Northern Ireland was established in 2001 after the report of the Independent Commission on Policing in Northern Ireland (the Patten Report). Its rank structure is similar to the English model (above); it has a Policing Board as its authority, and has additional accountability to a Police Ombudsman and an Oversight Commissioner. These additional features reflect the turbulent history of Northern Ireland.

The investigation of crime, and prosecutions

Since the Crown Prosecution Service, headed by the Director of Public Prosecutions, was established in

England and Wales in 1986, the responsibility for detecting and arresting or summoning suspects has been clearly separated from decisions about criminal proceedings against them. Whilst police can caution an offender or deal with them by fixed penalty notice, the Crown Prosecution Service conducts all criminal court proceedings against suspects dealt with by police in England and Wales (with the exception of specialist prosecutions such as cases dealt with by the Serious Fraud Office and some revenue and trading descriptions offences). All investigations, and the treatment of all suspects, are governed by the provisions of the Police and Criminal Evidence Act (PACE) 1984.

Scotland's legal system differs from the English in its law, judicial procedure and court structure. It has a system of public prosecutors, called procurators fiscal, headed by the Lord Advocate and independent of the police; the latter have no say in the decision to prosecute, and cannot even give a caution. All reports of crime, from police or other agencies, are sent to the local procurator fiscal and will be prosecuted in a district court, sheriff court or the High Court (see Chapter 2 for detail).

In Northern Ireland the system is closer to that of England and Wales, but minor summary offences may still be prosecuted by the police. More serious cases are reported to the Director of Public Prosecutions for Northern Ireland.

Other operational matters

There are many ways in which the police service deals with crime and other operational matters that cross force boundaries. These include, primarily, the Serious and Organised Crime Agency (SOCA), formed in 2006 from The National Crime Squad, the National Criminal Intelligence Service and some elements of HM Revenue & Customs and the Border and Immigration Agency. The SOCA is a national, executive non-departmental public body answerable to the Home Office, established to deal with the most serious categories of crime nationally.

In addition, forces may combine voluntarily, through the chief officers' associations (ACPO in England, Wales and Northern Ireland, and ACPOS in Scotland) to deploy officers strategically for major events, public order issues or emergencies.

It is also part of every police officer's daily duty, however, to serve any one who needs their help, and the majority of calls to the police service turn out not to be about crime, but other problems for which other agencies are simply not so readily available. These include traffic incidents, sudden deaths and mental health problems, in many of which doctors may become involved. In mental health cases, it will generally be an officer of inspector rank who will be responsible, especially if a medical opinion is required. In the rare event of medical assistance being needed at a major incident or emergency, procedures exist to designate police officers responsible for casualties, rendezvous points, body identification, etc. A doctor whose services may be called upon will need to identify such officers and work in accordance with the overall co-ordination they bring to the scene.

Police personnel

Recruitment to all UK forces firmly incorporates equal opportunities. Age limits, height limits and other former criteria have been largely abolished, and eyesight requirements have been much relaxed. Candidates accepted through a standardized, national process must become constables and are 'probationary' constables for their first two years of service, including considerable training. This includes not only their necessary professional knowledge, but skills including the proper handling of the diversity encountered amongst the public.

Promotion to sergeant and inspector, the principal supervisory ranks in a shift or local policing team, is by passing national exams and by selection. Promotion to higher ranks (chief inspectors and superintendents) is by selection in each force. Officers may also specialize in many ways, such as detectives, traffic, dog handlers or community relations. All forces have specialist units for offences against women, children or others defined as vulnerable people, and doctors may well meet them when treating victims.

Police support staff, who are not police officers but are employed by police authorities to help in each force, are now commonplace. A doctor will very often find caseworkers and other specialist support staff in custody areas, as well as scenes of crime officers, photographers etc.

Professional standards and complaints against police

Elsewhere in this book reference is made to doctors' ethical responsibilities towards persons in custody, including injuries that may result from the improper use of force by police. Such cases may lead to complaints or internal misconduct action against police officers and a brief outline of the system may be informative.

Throughout the UK, criminal cases must be proved beyond all reasonable doubt, as in external criminal prosecutions. Complaints and misconduct matters must be proved against officers on the balance of probability, but with a sliding scale of the burden of proof increasing with the seriousness of the alleged criminal act or misconduct. In England and Wales, criminal allegations (e.g. assault on a person in custody) are reported to the Crown Prosecution Service and misconduct matters

(e.g. incivility) may be reported to the Independent Police Complaints Commission, who also oversee serious criminal cases. Misconduct and complaint investigations are usually the responsibility of the deputy chief officer of each force.

In Scotland, criminal allegations are reported to the procurator fiscal. Her Majesty's Inspectorate of Constabulary may see fit to oversee cases in some circumstances (in Scotland only). The Police, Public Order and Criminal Justice (Scotland) Act 2006 established the Police Complaints Commissioner for Scotland (www.pcc-scotland.org) whose function is to respond to complainants dissatisfied by how their complaint against a police officer or staff member of a police force, police authority or policing agency was handled. The substance of the complaint is not investigated, nor may the Commissioner review a decision of the Crown.

In Northern Ireland, the Northern Ireland Human Rights Commission may oversee appropriate complaints cases.

Other forces

Apart from the principal forces of the UK described above, there are a number of others, distinguished by their function or jurisdiction. They include the Ministry of Defence Police (at or near military premises), British Transport Police (for all main line rail services and London Underground) and police for parks, ports or tunnels.

4

The practitioner's obligations

Michael A. Knight, with contributions by Michael Wilks and
C. George M. Fernie

Introduction

A forensic physician is called upon to undertake examinations in a wide variety of situations. Most people examined will be alive, and will therefore have certain rights, such as a right of confidentiality, and capabilities, which will include the capacity to give consent. It is the responsibility of the examining doctor to consider, in the individual case, where the boundaries lie among the (often conflicting) rights of the person examined, the processes of investigation and the interests of justice.

This chapter aims to define the responsibilities of the forensic physician solely in an ethical context. In dealing with the individual case, many of the ethical considerations outlined here will be modified. Some may even be discarded. It is essential, however, for the clinician to be aware of broad principles, so that he/she can decide how closely he/she wishes to adhere to them. He/she will need to bear in mind that to depart from them without good reason may invite the interests of the General Medical Council (GMC), and of the civil or criminal courts. The ultimate test of any action is whether the doctor is able to justify it to his/her peers.

Ethical principles define an accepted code of behaviour within a particular group, the group in this case being the medical profession. Ethical standards are not the same as moral standards, which represent principles accepted more widely within society. While ethical and moral behaviour will usually be within the law, there is no guarantee of compatibility between legal, moral and ethical behaviour.

It must also be stressed that doctors will bring their personal moral opinions, formed through education, cultural background and religious beliefs, to bear on individual ethical issues. For forensic physicians, it can be very easy, when dealing with detainees, for moral judgements about assumed guilt to interfere with impartiality. It is precisely because of this that absolute ethical principles are so important, as they provide a benchmark for doctors both in the clinical work of examining prisoners, victims or injured officers, and in acting as an impartial expert in relationships with the police, the legal profession and the courts.

An essential feature, not unique to forensic medicine, of the forensic physician's role is that of 'dual responsibility'. A doctor serving in the armed forces has responsibility both to the individual soldier and for the safety and efficiency of a wider group, such as a regiment. The company medical adviser has a responsibility to a sick employee, but has to pay regard to the interests of the employer. In all cases of dual responsibility there is a conflict between the confidentiality normally enjoyed by the patient and the wider interests of an institution. It should be remembered that the medical profession does not enjoy the absolute confidentiality found in the

Clinical Forensic Medicine, third edition ed. W. D. S. McLay. Published by Cambridge University Press. © Cambridge University Press 2009.

solicitor/client relationship and may be compelled to answer by the presiding officer of a court or be found in contempt.

In clinical forensic medicine this conflict is expressed in two distinct ways:

1. Most examinations have a dual content – therapeutic and forensic. In most cases, the doctor has a responsibility of care which may involve providing actual treatment, or a decision to refer for further care. In addition, many examinations involve the interpretation of clinical signs in an evidential context. Even the most minor of injuries may be the subject of detailed cross-examination in court, often long in the future. The doctor will be expected, using notes made at the time, to give an opinion on the appearance of the injuries, age and likely causation.

2. The doctor has a duty of confidentiality to the person examined. This is an essential feature of the doctor/patient relationship. However, the doctor also has an obligation to provide such details to the police as are necessary and appropriate for the investigation of crime, and, in the case of a person detained, for their safe care while in detention. This aspect of the dual relationship raises fundamental issues of confidentiality and consent.

Bearing in mind that as doctors we are subject to our own disciplinary codes, *the relationship between the forensic physician and the person examined will be one of doctor and patient.* Although this may have little parallel with a consultation, say, between a patient and a primary care physician, it is essential that we start by considering that the contact between the forensic clinician and examinees, be they prisoners, victims or police officers, is a modification of that ideal consultation. With that starting point we can then highlight the differences, and from this see how the relationship is modified.

Traditionally, the ethics of the doctor/patient relationship are framed by four main principles: autonomy, non-maleficence, beneficence and justice.

Autonomy is the capacity of people to choose freely and to control as far as possible what happens to them. Respecting this autonomy involves acknowledging the integrity of a person's choice, made according to his/her own values, conscience and religious convictions. In recognizing autonomy, the doctor implicitly agrees to two essential elements in patient care: the patient's ability to give or withhold consent, and the doctor's duty of confidentiality.

In clinical forensic practice, a prisoner's autonomy is clearly restricted by his/her loss of liberty. It may also be impaired by illness, intoxication and drugs, all of which restrict the capacity to make free choice. The loss of liberty also makes prisoners fearful and vulnerable, and often more acquiescent. It is part of the doctor's responsibility to recognize this, and take on a more interventionist, or advocate's, role. The prisoner who is so drunk that he/she cannot appreciate the severity of a laceration, or the drug misuser whose request for medication should be denied because his/her recent drug history cannot be validated, are examples where free choice can be properly overridden. But it is essential not to confuse loss of liberty with loss of autonomy. Refusal to be examined or to be treated, if made in an informed way, must be respected. To take action in opposition to such refusal may lay you open to a charge of assault.

There are, however, situations in which consent can be overridden by police, most notably in the case of intimate searches and DNA sampling. These are dealt with in detail later.

Non-maleficence reminds us that, while the price of doing good may be to do harm, there should be both a minimization of harm and an outcome in which there is a balance in favour of good. In practical terms it is a principle that obliges the doctor to respect a patient's dignity and privacy.

Beneficence is a wider concept than simply doing good. We are doctors because we seek to care. As civilized humans, we adopt the assumption that our society is essentially compassionate, and that those with more will try to help those with less. In the context of forensic medicine, those with less include people with less information and, crucially, with less liberty.

The final principle is *justice*, here referring to inequalities in access to health care in the acute custodial setting, although this is less of an issue than with prolonged imprisonment. Bear in mind the GMC's guidance contained in *Good Medical Practice* [1] on ensuring 'The investigations or treatment you provide or arrange must be based on the assessment you and the patient make of their needs and priorities, and on your clinical judgement about the likely effectiveness of the treatment options. You must not refuse or delay treatment because you believe that a patient's actions have contributed to their condition. You must treat your patients with respect whatever their life choices and beliefs. You must not unfairly discriminate against them by allowing your personal views to affect adversely your professional relationship with them or the treatment you provide or arrange.'

We all have a moral obligation to act fairly in respecting rights, to obey laws and to act in accordance with general moral principles. As forensic physicians, each of us will bring our own moral perspective of justice to bear on any particular case. We cannot help it, nor should we be concerned about it. What matters is how it affects our actions. To bring personal moral judgements to bear on our management of individual cases undermines our capacity to be impartial, and is unethical. The forensic physician is called upon to perform a wide range of duties. These responsibilities should, and normally will, be clearly set out in the contract held with the police authority.

These duties have traditionally been grouped in accordance with their specialist (forensic) content, a higher fee being paid for those duties requiring more skill. A lower fee is paid for those examinations that have more therapeutic content, such as an examination for fitness to detain. These distinctions are less clear in practice, for, as has been said, many examinations have both therapeutic and forensic content. In recent years, forensic physicians have felt that an examination to determine fitness for interview, as an example, may have important implications for the integrity of statements and confessions given at interview, and that its importance should be given more significance.

In the course of your duties, and apart from the clinical and forensic responsibilities, you will have a professional relationship with a wide variety of people and disciplines. These include solicitors, barristers, social workers, lay visitors, court officers and criminal justice units. The degree of confidentiality of information held by the doctor will always influence the extent of disclosure to these different groups.

The legal framework

Let us now consider those laws and legal processes relevant to forensic practice. The most important is the Police and Criminal Evidence Act 1984 (PACE), operative in England, Wales and Northern Ireland. Under this Act, the Home Secretary is required to issue Codes of Practice regulating police practice in a number of areas. Code C relates to the detention, treatment and questioning of persons by police officers. In this context 'treatment' refers to overall care, and embraces more than the medical aspects of detention. This Code determines, and tightly regulates, the work of the custody officer in the care of detained persons. Scrupulous attention is required if prisoners' rights are not to be disregarded or overridden, and a knowledge of this Code is an essential requirement for a good working relationship to be established between the custody officer and the forensic clinician.

Code C has been amended, now using the term 'appropriate healthcare professional', to include professional groups such as nurses or paramedics who are used in the first instance in some forces to attend detained persons needing medical care. Such forces will also have forensic physicians available to them for guidance, or for the examination of more complex cases, for example those involving sexual offences or mental health.

A 'healthcare professional' is defined under PACE Code C Notes for Guidance 9A thus: 'A healthcare professional means a clinically qualified person working within the scope of practice as determined by their relevant professional body. Whether a healthcare professional is 'appropriate' depends on the circumstances of the duties they carry out at the time.'

For the remainder of this chapter the term 'doctor' will be used for simplicity, but it should be assumed, unless otherwise stated, that the terms 'doctor' and 'healthcare professional' are interchangeable.

Paragraphs 9.2 to 9.14 of Code C deal specifically with medical treatment. Familiarity with these paragraphs will enable the doctor to give advice to the custody officer which is either consistent with, or complementary to, his normal responsibilities.

Code D defines police procedures in relation to the identification of persons. In particular it contains references to the mentally impaired, appropriate adults and the taking of samples, both intimate and non-intimate.

Other laws and regulations that bear on the work of the forensic clinician include the following:
- The Misuse of Drugs (Notification and Supply to Addicts) Regulations 1973
- The Public Health (Control of Disease) Act 1984
- Human Rights Act 1998
- Data Protection Act 1998

The detention of an individual against consent raises questions of personal liberty and human rights. The Declaration of Geneva (1948) is an international statement of the duties and responsibilities of doctors. This has most recently been amended by the World Medical Association at the General Assembly in October 2006. It has been adopted by some medical schools as a benchmark for doctors, replacing the Hippocratic Oath as a basic set of principles to acknowledge the student or graduate's commitment to medical practice. Acceptance of the fundamental ethical principles of autonomy and justice requires doctors to be alert to potential or actual abuse of prisoners, and to ensure that appropriate representations are made.

Consent

A general principle of English Law is that a patient always has the right to withhold consent to medical treatment, even where such a refusal may involve declining life-saving treatment. In his judgment in *Re T* [1992] 4 All ER 649 Lord Donaldson, the Master of the Rolls, stated, 'Doctors faced with a refusal of consent have to give very careful and detailed consideration to the patient's capacity to decide at the time when the decision was made. What matters is that the doctors should consider at that time he had a capacity which was commensurate with the gravity of the decision he purported to make. The more serious the decision, the greater the capacity required. If the patient has the requisite capacity they are bound by his decision. If not, they are free to treat him in what they believe to be his best interests.'

This illustrates two essential questions facing the doctor:
- Is the consent for therapeutic or forensic examination?
- Is the consent informed 'valid', in other words fully understood in the context of the medico-legal process?

In almost every case, examinations of prisoners, victims and officers will have both therapeutic and forensic content. The proportion of one compared to the other may be small, but it will nearly always be there. One of the most important reasons for keeping accurate and comprehensive notes is that information, derived from what at the time was a therapeutic examination, may have to be reinterpreted – often months later – in the form of a statement or in evidence in court.

In respect of prisoners, s9 of Code C of PACE lists circumstances in which the custody officer is obliged to seek medical assistance whether or not he/she is asked to do so by the detainee; he/she will do so when the detainee appears to be suffering from a physical or mental illness, or is injured, or 'appears to need clinical attention' (para 9.5).

In these circumstances there may be limited consent, or none at all, for the examination, and the doctor has to proceed on the basis of *implied* consent, that is, on the assumption that a person suffering from an illness would wish to have that illness treated, particularly if there was a risk to life. The doctor can proceed as far as is therapeutically necessary, and, during the course of the procedure, will gather information that may be of forensic value, and useful to the investigation of crime. The doctor, by virtue of his/her position as a clinician advising the police, is free to give an opinion on the forensic content of his/her examination, but is not free to take samples or undertake intimate searches without consent.

The custody officer is obliged under para 9.7 of Code C to seek medical advice if the detainee appears to be suffering from an infectious disease, or, under 9.9, if a detained person has in his/her possession, or claims to need, medication relating to a heart condition, diabetes, epilepsy or a condition of comparable seriousness. In these circumstances, the doctor will obtain consent for an examination to assess the prisoner's fitness for detention, and there is unlikely to be any forensic content.

When a person in custody requests the presence of a doctor, and therefore has some expectation of examination and treatment, there will be an assumption of implied consent. Such a right of request exists under para 9.8 of Code C, and includes the right to be examined by a medical practitioner at the prisoner's own expense. There are those, such as Robertson [2], who feels that 'normal doctor/patient rules clearly do not apply in this situation.' However, most doctors will try to apply the normal rules that govern the doctor/patient relationship to the best of their ability in what is an abnormal clinical situation.

More detailed issues of consent apply where the doctor is called to examine a detainee in order to assist and advise the police on the collection of evidence with respect to an alleged crime. Such evidence will be obtained by an examination to assess the presence – or absence – of injuries, and to interpret the significance of the findings. It may also involve the taking of samples, the analysis of which may confirm or refute an allegation, for example following an allegation of sexual assault. In these circumstances the doctor is obliged to be specific about his/her role, and to emphasize that his/her responsibilities to the police include the interpretation of relevant clinical findings in an evidential context, but that his/her responsibilities to the prisoner/patient include keeping confidential those matters that are not, in the doctor's opinion, immediately relevant to the case. The term 'immediately' is important, as it reminds us that in later statements or evidence in court, you may not be free to judge the relevance or 'materiality' of the findings. This is dealt with later in the section on disclosure.

Since the consequences of acting without consent may be damaging to the doctor, both in terms of the law, and in the eyes of the GMC, some forensic clinicians prefer to obtain consent from prisoners in writing. Consent forms need to make clear that the subject understands the nature and purpose of any examination or investigation undertaken. It is arguable whether consent in writing offers a greater protection to the doctor than that given verbally. There is therefore no requirement that consent should be written, but the fact that consent has been given orally should always be recorded in your private notes. Oral consent should ideally be witnessed, for example by a police officer or detention officer/custody assistant.

The only situation in which a forensic sample can be taken *without consent* is under the provisions of the Police Reform Act 2002. If a person is involved in a road traffic collision, as the result of which he/she is thought by a constable to have become incapacitated, the forensic physician can take a blood sample which is then stored appropriately. If the person dies, the sample becomes the property of the coroner. If the person survives, on recovery their consent will be sought for analysis of the sample; a refusal at that stage will generate an automatic conviction. If consent is given for analysis of the sample, the result of the analysis will dictate conviction or otherwise in the usual way.

Intimate and non-intimate samples

Sections 62 and 65 of PACE define intimate and non-intimate samples. However, PACE was amended by s58 of the Criminal Justice and Public Order Act 1994, and intimate samples are now defined in Code D (6.1(a)) as follows: 'An intimate sample means a dental impression or a sample of blood, semen or any other tissue fluid, urine or pubic hair or a swab taken from any part of a person's genitals or from a person's body orifice other than the mouth.'

Non-intimate samples are defined under Code D (6.1(b)) thus: '. . .

(i) a sample of hair, (other than pubic hair) which includes hair plucked from the root;

(ii) a sample taken from a nail or from under a nail;

(iii) a swab taken from any part of a person's body other than a part from which a swab taken would be an intimate sample;

(iv) saliva

(v) a skin impression which means any record, other than a fingerprint, which is a record, in any form and produced by any method, of the skin pattern and other physical characteristics or features of the whole, or any part of, a person's foot or any other part of their body.'

In redesignating mouth swabs as 'non-intimate', the Criminal Justice and Public Order Act followed the example set in Northern Ireland, where the status of saliva and mouth swabs was moved from the intimate to the non-intimate category by Schedule 14 to the Criminal Justice Act 1988.

Section 6 of Code D to PACE describes the circumstances in which these samples can be taken:

Intimate samples may only be taken if an officer of the rank of inspector or above authorizes the taking of such samples, which he may only do if he has reasonable grounds '. . . to believe such an impression or sample will tend to confirm or disprove the suspect's involvement in a recordable offence . . .', and 'with the suspect's written consent'. (Code D 6.2(a)).

'Dental impressions can only be taken by a registered dentist. Other intimate samples, except for samples of urine, may only be taken by a registered medical practitioner or registered nurse, or registered paramedic.' (Code D 6.4).

Non-intimate samples can only be taken with the consent of the detained person, unless para 6.6 of Code D applies. Paragraph 6.6 gives a range of conditions under which non-intimate samples may be taken without consent, including the inspector's authority and the circumstances of the arrest and detention.

Paragraph 6.7 indicates clearly that 'Reasonable force may be used, if necessary, to take a non-intimate sample from a person without their consent under the powers mentioned in paragraph 6.6.'

Forensic physicians or other healthcare professionals may be asked to assist in the taking of non-intimate samples, but should only do so when the detainee has given informed written consent to the procedure; they should **never** be involved in taking **any** samples by force. The most common non-intimate sample to be taken by force is a buccal swab for DNA, and that is a matter for the police alone.

By redefining mouth swabs as non-intimate, the need for the attendance of medical personnel, and for consent to the taking of samples, has been avoided, thereby opening the way to the use of DNA in the identification of a perpetrator of a crime, and to the establishment of DNA databases.

It should also be noted that para 6.3 of Code D of PACE states, that: 'Before a suspect is asked to provide an intimate sample they must be warned that if they refuse without good cause, their refusal may harm their case if it comes to trial.' While it is not part of your obligation to interpret the law, you will be aware that the operation of this clause increases the prisoner's vulnerability, and therefore heightens the need for an unambiguous statement of your role. In contentious cases you may wish to supplement the prisoner's written consent in the custody record with your own consent form.

Intimate body searches

Section 55 of PACE 1984 allows for intimate body searches to be carried out under certain circumstances. These powers present the medical practitioner with a considerable ethical dilemma. The Act distinguishes between two groups of material for which an intimate search can be authorized. Referring to detainees, s55(a) deals with '. . . anything which (1) he could use to cause physical injury to himself or others; and (2) he might so use while he is in police detention or in the custody of the court . . .'. This section is designed to cover items such as weapons, sharp implements and other similar dangerous material. Section 55(b) deals specifically with drugs.

Intimate searches are dealt with in Annex A of Code C to PACE. Such a search is defined in para A 1 thus: 'An intimate search consists of the physical examination of a person's orifices other than the mouth.' The paragraph continues, 'The intrusive nature of such searches means the actual and potential risks associated with intimate searches must never be underestimated.'

The difference between the two subsections determines the difference in the location and type of search, and who is authorized to undertake it. A search for a weapon may be carried out at a hospital, surgery, other medical premises or a police station. An intimate search for drugs may not be carried out at a police station, and therefore must be performed on 'medical premises' as above, and must be carried out by a registered medical practitioner or a registered nurse. (Code C Annex A, A (a) 4).

However, in extremis, a search for a weapon or similar item (not drugs) can be carried out by a police officer providing that police officer is of the same sex as the examinee, and authority has been obtained from an officer of at least inspector rank.

Class A drugs, as defined under the Misuse of Drugs Act 1971, comprise a wide range of substances, including the opiates, but excluding cannabis.

A medical practitioner seeking to conduct an intimate search, properly authorized under s55, would, in the first instance, seek the consent of the detainee. The dilemma for the doctor arises if such consent is refused. Zander [3] correctly points

out that a doctor or nurse cannot be compelled to carry out searches of body orifices where there is no consent. However, he goes on to say, '. . . consent to such a search by the suspect is not essential and force could therefore be used to carry out the search – presumably even if it is being carried out by a medical practitioner or nurse'. This view was supported by a Home Office draft circular [4] which held that 'In s55 of PACE there is no mention of consent or the absence of consent in respect of constables or qualified persons. Under this section, therefore, a qualified person is empowered to act without the consent of the person concerned. It was not the intention that the power of a superintendent to authorise a medical examination should be frustrated because the suspect could not be restrained.' There is, therefore, an expectation that medical personnel will be asked to carry out searches of body orifices without consent, despite both the ethical difficulties this would cause, and the potential harm and technical difficulties inherent in such a procedure.

The Home Office Circular continues (para 37): 'Provided suitably qualified persons conducting intimate searches do not use unreasonable force, or cause injury through negligence, they will, in the Secretary of State's view, be protected from complaints arising from searches. On normal principles if a procedure is provided by Act of Parliament for carrying out that which would normally be unlawful, then those acting under the procedure will have a defence to any proceedings, civil or criminal, brought against them.'

It appears that doctors conducting such searches without consent, despite the 'assurances' given by the Home Office, would be inviting proceedings under all three elements of the so-called 'triple jeopardy', criminal proceedings for assault, civil proceedings for the tort of battery, and disciplinary proceedings before the GMC. To date, these matters have not been tested before any of these Courts or Tribunals.

The British Medical Association (BMA) jointly with the Royal College of Nursing (RCN) [5] provided guidelines for doctors and nurses with regard to intimate searches: 'In the surroundings of the police station where a refusal to perform an intimate search may imply guilt, it is very unlikely that the health professional will be able to obtain freely the consent of the suspect to perform an intimate search. However, except on very rare occasions, an intimate search should not be performed without the subject's acquiescence having first been obtained.' In relation specifically to searches under s55(1)(a), the guidelines insist that: 'We are not convinced that there are sufficient grounds for an intimate search if a non-acquiescing subject is believed to have concealed upon him an object or substance which will not harm others but only himself', echoing the definition of the 'appropriate criminal intent' under s55(17)(a) of the Act.

Havard [6] gave similar guidance: 'Doctors should not undertake such (intimate) samples unless the person consents, and they are not required to do so under the Act. Refusal to consent may provide corroboration of evidence subsequently given in court and adverse inferences can be drawn from refusal when there is no good cause for it.' (A view now confirmed by PACE Code C Annex A, A (a) 2B.)

In the same year the BMA resolved that: '. . . no medical practitioner should take part in an intimate body search of a subject without that subject's consent'. This view was confirmed in joint guidance from the BMA and the Association of Forensic Physicians (AFP), last updated in 2004 [7].

In 2005, the Codes were amended to include the requirement for detained persons to consent to examination by X-ray or ultrasound scan. Such examinations can be requested if an officer of inspector rank or above considers that the detainee may have swallowed a Class A drug, and was in possession of that drug with the intention of supplying it to another or to export it. (Code C Annex K).

Capacity

In assessing a detainee's fitness for detention and/or interview, the doctor will make judgements about that person's ability both to give consent, and to understand and answer questions put to him/her at formal interview. This raises the issue of capacity, which has been extensively covered in a publication issued jointly by the BMA and the Law Society [8], updated in 2004. What matters to the clinician in advising the police is whether or not a person detained has the capacity to give consent, and to understand the procedures applied to him/her. If the doctor is content that a detainee is fully aware, and therefore fully capable, then the interview may proceed, and consent for investigation and examinations, whether performed by the police or by the doctor, will be valid. It must be remembered that any suggestion that a person detained did not understand what was happening to him/her might have serious consequences later on if the matter proceeds to trial. The doctor may wish to set a time limit on the extent of the fitness for interview, or may give directions regarding reassessment.

Appropriate adults

The Codes of Practice to PACE recognize a range of circumstances in which an appropriate adult should be present during the cautioning, searching, interviewing or charging of vulnerable suspects, in particular juveniles and persons who are mentally disordered. The appropriate adult should be present throughout the custodial process for the following groups of detainees:

A person of any age who is mentally disordered or otherwise mentally vulnerable. (Code C 1.4)

Juveniles i.e. those under seventeen years of age, or who *appear* to be under seventeen. (Code C 1.5)

A person who appears to be blind, seriously visually impaired, deaf, unable to read or speak. (Code C 1.6)

The concept of 'mental vulnerability' was introduced to Code C in 2004, and refers to 'detainees who, because of their mental state or capacity, may not understand the significance of what is said, or of questions or of their replies'. Code C 1.7 indicates a 'hierarchy' of persons who can act as an appropriate adult.

Confidentiality

The principle of medical confidentiality extends back to the Hippocratic Oath, but is stated in guidance from the GMC [9]: 'Patients have a right to expect that information about them will be held in confidence by their doctors.'

An action for breach of confidentiality has always been possible under civil law. In the controversial case of *AG* v. *Guardian Newspapers Ltd* (2) [1988] 3 All ER 545 (the so-called Spycatcher case) the general principle was stated by Lord Gough: 'I start with the broad general principle . . . that a duty of confidence arises when confidential information comes to the knowledge of a person (the confidant) in circumstances where he has notice or is held to have agreed, that the information is confidential, with the effect that it would be just in all the circumstances that he should be precluded from disclosing the information to others.'

While the view of the GMC, and the likely view of the civil courts, would be severe censure of a doctor who knowingly disclosed confidential information about a patient to a third party, it must be stressed that, in the matter of medical records, there is no absolute privilege. However, it is essential that forensic physicians start from the basis of absolute confidentiality, and develop a view, in the individual case, on the extent of legitimate disclosure, whether informally to a custody sergeant or investigating officer, or formally in a custody entry, statement or report.

A major bearing on the extent of confidentiality that can be accorded to a detainee lies in the dual role of the forensic examiner, referred to earlier. By virtue of being required by the police to attend in both a therapeutic and forensic capacity, the doctor is necessarily expected to make a report to the police. In relation to a detainee's fitness to be detained, the information given must be relevant to that person's likely period of detention, the sole purpose of the information being to safeguard that person's wellbeing while in custody. In relation to an examination for evidential purposes, the doctor's duty is to provide to the police that information that he/she feels is material to the investigation. At this early stage he/she should not impart information that does not seem relevant. The relevance of information held may change, and further information may need to be disclosed, but this occurs at a later stage, and is governed by legally enforceable procedures on disclosure.

Confidentiality in the custodial situation

A major conflict for the doctor examining a detainee is in balancing confidentiality with personal safety. It is by no means uncommon for doctors to be threatened or assaulted by prisoners. Sensible guidance on this issue is set out in the joint BMA/AFP booklet on the health care of detainees [7]. The advice can be summarized as follows:

- It is good practice for a prisoner to be accompanied by an escort, usually a police officer.
- The escort should remain within calling distance, but out of earshot.
- A doctor should never examine a person (including police officers) of the opposite sex without a chaperone present.
- Essentially, there must be a balance between the individual's right to privacy and the safety of the forensic physician.

The doctor will be required, or expected, to make records of his/her examination. In many instances a note will be made in the custody record giving a brief summary of the advice given regarding a person's detention. In addition to a station-based record, the doctor will keep private notes. These may include written notes and body diagrams. A doctor should be entirely free to keep those records he/she thinks appropriate. In general, forensic physicians are advised not to take photographs in the course of their duties. In cases which are sufficiently serious to warrant recording by photographs, a trained police scene of crime officer should be available to take photographs of a professional standard which become part of the evidence in the case.

When making private notes it is essential that the record is complete. Although these notes do not have absolute privilege, it is bad practice, and unhelpful both to the investigation and to the case in court, for potentially relevant information to be omitted. The doctor may well feel that certain matters are irrelevant to the case, but in the absence of an overview of the entire investigation and evidence, such a judgement may well be flawed.

Section 1 of *Confidentiality* [9] states clearly the view taken by the GMC on security of records: doctors who are responsible for confidential information must 'make sure that the information is effectively protected against improper disclosure at all times'.

It is difficult to comply with this apparently straightforward principle in the abnormal clinical situation between a doctor and a detainee to whom PACE applies. Paragraph 9.16 of Code C requires that 'If a medical practitioner does not record his findings in the custody record, the record must show where they are recorded.' However, the paragraph goes on to indicate that '. . . information which is necessary to custody staff to ensure the effective ongoing care and wellbeing of the detainee must be recorded openly in the custody record.'

Paragraph 2.5 of Code C states: 'The detainee, the appropriate adult or legal representative shall be permitted to inspect the original custody record after the person has left police detention . . .' Paragraph 2.4 A states that: 'When a detainee leaves police detention or is taken before a court, they, their legal representative or appropriate adult shall be given, on request, a copy of the custody record . . .'. There therefore exists a wide variety of people who may have legitimate access to a record containing clinical material. When making entries, doctors should be aware of the possible circulation of the record used.

Data Protection Act 1998

This ensures that information relating to an individual is obtained fairly, kept up to date and stored securely. The individual whose data are stored has rights of access enabling him/her to check the accuracy of the information. No information referring to those in custody, whether held by the police or the doctor, should be held on computer without appropriate registration under the Data Protection Act 1998. This Act now encompasses the provisions previously set out in the Access to Health Records 1990, which now only applies to deceased persons.

With appropriate consent in place, the forensic clinician is free to share information with the police, whence it will be disseminated to other agencies such as the Crown Prosecution Service, and prosecuting and defending counsel. This principle also applies to the victims of crime. However, we here must enter a note of caution. In the earlier section on consent, the doctor was invited to consider, when obtaining consent, how extensive that consent is, and therefore how free the doctor is to disclose the information obtained. It must be remembered that the consent of a detained person, or of a victim of assault, may not be fully 'informed'. This is particularly true when we consider the victim of a serious sexual assault, who will be tired, frightened and confused, and who may be under the influence of alcohol or other substances. Such a person may be incapable, at the time, of making decisions regarding the dissemination of highly confidential information. In such a case, 'best practice' dictates that a further approach is made at a later date to obtain detailed and informed consent to disclosure.

Disclosure

Several high-profile cases, including *R* v. *Saunders* (unreported) (the 'Guinness' case), *R* v. *Ward* [1993] 1 WLR 619; 2 All ER 577 CA and *R* v. *Keen* [1994] 1 WLR 746 have highlighted the issue of 'unused' or 'undisclosed' material. A firm onus is placed upon the prosecution to identify evidential material which, though not forming part of the prosecution case, should nevertheless be disclosed to the defence.

Such material will include the hand-written record, and private notes, made by a doctor following an examination. It may also include other confidential information, such as reports from probation officers, social services and health carers. The issue of disclosure was refined in *R* v. *Keane* (1994) 99 CrAppR1 by Lord Taylor of Gosforth CJ (page 752): 'The prosecution must identify the documents and information which are material . . . Having identified what is material, the prosecution should disclose it unless they wish to maintain that public interest immunity or other sensitivity justifies withholding some or all of it. . . . If in an exceptional case the prosecution are in doubt about the materiality of some documents or information, the court may be asked to rule on that issue.' The court then has the responsibility of conducting a balancing act in deciding between the rights of the defendant for a fair trial, and the rights of the keeper (here, the examining doctor) of the material to maintain confidentiality.

Firm guidance was issued by the Crown Prosecution Service in 1995 to Branch Crown Prosecutors that police surgeons' hand-written notes should be regarded as 'unused material', and should be passed to the defence, provided that the materiality test, as stated in *R* v. *Keane*, is met. Consequently, forensic physicians are now often approached by both police and Crown Prosecutors to disclose their hand-written notes, either immediately following an examination, or shortly afterwards. These notes may contain highly sensitive information, which the source may wish to keep confidential at all costs. Examples of such material include a previous history of sexual abuse in a victim of rape or a history of infidelity of which the partner of the victim was unaware.

There is a clear conflict between the need for the doctor to respect confidentiality, and the requirement to disclose. If a doctor accedes to a general request from the police to disclose, he faces severe penalties from the GMC. The GMC's stance remains unchanged, and is set out in the 2004 edition of *Confidentiality* [9]. At para 22, it states: 'Personal information may be disclosed in the public interest, without the patient's consent, and in exceptional cases where patients have withheld consent, where the benefits to an individual or to society of the disclosure outweigh the public and the patient's interest in keeping the information confidential. In all cases where you consider disclosing information without consent from the patient, you must weigh the possible harm (both to the patient, and the overall trust between doctors and patients) against the benefits which are likely to arise from the release of information.' Further 'In cases where there is a serious risk to the patient or others, disclosures may be justified even where patients have been asked to agree to a disclosure, but have withheld consent.' Specifically, 'Disclosure of personal information without consent may be justified in the public interest where failure to do so may expose the patient or others to risk of death or serious harm.'

The suggestion that 'You should inform patients that a disclosure will be made, wherever it is practicable to do so' may be more problematic in the custodial setting but it should be possible to comply with documentation in the patient's record any steps you have taken to seek or obtain consent and your reasons for disclosing information without consent. While stating that '. . . disclosure is necessary for the prevention or detection of a crime', the GMC is quite clear, in para 20, that: 'You must not disclose personal information to a third party such as a solicitor, police officer or officer of a court without the patient's express consent.'

The doctor's position in relation to the GMC is therefore unequivocal. In the absence of consent, he should not disclose unless directed to do so by a court. If he does disclose without consent, he faces the possibility of disciplinary procedures for impairment of fitness to practise.

In an attempt to resolve this dilemma, and following the publication of a Government consultation paper on disclosure, the BMA set up a

5

The doctor in court

Peter J. Franklin

The word forensic derives from the Latin word forum. In Rome, issues of the day were debated in public in the forum. Today, disputed matters such as arise from contracts, or employment, between citizens or companies, even involving the state, may be determined after public debate; these now occur in courts. The word forensic means related to a court, but it has come also to imply trace evidence capable of analysis in the laboratory (forensic science – see Chapter 16). It is the function of a court to hear conflicting evidence about the matter in hand and to determine which argument is (nearer to) the truth.

Types of evidence

The vast majority of people who appear in a criminal court to give evidence are led by the prosecution through a factual account of something that they have witnessed. After presentation of this evidence, the witness is questioned about it by the defence and alternative explanations may be offered for consideration by the witness and the court. When discrepancies are identified, the prosecution has a final opportunity to redress the balance by asking more questions. The court, too, may question the witness. In the case of witnesses for the defence, the same process of examination, cross-examination and re-examination applies. Elaborate

rules have developed to ensure that evidence is presented and challenged in a fair way. To witnesses these rules are arcane, and often seem designed to prevent evidence coming before the court, but most have stood the test of time. A witness may find his/her evidence interrupted while judge and advocates debate what may or may not be heard by a jury. The admissibility of hearsay evidence is a good example. The witness's manner of presenting evidence may add to, or detract from, the value that the court will attach to that evidence.

As a rule, lawyers and members of juries hold doctors to be honest, trustworthy, upstanding people who are capable of proper observation and then reflection upon what they have seen. As a medical witness, your aim, as you prepare a statement for court and later attend to present the evidence orally, is to marshal facts and opinions in a clear, concise manner for consideration by lay people. Doctors are among those allowed to offer *professional evidence*, that is to say – unlike *witnesses of fact* – they are likely to be asked to offer an opinion to the court based on what they have been told, what they have observed and what they concluded. A simple example could concern the description of an area of bruising, after which the witness is asked to state how and when it could have been caused. It can assist the court to know that a particular injury is unrelated to the incident under consideration.

Doctors giving *expert evidence* may not have examined the patient at all. They will have been sent a collection of papers, including witness statements, the doctor's reports and maybe copies of the doctor's original notes to peruse, and they will have been asked particular questions arising from these papers. They will prepare a report designed to test the observations, skill and opinions of the examining doctor, and to assist in cross-examination. They may sit in court or be called to testify in person.

Types of court

Although *civil courts* decide the matter under consideration 'on the balance of probability', forensic physicians provide evidence mainly for *criminal courts* where (in England and Wales) they appear before magistrates or in a Crown Court. Decisions in criminal courts are reached when matters are 'beyond all reasonable doubt'. Another forum often visited by doctors is the coroners' court. These courts are described in Chapters 1 and 18 respectively; Scottish procedure is outlined in Chapter 2.

Procedure

Forensic physicians work mainly at the behest of the police. The 'forensic' element of their work may be considered minor in comparison with their responsibilities for the care of those detained in police custody, but that seemingly mundane task can and does have evidential implications. That being so, it behoves every forensic physician to be meticulous in documentation, for only then may statements (see below) be completed fully and competently. You should also confirm that your statement is based upon your contemporaneous notes. It is a truism that the better the statement the less likely is a subsequent court appearance. The internal administrative structure varies from police force to police force, but requests for information come from the criminal investigation department, traffic officers, discipline department

and, of course, the Crown Prosecution Service. Statements prepared for court are given in terms of s9, Criminal Justice Act 1967, but further information may be available from, for instance, the custody record, correspondence and informal information given to the police.

Section 9 statement

The purpose of a statement is to provide credible information for the court. Much evidence is agreed between the parties, so that the provision of a statement acceptable to defence, prosecution and bench helps to clarify the issues, saving time and expense by obviating the witness's attendance. The statement begins with a standard format (see Box 5.1), but is not invalidated by the omission of the statutory provisions; in any case, these change from time to time. You may wish to say within the statement that you have produced it by referring to your original notes of the consultation.

> **Box 5.1** Statement of witness
>
> (Criminal Justice Act 1967, s9)
> (Magistrates' Courts Act 1980, ss5A(3a) and 5B)
> (Magistrate Court Rules 1981, r70)
> Statement of Dr Peter John Franklin, MB, BS.
> This statement (consisting of . . . pages, each signed by me) is made true to the best of my knowledge and belief and I make it knowing that, if it is tendered in evidence, I shall be liable to prosecution if I have wilfully stated anything in it which I know to be false or do not believe to be true.
>
> Dated the 15th day of March 2008
> Signed

There follows a preamble which explains who is writing the statement and how experienced is the author. You need to explain who you are, including relevant qualifications and experience. For example, if the case is one of sexual assault and you hold the qualification of MRCOG, put that in, with an explanation. Similarly, in a case pertaining to mental illness, you should indicate that you are approved under the Mental Health Act 1983 as amended by the Mental Health Act 2007. You could then say how much relevant experience you have working as a forensic physician. The purpose of this is to allow the court to assess how useful your evidence is likely to be and how much weight should be given to it.

The statement is more easily understood when broken into discreet paragraphs, each numbered sequentially. Pages are also numbered, making it easier to be taken to a particular point when in the witness box. Next comes an explanation that the patient gave consent for the consultation and a subsequent report to be produced for court. Then comes the reason for the consultation, the venue, the time it started and finished, and who was present.

It is proper to include the history – or histories (and by whom they were given) – for that is how doctors always work. We take a history and, after an examination where we test aspects of the history and consider differential diagnoses, we reach a working diagnosis. However, the court may decide not to allow the inclusion of the history, as it is 'hearsay' evidence. In a case of alleged sexual assault you may have in your notes sensitive confidential information that you believe the patient would like to be kept secret. In that case, you may refer to further information that you have which you believe is not relevant to the case. This means that you will be called to court to explain what the information is. You may try to reveal the facts only after the court has been cleared, but if the judge tells you that the information is relevant you will disclose it. In this way, you will have done all that is reasonable to maintain the patient's confidentiality. Any notes or personal data, and copies of statements and reports, whether in documentary or electronic form, are covered by data protection legislation (see Chapter 4). You are advised to keep your notes forever, even after retirement, for a sight of them, or a statement, can be requested at any time, maybe years after your consultation. It remains uncertain, though, how you arrange to dispose of this material after your death, as notes may still be relevant to a court hearing. You may ask a young colleague to hold them and to notify the police that they remain available.

Findings on examination are detailed in a logical sequence. Attention must be drawn to any inconsistencies between the history and the examination. Lay people might expect that following a sexual assault, particularly of a child, the medical examination would be highly significant. Experience will show that this is not necessarily so. This needs to be explained: it is often the case that all one can say is, 'My findings neither confirm nor refute the allegation.' Such a remark expresses the witness's opinion, and concludes the statement.

There are dangers in dictating a report or a statement to a police officer, for such a procedure inhibits the normal flow of a medical report, and it is better to ask the police officer to call back in a day or two when you have had ample time to prepare a proper report with which you are comfortable. An excellent habit is to prepare a statement one day and then return to it another day and reread it before putting it in its final format: mistakes are more readily found. Finally, it is helpful to reserve the word 'statement' for a document to be used in court, thereby concentrating one's mind on its ultimate purpose.

In court

Completion of a section 9 statement renders the witness liable to a subsequent court appearance. Any witness summons carries the defendant's name and the date of the alleged offence, but you may have examined the complainant on a date some days after the alleged offence. You must familiarize yourself with the local arrangements for ascertaining the necessary information. You should then look out your own notes, reports and statements to refresh your memory of the case well in advance of any court appearance. In addition, revise your knowledge of the relevant clinical forensic medicine. Consider the questions likely to be raised and how you will respond. You are a professional witness whose job it is to assist the court with difficult technical medical matters that lay people cannot readily understand without assistance. As part of that explanatory process, your statement must be written in plain English; wherever technical terms are essential these should be accompanied by the most appropriate lay term. You are neither a defence nor a prosecution witness. Despite a prosecution decision not to call you, the defence may wish to test your evidence and insist that you attend court. You should keep court staff aware of any planned absence, but your obligation is to attend if and when summoned. A failure to do so is a contempt of court, laying you open to severe penalties ranging from a public apology to the court to a swingeing fine. In practice, courts are understanding of the pressures on a doctor's time; most medical witnesses can be contacted by telephone to arrange a suitable time to give evidence.

When the time comes to attend court, men should always dress in a suit with a discreet tie. Ladies should be equally formally dressed, but it is important for witnesses to feel comfortable. If you are unfamiliar with its layout, ask to see the inside of the court before you enter. Only expert witnesses may be present in court to hear any of the evidence before they give theirs. Your time should be totally dedicated to the court, with no responsibilities to work elsewhere.

You are likely to have to pass through security, so leave behind belongings such as pager and telephone. Try to park with an abundance of time paid for, to eliminate any worry about a parking fine when you ought to be concentrating on the evidence.

When you enter the witness box you will be asked to swear on a holy book taken in the right hand, use some religiously significant ritual or affirm that you will 'tell the truth, the whole truth and nothing but the truth'. During this procedure you have the opportunity to gauge the volume and speed at which you will speak. You should address your replies to the judge (see Box 5.2 for terminology) or to the jury rather than to the lawyer who is talking to you. As you engage in a conversation with the lawyer it becomes difficult not to face him. You can try standing with your feet facing the judge and then turning your shoulders to the lawyer. Although

this is a little uncomfortable, when you become anxious, and you forget that you should be facing the judge, your body will return to align with your feet and you will find yourself facing where you ought to be facing. You should speak loudly enough for all of the court to be able to hear you. You should speak slowly enough for the judge to make notes without asking you to stop. To do this, you need to be watching his/her pen as he/she writes.

Box 5.2 Correct terms of address in court	
Judicial officers in court should be addressed as:	
All Higher Court Judges	
(House of Lords/Court of Appeal/Divisional Court)	My Lord/My Lady
High Court Masters & Registrars	
Master (whether male or female)	Master
Registrar	Registrar
Circuit Judges	
Central Criminal Court (and some provincial courts)	My Lord/My Lady
Circuit Judges	
Crown Court	Your Honour
All other Courts* and Tribunals	Sir or Ma'am
Note: *In Northern Ireland, magistrates are addressed as 'Your Worship'.	

The prosecution lawyer will lead through your statement, starting with your name, address and professional qualifications. This allows you to explain to the court just how relevant is all of your experience and why, therefore, the court should pay particular attention to your evidence.

As you are taken through the rest of your statement, you may need to refer to your original, contemporaneous (thorough and complete) notes, but you must ask the permission of the judge or magistrates. This is unlikely to be refused. You are liable to be asked whether the notes were made at the time. The court needs to know that they are accurate and not subject to any possible weakness caused by a poor memory, if they were made later.

The process of eliciting your evidence by the lawyer who called you is described as the *examination in chief*. You will be asked to explain why you have reached the conclusions that you have. When the prosecution lawyer has finished going through your statement the lawyer for the defence will rise to *cross-examine* you on what you have said. He/she will, of course, offer different explanations for what you have described. If any point is valid, it is right to concede that that explanation is reasonable, but may not be the whole truth. An example: 'Yes, it is true that that bruise on the front of the leg might have been caused by an accidental fall. Indeed, all of the 17 injuries that I have described might have been caused by accidents but I still prefer the explanation I have already given that the overall pattern of injuries of different ages is consistent with 'non-accidental injury.'

When the defence has finished, you may be *re-examined* by the prosecution. Under the rules of evidence no new matters may be introduced at this stage. The prosecution is only allowed to revisit matters already aired. When these matters have been exhausted the judge may have questions for you of his/her own. So, look to the judge for permission to leave. When you do leave, you are likely to be released from the court, but you might be expected to stay around in case the court needs further medical advice and assistance from you.

In answering questions, try always to be brief. If you can honestly and safely reply with a simple 'yes', that is fine. If you are unclear what is being asked, ask for the question to be repeated. If you do not know the answer then say, 'I do not know.' This is not an admission of ignorance, but of honesty. It is tempting, always, to try to assist the court wherever you can, but you are strongly advised to stick within your areas of knowledge.

In time, you may become comfortable in court, but you will never be as comfortable as the lawyers. Some may try to discredit you and, therefore, your evidence, perhaps by suggesting that you are 'only' a primary care physician. A lawyer may try to belittle you by saying, 'Ah yes, doctor, but that is only your opinion.' You need not respond, because an opinion is what has been requested of you. Do not allow yourself to be provoked into an impolite riposte. When well prepared, you can rise above any lawyerly sarcasm. Another technique to recognize and guard against is the use by lawyers of lengthy questions containing multiple elements, some of which you accept, but others put a contrary slant. You are quite entitled to ask for a question to be rephrased, if need be by appealing to the judge.

The expert

With postgraduate training and relevant experience, including a postgraduate qualification, you may offer your services to lawyers as an expert. The use of experts has become controversial, but the defence is entitled to seek an opinion on which to base a valid challenge to the evidence provided by the prosecution doctor. You may quite properly agree with many of the points but if there is a reasonable, alternative explanation it is right for the court to hear it. Expert witnesses have the disadvantage that they have not seen the patient, but they do have the advantage of seeing many more of the relevant papers than the examining doctor. They are better placed to put the evidence that they have seen in perspective. They are likely to see different histories, and these may readily suggest sensible explanations to put before juries. From the solicitor's point of view, an expert's opinion allows different fields for cross-examination to be explored. As is made clear in the 'expert declaration' below, no spurious ground may be advanced; no defence expert need be afraid of agreeing entirely with the prosecution case. Guidance for expert witnesses is available on the BMA website [1].

The expert report can follow whatever format the expert chooses to use but, instead of the formal s9 introduction, there must be a declaration of truth at the end. The suggested format is given below.

EXPERT DECLARATION

1. I understand that my overriding duty is to the court both in preparing reports and in giving oral evidence. I have complied and will continue to comply with that duty.
2. I have set out in my report what I understand from those instructing me to be the questions in respect of which the opinions are required.
3. I have done my best, in preparing this report, to be accurate and complete. I have mentioned all

matters which I regard as relevant to the opinions I have expressed. All the matters on which I have expressed an opinion are within my field of expertise.

4. I have drawn to the attention of the court all matters of which I am aware, which might affect my opinion.

5. Wherever I have personal knowledge, I have indicated the source of factual information.

6. I have not included anything in this report which has been suggested to me by anyone, including the lawyers instructing me, without forming my own independent view of the matter.

7. Where, in my view, there is a range of opinion, I have indicated the extent of the range in the report.

8. At the time of signing the report I consider it to be complete and accurate. I will notify those instructing me if, for any reason, I subsequently consider that the report requires any correction or qualification.

9. I understand that this report will be the evidence that I give on oath, subject to any correction or qualification I may make before I swear to this veracity.

10. I have attached to this report a summary of my instructions.

STATEMENT OF TRUTH

I confirm that insofar as the facts in my report are within my knowledge I have made clear which they are and I believe them to be true, and the opinions I have expressed represent my true and complete professional opinion.

Fees

You are advised to check with the BMA website [2] for current fees. The police pay for a section 9 statement (responsibility to pay for work as a witness passes to the Crown Prosecution Service after the police investigative phase ends). It is proper to wait until a statement is requested. It is wrong to produce one on every patient you see. If the defence asks for a copy of your notes or a statement or report, you may charge them a reasonable fee for this. It is courtesy also to tell the police and prosecuting authority that this copy has been requested by the defence.

In England and Wales in criminal matters, fees for your attendance, including travel to and from court, are paid from central funds. As a professional witness, the fees are determined by the Lord Chancellor's office. If called by the Crown, the time away from your practice is split into two-hour periods: you may claim in accordance with the time absent. If you need to employ a locum to cover your work, you may claim for that instead, not in addition. Claims must be supported by appropriate receipts. If you attend court and do not give evidence you can still claim, but you need to ensure that the prosecuting caseworker or court know of your attendance. Cancellation fees may be paid if you cannot mitigate your costs, but will have to be argued on a case-by-case basis.

An expert witness in criminal matters can submit reasonable fees for considering papers, examining a person, preparing a report and for attendance at court, subject to the constraints of the Legal Services Commission, taxation or any instructing private individual. It is prudent to get written instructions and confirmation from instructing solicitors or the Crown that they will meet your costs before any work is commenced. Payment for attendance at court as an expert witness, together with travel expenses, should be sought from the court, and is subject to guidance from the Lord Chancellor's office.

REFERENCES

1. www.bma.org.uk/ap.nsf/Content/Expertwitness (updated October 2007)
2. www.bma.org.uk/ap.ns/Content/medicolegal

FURTHER READING

Ward R, Wragg A, eds. (2005) *Walker and Walker's English Legal System*, 9th edn. Oxford: Oxford University Press. ISBN 0406959536.

6

Custody medicine: physical conditions

Jeanne Herring

Introduction

Forensic physicians (FPs) attend police custody suites to advise on immediate medical care for detained persons (DPs) and on any need for ongoing care during the detention period. They may be asked to assess adults' or juveniles' fitness for detention following arrest, to conduct a mental health assessment where custody is the place of safety, to examine children brought to a place of safety under a Police Protection Order, to advise on those detained by Immigration and to give medical guidance for those on remand or sentenced. Detained persons may need to be interviewed and/or charged and are commonly held overnight for court.

Guidance for the police in England, Wales and Northern Ireland is provided in the Police and Criminal Evidence Act 1984 (PACE). Revised Codes of Practice under the Act are published from time to time by the Stationery Office in, respectively, London and Belfast. Medical advice should be sought for those:

- apparently suffering from a physical or mental illness;
- needing assessment of problems related to substance misuse including alcohol;
- who require medication;
- injured before or during arrest;
- who may be suffering from an infectious disease;
- who request a doctor;
- discharged to custody from hospital.

The Police and Criminal Evidence Act 1984 allows for clinical attention to be given by an appropriate healthcare professional (HCP) but, as this chapter is written primarily as guidance for doctors working in the custodial environment, it is written in the second person. Health care is increasingly provided by multidisciplinary teams who may seek FP guidance by telephone or the doctor may be called to attend following an initial assessment by an HCP colleague. A clear understanding of the different roles and responsibilities for each aspect of DP care is essential (*Good Medical Practice*, p. 22) [1] and may be assisted by agreed written working guidelines. Team working does not lessen the doctor's personal accountability for the professional conduct and care given. There is a need to ensure that communication is effective, both within and outside the team, and respects guidance on confidentiality (see Chapter 4). Clinical governance procedures should be in place to monitor and review the team's performance and deal supportively with any problems raised (*Management for Doctors*, p. 16) [1].

Principles

The health, safety and wellbeing of the DP are paramount [2] and this may at times override forensic

Clinical Forensic Medicine, third edition ed. W. D. S. McLay. Published by Cambridge University Press. © Cambridge University Press 2009.

considerations. Detained persons have the right to request a doctor of their own choice although there is no obligation on that doctor to attend. Your duties are to conduct adequate assessments, provide suitable treatment or investigations when necessary, work within your own competence and keep good records. Effective communication is essential, including DP, police and HCPs, even those who may care for the person outside custody. At all times you must be aware of seeking appropriate consent to treatment. In respecting confidentiality, carefully consider the disclosure of only relevant information necessary for DP care and be prepared to justify these decisions if later challenged (*Seeking Patients' Consent* and *Confidentiality*) [1]. The DP should understand that he is not obliged to consent nor is there an absolute privilege of confidentiality.

Except in emergency situations, juveniles should have a parent or responsible adult present. When a DP of the opposite sex is examined, consider a chaperone of the same sex.

Consultation problems within custody

During the consultation its purpose may change from therapeutic to evidence gathering; in that event, be open about this, seeking and recording appropriate consent.

The effectiveness of any doctor/patient consultation is based on consent and trust, which facilitate reliable history taking, thorough examination and a considered management plan shared with the patient. In an emergency the doctor can treat only for that condition on the 'best interests' principle. Many DPs have multiple morbidities, and in any consultation combinations of physical illness, mental illness and injury are common. In addition, recent drug consumption has been demonstrated for one or more illicit drugs in 69% and two or more substances in 36% [3]. Co-morbidities and specific risks in the custody consultation elevate the potential for death in custody. If an enquiry investigating such an event revealed sub-optimal treatment the FP could face criminal proceedings.

Custody presents many barriers to favourable communication and treatment, and this may begin when the doctor is initially briefed with a version of events necessarily viewed from a police perspective. You may be advised on any clinical conditions by an HCP, and the one or two steps removed history introduces a potential for error and even prejudice. You may feel more or less subtle pressure to resolve matters in the best interests of the criminal justice system and not in the DP's best medical interests.

History taking may be unreliable as DPs can be intoxicated, lack awareness of their condition, give false information to obtain prescription medication or to try to force diversion on medical grounds. In some DPs, mental health problems, learning disabilities or language barriers impede communication. Anxiety levels may be heightened, causing distraction and reducing concentration during the consultation for both parties. Privacy may enhance truthful history sharing, especially in relation to illicit drug misuse, but police advice regarding doctor safety must be fully considered. Risks of violence towards HCPs working with those with a history of violence, intoxication and those with personal problems are well documented [4]. The FP normally lacks previous medical knowledge of the DP and has no access to records held in other parts of the health service. It is prudent to verify a history, preferably with the consent of the DP, that would require a prescription of drugs, particularly if these are misused in the community, but this can be impossible outside daytime hours.

Thorough examination can be limited by lack of or changing capacity to consent, intoxication, verbal or physical hostility and poor compliance and concentration. Clinical conditions may be imperfect and not infrequently examinations take place in poorly lit cells with the DP lying on the floor surrounded by blood or other body fluids (always treated as high risk) hindering the ability to make a comprehensive examination. Sterilization equipment is rarely available, limiting safe management of wounds to basic care only.

There is a short time window for treatment plans, and DPs are commonly reluctant to agree management plans if they seek diversion, or mistrust the doctor. A humane, honest and non-judgemental approach with an emphasis on reassuring the DP of your independent role, and your desire to provide good health care and advice to custody carers to enable them to provide safe supervision in the DP's best interests is usually rewarded. Lack of co-operation may subside as anger at incarceration lessens, intoxication resolves and the DP reconsiders the need for medical assistance, so a further consultation may be advisable at a later stage.

Research indicates that episodes of deliberate self-harm (DSH) occur soon after arrest, particularly in those with a previous history of DSH and a past psychiatric history and also in those withdrawing from drugs. The young appear to be especially at risk from these factors [5]; you must fully consider this in advising staff on the level of cell supervision. A survey of 600 doctors in Scotland [6] revealed that one in three doctors had experienced physical or verbal abuse at work in the past year. The Emergency Workers (Scotland) Act 2005 was introduced to increase penalties for individuals who assault public sector workers such as hospital doctors and those attending emergency situations in the community.

Cell facilities, sanitation and freedom to access fluids and food are limited in comparison to the DP's home conditions. Disabled DPs will need special consideration, as few custody suites have suitable disabled facilities.

Police staff lack clinical training, so that you must only expect delivery of a standard of care provided by a lay person. You need to advise fully in writing any potential health needs or risks, with guidance on how these should be managed. Check that this has been fully comprehended (for instance, the risk of hypoglycaemia in diabetics and its management). Bring to the attention of the custody officer any need for medical review, and how this interfaces with the criminal justice process. Although nurses or paramedics may be available in some suites, the administration of medication in many areas is by non-clinical staff, increasing the potential for error.

Detained persons may themselves request review, but if you feel that a clinical change or a time-related risk may develop (such as epilepsy or alcohol withdrawal) give guidance, verbally and in writing, when a further assessment should occur. If you cannot make a thorough assessment initially, always raise the possibility of further review.

When care is dangerously compromised and might cause deterioration in clinical condition, act with caution and recommend that the DP is not fit to be detained, or refer to hospital. You may need to review a decision by a hospital HCP unaware of the limitations of custody and the lack of clinically trained staff on site to deem fit and discharge a DP from Accident and Emergency (A&E) back to custody.

Consider cell conditions (for example ambient temperature and ventilation) and supplies (such as blankets and pillows) and that the DP is allowed sufficient sleep or rest. Personal hygiene, specific dietary and fluid requests should be brought to the attention of the custody staff. Suggestions for access to fresh air and paradoxically a cigarette break (stations became non-smoking in July 2007) may resolve tension and reduce unnecessary medication or DSH attempts induced by frustration.

In summary, be alert to the host of difficulties that introduce risks specific to custody consultations, and be confident that risks have been managed in a safe and appropriate manner and that the necessary information for ongoing care has been shared with staff. A review should be advised if the level of risk remains high or might reasonably be predicted to escalate as detention progresses.

Notes or pro formas

Clear, concise, contemporaneous notes and, when suitable, use of body diagrams to document injuries are essential. These are the foundation for comprehensive and unambiguous statements that may prevent court appearances at a later date. Example pro formas for most clinical situations may be found on the Faculty of Forensic and Legal Medicine (FFLM) website [7]. Your personal notes should be retained and stored safely. For computerized records, registration under the Data Protection Act 1984 is required.

In many suites there are now National Strategic Police Information Systems (NSPIS) computerized custody records incorporating a medical section. Entries need sufficient information, given in lay terminology, to allow custodians to care for the DP, but non-pertinent information should be retained in you own notes. Some NSPIS domain fields are compulsory, but you may feel unable to give a sound opinion after a limited consultation, and a system should be developed in each FP group to avoid confusion. An example is the need to give a time when the DP will be fit for interview, although heavily intoxicated at the time and a full assessment has not been possible.

If a DP refuses to permit disclosure of medical information that the doctor deems essential for his safety, inform him of the intention to disclose and the reasons why this is necessary. There must also be sufficient baseline information to assist the next doctor or HCP to monitor the situation and provide continuity of care. It may be that some information should be shared with other HCPs and not the police; this may be left in sealed, named envelopes.

Medication

You have a duty to care for DPs to the same standard as people not in custody, including the continuation of appropriate medication prescribed prior to detention. The Medicines Act 1968 permits doctors to prescribe a prescription only medicine (POM) to a DP in their care: this must be on a private prescription. It is important to ensure that record keeping for prescribing and administration of medication is kept accurate to date and time, and that the instructions guarantee the intended DP is given the correct medication, in the correct dosage, at the appointed time. Bear in mind that prescribed medication regimes prior to detention have been carefully evaluated and continued only when appropriate and safe. Always consider the risks

and benefits of prescribing to any DP under the influence of drugs or alcohol.

Parenteral POMs may only be administered by a medical practitioner or an appropriately trained HCP acting on the instructions of the FP, and it is recommended that the FP or HCP supervise the self-administration of insulin to prevent an overdose in the attempt to seek diversion. Self-administration of adrenaline by Epipen may be authorized after you have assessed the risks of anaphylaxis in custody against the potential for harm to self or others from the device.

All doctors must comply with the Misuse of Drugs Act 1971, the Misuse of Drugs Regulations 2001 and PACE 1984 (in Scotland, the Criminal Procedure (Scotland) Act 1995) in respect of controlled drugs, keeping them in a locked receptacle with a record of when they are used. No police officer may administer or supervise the administration of controlled drugs listed under the Misuse of Drugs Regulations 2001 Schedule 1, 2 or 3; this should be under the personal supervision of the registered medical practitioner authorizing their use. These include methadone mixture, methadone tablets, buprenorphine and temazepam.

It is important to note a history of allergy to medication and dressings. Local prescribing policies may be informed by a prescribing group directive (PGD) but, although nurses may supply under a PGD, police officers and custodians are not permitted to do so.

Medication may be obtained from the DP's property, be brought in from home, obtained from the custody drug supplies provided by the police or be dispensed from the doctor's bag. You may also obtain medication from a local pharmacist on a private prescription; controlled drugs should be issued on a FP10CD personalized prescription. Take particular care with methadone to inform the regular pharmacist and prescribing doctor so that, if released, the DP does not take a double dose with potential fatal effects.

Administration of medication in custody should be from a secure location, either the FP's bag or a secure cupboard with limited access. You should be confident that medication dispensed from your own bag is in date and in good condition; it is recommended that a note be kept of name of supplier and batch number.

When medication is brought in from home it is important to verify that it bears the correct name and dosage, it was recently dispensed and that the quantity remaining is consistent with the date issued and dosage regime. Detained persons with opiate or benzodiazepine dependence may self-medicate with POM at levels that far exceed guidance on safe prescribing. If the medication preparation and regime cannot be verified as appropriate and safe it should not be continued. Special care should be extended to liquid preparations, and it may be safer to obtain a new prescription.

If you leave medication for a DP this should ideally be in individual dose, self-closing tablet bags that bear the DP's name, medication name and strength and quantity required at stated times. Mark clearly on the envelope and record the total quantity of each tablet you leave. Leave written instructions for administration or on the NSPIS medication record. The total number or quantity should be recorded so that it is possible to check at any time how many have been used. Bring any potential serious side effects that might occur to the attention of staff, as well as the need to administer with or without food.

Ideally two police (or civilian) officers should administer medication and they must observe the DP taking the medication to avoid hoarding. Refusal to take any should be reported to the FP. You may also authorize medication to be left in the cell with the DP, particularly asthma inhalers or angina sprays, if the person is not assessed as high risk of DSH and the device has been checked for tampering.

Leave instructions about disposal of unused medication when the DP is released or transferred or give authority for it to travel with him to court or prison.

Liaison with custody staff on arrival

The problems that can hinder a consultation have been considered previously, but to give appropriate advice it is essential for you to be fully briefed in relation to the medical guidance required. It is desirable, despite time constraints, to record on arrival this information:

- why FP has been called (physical, mental illness, medication or injuries);
- reason for arrest (e.g. special medical care may be advised for those detained under the Terrorism Act 2000, see FFLM website [7]);
- details of arrest (behaviour of the DP, whether restraint or force used);
- if medication, prescriptions, containers or medical information in possession at arrest;
- suggestion that illicit drugs have been used or were found on or near the DP;
- information from other sources, e.g. relatives, family, friends, carers, hospital or primary care physician;
- police information on Police National Computer (PNC) and risk assessment;
- is request to assess fitness for detention, charge, interview or transfer or any combination of these? (NSPIS requires a response to all questions for each consultation);
- anticipated length of detention (caution: further charges may be brought, so you should consider the need to give guidance on any necessary medical review, e.g. epilepsy);
- details of any previous FP or HCP assessments relevant to this detention;
- estimated time to interview (caution: may differ from estimated time);
- forensic samples or specialized forensic assessments required;
- home circumstances (if release considered).

Consultations in relation to specific medical conditions

The following section describes the impact of common medical conditions on fitness for detention. If you would not feel it safe to manage the person with this condition at home, consider a recommendation for hospital transfer.

You will also need to consider how these conditions affect fitness for interview. A DP may be unfit for interview when:

(a) Conducting an interview could worsen any existing physical or mental illness to a significant degree.

(b) Anything said or done by the DP at the time of detention may be considered unreliable in subsequent court proceedings *because* of the physical or mental state of the DP.

Clear schemata for assessment of fitness to interview exist [8].

Asthma

You must be aware that patients with severe asthma and one or more adverse psychosocial factors (such as psychiatric illness, alcohol or drug abuse, denial, unemployment) are at risk of death [9]. Detained persons with life-threatening asthma are not fit to be detained. The flow diagram in Fig. 6.1 has been compiled with guidance from published sources [10].

Diabetes

This may be Type 1 insulin-dependent diabetes mellitus (IDDM) or Type 2 non-insulin-dependent diabetes mellitus (NIDDM). Record a clear history, noting duration of diabetes, medication, episodes of hypo- or hyperglycaemia and hospital admissions. Diabetics may have disease complications or co-morbidities with the potential to cause vulnerability during detention or interview, and these should be actively sought and recorded. These include cardiovascular, renal, visual, neurological and skin problems. Risks of complication are increased in those with poor disease control, a frequent situation for many detained in custody. South Asian or Afro-Caribbean racial groups have a higher risk of diabetes and complications. Co-morbidity with substance misuse, especially alcohol, is common, and mental illness, in particular depression, has a higher incidence in diabetics; these should be fully considered in advice for care during detention and interview.

You should have the means to test blood glucose, preferably with a quantitative portable meter that also indicates if ketones are present, and you should always consider a baseline blood glucose estimation. Results should be shared with other HCPs for ongoing care.

Oral hypoglycaemics and insulin should normally be continued after careful evaluation for safety. In relation particularly to IDDM, check that regular meals are available and the DP has access to rapidly absorbed carbohydrate-rich food if needed. Ensure that custody staff have been informed of the features of hypoglycaemia (sweating, pallor, anxiety and confusion) and advised that, if a diabetic's condition deteriorates, it is safer to assume this is related to hypoglycaemia and to offer or administer glucose swiftly. This may prove life saving and would not adversely affect hyperglycaemia. You must then be informed, even if recovery is complete, as therapy alterations may be necessary. Hypoglycaemia can also occur as a complication of heavy alcohol use and stimulant drug ingestion.

Some DPs with IDDM may use a syringe or pen device as a weapon on themselves or others. It is also possible for them to seek medical diversion by administering an overdose and, therefore, you should consider supervising the self-administration of insulin. The DP might also inject insulin, then refuse food to create a hypoglycaemic episode; if this is a concern, suggest giving food and then insulin rather than the reverse procedure. Refusal to administer insulin would indicate the need for detailed contemporaneous notes advising the DP of potential short- and long-term risks and a care plan to advise frequent reassessments.

The possible impact of impaired blood sugar on cognitive function, concentration and memory and recall needs to be considered in relation to fitness for interview. After an episode of hypoglycaemia conduct a full mental health assessment after recovery to exclude impaired intellectual functioning. It has been recommended that blood glucose should be kept above 6 mmol/L for a diabetic person to give a statement or be interviewed [11].

Management of Asthma in Custody

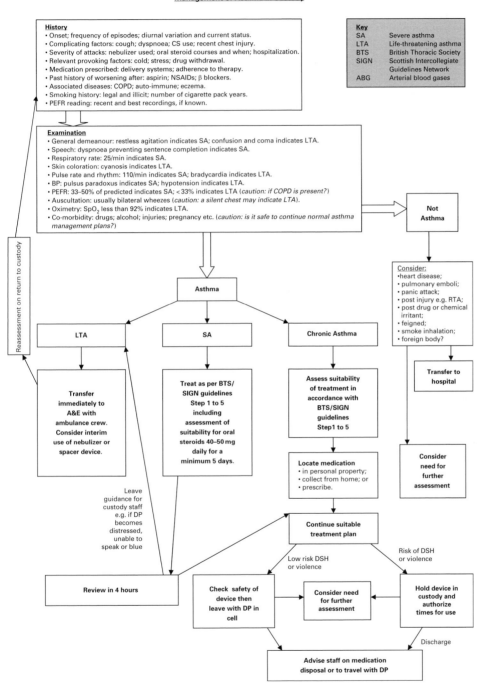

Fig. 6.1 Management of asthma in custody.

Detained persons with rising blood glucose need careful monitoring; if necessary, custody staff should be given instructions to rouse and check responses overnight. Normally it is advisable for DPs with IDDM and any NIDDM persons with other co-morbidity or complications to be reviewed by the FP or HCP every day.

The flow chart shown in Fig. 6.2 has been compiled with reference to current guidance [11, 12].

Epilepsy

Many epileptics in custody are well controlled and reliably manage their condition. Others, however, may have a chaotic non-adherence to therapy, complications of other conditions such as substance misuse, psychiatric illness or recent injury. Some DPs state they suffer from 'fits' but these may be in relation to alcohol or benzodiazepine withdrawal [13]. False claims of fits or seizures may be made in an attempt to seek medication and pseudo-seizures may be feigned as an attempt to avoid the criminal justice system. Fits may also occur in acute drug intoxication, especially following drug-stuffing and rupture of the package. It may be difficult to verify the therapy history, and all these factors mean a cautious and meticulous history should be taken to include:

- type of epilepsy, e.g. partial simple or complex, generalized or temporal lobe;
- frequency of fits;
- date of most recent fit;
- note of relevant provoking factors, e.g. stress or sleep deprivation;
- details of medication and dose regime;
- when medication was last taken and when next dose is due;
- associated head injury (old or recent);
- substance misuse;
- mental health disorder including learning disability;
- intracranial lesions as a cause of epilepsy, e.g. tumour.

Careful examination is needed for all epileptics to assess neurological and mental state. Intoxication with alcohol or other central nervous system depressants or concomitant head injury need to be excluded before authorization is given to continue any legitimate medication in the person's property. Intoxicated DPs may need to be reviewed to check for sobriety before medication is recommended.

A claim that the person has epilepsy, but is treated with benzodiazepines only, should be regarded with scepticism (except clobazepam, recommended in the BNF as an adjunct in epilepsy with associated anxiety state). Clonazepam is the only benzodiazepine used as a long-term anticonvulsant in all forms of seizure, in particular myoclonus and absence attacks.

Missing a single dose of anticonvulsant overnight should normally have little adverse effect as many of these drugs have a long half-life. Carbamazepine and sodium valproate, however, both have a short half-life of about 12 hours and should be recommenced as soon as practicable, and administered in divided doses up to four times daily to avoid side effects. Phenytoin is the only drug likely to cause toxicity if a high dose is suddenly administered, so await verification or commence with a lower dose if the DP claims to take a dose you consider high. Custody staff should have the necessary skills to administer first-aid if a known epileptic has a fit during detention, and the doctor should then be called to review the DP. Following a single fit, it would normally be safe for the patient to remain in custody, but unconsciousness longer than 10 minutes, second fit or 'first-ever' fit, status epilepticus or fit related to head injury indicate immediate hospital transfer.

Status epilepticus should be treated with intravenous or rectal diazepam (never intramuscular) with good airway attention and then hospitalization for a period of observation afterwards.

Epileptics may suffer from cognitive impairment as a result of their condition or therapy, and their intellectual function, memory and concentration need to be assessed as well as assessment for personality disorders that might render them vulnerable in interview. An appropriate adult might be afforded to such cases.

Management of Diabetes in Custody

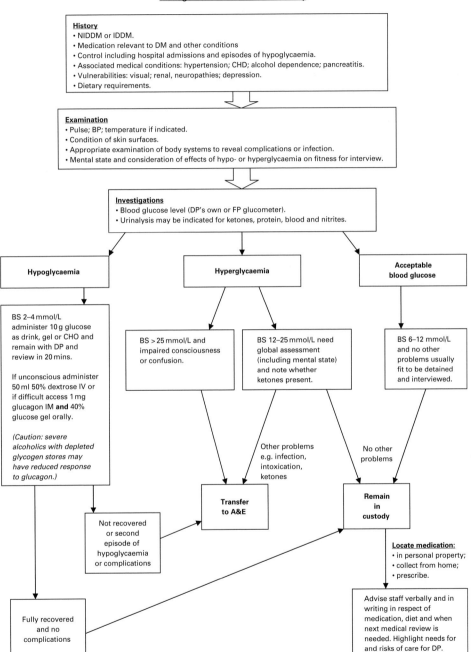

History
- NIDDM or IDDM.
- Medication relevant to DM and other conditions
- Control including hospital admissions and episodes of hypoglycaemia.
- Associated medical conditions: hypertension; CHD; alcohol dependence; pancreatitis.
- Vulnerabilities: visual; renal, neuropathies; depression.
- Dietary requirements.

Examination
- Pulse; BP; temperature if indicated.
- Condition of skin surfaces.
- Appropriate examination of body systems to reveal complications or infection.
- Mental state and consideration of effects of hypo- or hyperglycaemia on fitness for interview.

Investigations
- Blood glucose level (DP's own or FP glucometer).
- Urinalysis may be indicated for ketones, protein, blood and nitrites.

Hypoglycaemia

Hyperglycaemia

Acceptable blood glucose

BS 2–4 mmol/L administer 10 g glucose as drink, gel or CHO and remain with DP and review in 20 mins.

If unconscious administer 50 ml 50% dextrose IV or if difficult access 1 mg glucagon IM **and** 40% glucose gel orally.

(Caution: severe alcoholics with depleted glycogen stores may have reduced response to glucagon.)

BS > 25 mmol/L and impaired consciousness or confusion.

BS 12–25 mmol/L need global assessment (including mental state) and note whether ketones present.

BS 6–12 mmol/L and no other problems usually fit to be detained and interviewed.

Other problems e.g. infection, intoxication, ketones

No other problems

Transfer to A&E

Remain in custody

Not recovered or second episode of hypoglycaemia or complications

Fully recovered and no complications

Locate medication:
- in personal property;
- collect from home;
- prescribe.

Advise staff verbally and in writing in respect of medication, diet and when next medical review is needed. Highlight needs for and risks of care for DP.

Fig. 6.2 Management of diabetes in custody.

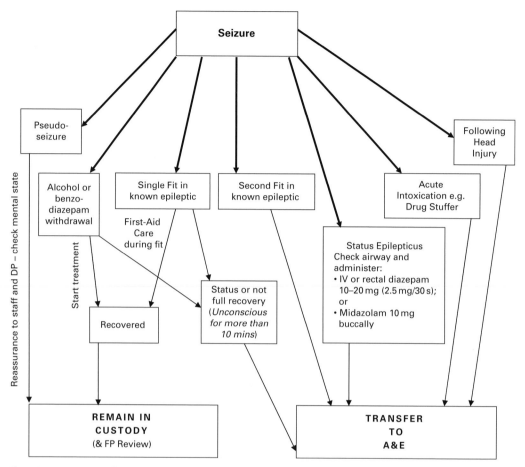

Fig. 6.3 Management of seizures in custody.

A flow chart for the management of seizures in custody is shown in Fig. 6.3.

Heart disease

The most common cardiac conditions encountered in the custodial setting are hypertension, angina, cardiac failure and stable dysrrhythmias. A full history, examination of the cardiovascular system including blood pressure (BP), pulse and auscultation of the heart and chest should be performed for baseline measurements. Regular medication can normally be continued after drug or alcohol intoxication has resolved. Stimulants and solvents have both been reported to cause death from dysrrythmias and referral to hospital may be advisable in cases where there is pre-existing cardiovascular disease.

Detained persons may be allowed to keep their angina sprays (glyceryl trinitrate; GTN) or tablets with them, after checking for concealed items, unless there is a significant risk of self-harm from the device. They should be told to advise staff of frequency of usage and immediately if chest pain does not settle so hospital transfer can be organized.

You must assess immediately any symptoms of acute chest pain and/or breathlessness for possible hospital diversion, but this referral may be urgent and precede the arrival of the doctor. It may be appropriate to advise staff to administer 300 mg aspirin (if non-allergic) and GTN spray over the telephone. If you are in the custody area at the time, remain until the ambulance arrives in case emergency intervention is required; this reassures both DP and staff. Management of acute chest pain in custody needs caution: arrange hospital transfer if there is any doubt about the causation of chest pain.

Deep vein thrombosis (DVT)

Intravenous drug misuse is an important risk factor in the community for DVT [14]. Detained persons' compliance with anticoagulant therapy is commonly chaotic. Take a careful history and, in acute cases, consider the use of clinical prediction scores such as Wells [15]. A score > 2 suggests referral for D-dimer testing, ultrasound and commencement of low molecular weight heparin. In the case of DPs with chronic conditions, note when the last INR (international normalized ratio) blood test was taken and the result. Recommend continuation of anticoagulant therapy for stable uncomplicated cases but those whose therapy has lapsed or who have complications should be considered for transfer to A&E. Blood tests for INR can be performed during detention if necessary.

Sickle-cell disease (SS)

Most DPs with this disease are aware of their illness, vulnerabilities and what to expect during a crisis. Advise custody staff of the features of a sickle crisis and the need for immediate hospital transfer. Cold, stress, rapid cooling after exercise as in a pursuit, lack of adequate analgesia, dehydration and infection are all known to precipitate a crisis, which might be relevant in custody. Staff should be advised to supply adequate warmth with blankets, fluids and analgesia for these DPs.

Those with homozygous SS may suffer from poor growth, end organ damage (eye, lungs, kidney and brain), drug dependence (including iatrogenic) as well as social, psychological and emotional problems. Any of these increases vulnerability during detention and interview, so needs careful consideration.

Pregnancy

Female DPs, seeking diversion, may spuriously claim to be pregnant, but irregular or absent menses are frequently found in substance misusers. You have to consider fitness for detention individually if pregnancy is confirmed. A pregnancy test may be performed in the first trimester to confirm the diagnosis, and urinalysis may be helpful. Examination should include pulse, BP, abdominal examination, auscultation of the fetal heart and examination of the relevant major body systems. Complications such as vaginal bleeding, lack of fetal movements, abdominal pain, pre-eclampsia, hyperemesis and substance misuse need full evaluation to decide whether further detention is safe. Encourage contact and refer to the relevant agencies if the woman has not yet engaged with health care.

Injuries (see also Chapter 10)

Core competencies of the FP include documentation, management and interpretation of injuries in DPs, alleged victims and police officers. Make an accurate record in contemporaneous notes with use of body diagrams when indicated. After examination, you should be able to provide immediate care for injuries and understand when it is necessary to refer for secondary care. You should be able to suggest possible aetiology and estimate the age of an injury.

History when relevant should include:
- time when injury alleged to have been sustained;
- weapon used?
- treatment given;
- pre-existing illness or injury;
- regular medication, e.g. anticoagulants, steroids;

- drugs or alcohol (pain perception at time of injury and examination may be affected);
- dominant hand of victim and alleged assailant;
- clothing worn at time of injury and any damage;
- environment where injury occurred, e.g. gravel, bushes;
- body position of victim and alleged assailant at time of infliction.

Examination for each injury should consider:

- skin colour (some reveal certain injuries less easily, e.g. bruises in black skin);
- description (forensic terms but also with lay nomenclature for statements);
- size (metric) and shape;
- site (preferably relevant to fixed bony landmarks);
- coloration;
- observations, e.g. tags;
- patterns, e.g. brush abrasions, teeth-marks in bites;
- swelling and/or tenderness (distraction test to enhance objectivity);
- foreign bodies, debris, body fluids;
- features of healing if present.

Consideration following assessment might include:

- drawings;
- possible use of photography;
- are forensic swabs needed?
- nature of injury and broad causation, e.g. laceration caused by blunt trauma;
- possibility of associated injury, e.g. bony or nerve damage;
- broad estimations of age of injury;
- compatibility with alleged causation;
- possible transient injuries that may have resolved, e.g. erythema, handprint from slap;
- skin colour effect on injury appearance, e.g. black skin;
- possibility of self-infliction or embellishment to injury;
- record of advice or treatment given;
- is review necessary?

Treatment of injuries: consider basic general principles for wound management, remembering that initial treatment should always be in the best interests of the injured person. Forensic duties are second to this, but when harmful complications are unlikely, forensic evidence and samples may be collected prior to treatment.

Cleansing: this should normally be undertaken with soap and water or normal saline with good attention to hygiene. Where possible, remove debris in lesions to avoid traumatic tattooing.

Skin closure and dressings: leave simple wounds such as abrasions or minor lacerations undressed or covered with a non-adhesive dressing. Assess carefully the risk of self-harm prior to application of any dressing that might be used as a ligature.

Larger lacerations or incised wounds may require skin closure with strips, tissue adhesive or sutures. Only undertake suturing of wounds in custody when sterile equipment is available and there are systems for disposal of sharp waste materials. Lacerations caused by dog bites are normally not closed, but appropriate antibiotic cover must be considered, as reports indicate wound infection occurs in 2–30% of cases [16].

Referral to secondary care: the extent of some wounds, possible damage to underlying structures and inadequate facilities or supplies in custody might necessitate referral to hospital. Examples include stab wounds (it is always difficult to estimate depth), where glass is involved, and where you suspect complications such as fracture or deeper tissue damage to organs. Referral is not urgent for simple non-displaced minor fractures where X-ray assessment would not alter clinical management, such as nose fracture without marked discomfort.

Medication: some injuries such as human and animal bites or closed-fist injuries may need appropriate antibiotics (remember the possibility of allergy). Be wary of prescribing analgesics or anti-inflammatory medication to the

Table 6.1. Glasgow Coma Score

Eye opening (E)	Verbal response (V)	Motor response (M)
4 = Spontaneous	5 = Normal conversation	6 = Normal
3 = To voice	4 = Disorientated conversation	5 = Localizes to pain
2 = To pain	3 = Words, but not coherent	4 = Withdraws to pain
1 = None	2 = No words . . . only sounds	3 = Decorticate posture
	1 = None	2 = Decerebrate
		1 = None
		TOTAL = E + V + M

intoxicated or anyone with a history of allergy. Document refusal to accept such medication and the reasons why. Also be aware of the tetanus status of the DP, of national policies and when to refer to A&E for immunoglobulin. Blood-borne pathogens are considered in Chapter 14.

Review: if you need to review, re-dress or revisit antibiotic cover when the person is not intoxicated or less hostile, document the time for this clearly. Any advice for follow-up care in the community on release from custody should also be documented.

Head injuries: the assessment of DPs with head injury is fraught with difficulties. Your underlying objective is to determine level of consciousness and to make an informed decision on how safe it for them to remain in custody.

Attempt to find out from the DP or witnesses present at the time how the injury occurred. This allows you to judge better the severity of the impact and the underlying risk of a serious head injury. The exact mechanism – how, where, weapon, speed of impact – assists an informed judgement, but full details may be elusive. Note relevant medical history and any history of recent and/or chronic drug or alcohol use. This history may be difficult to obtain from patients with learning difficulties or mental illness, so try to obtain information from family and friends.

Examine the head and any wound. Take baseline BP, pulse and neurological examination.

Blood sugar should be measured in all cases of impaired consciousness and assess in conjunction with a Glasgow Coma Scale (GCS – Table 6.1).

'Red flags' where the DP should be immediately considered for diversion to hospital [17] have been well documented:

- impaired consciousness (GCS < 15/15) at any time since the injury;
- focal neurological symptom or sign;
- suspicion of a skull fracture or penetrating injury;
- amnesia for events before or after the injury;
- persistent and severe headache since the injury;
- vomiting since the injury;
- seizures since the injury;
- high-energy head injury, e.g. road traffic accident (RTA) or fall from a height;
- current drug or alcohol intoxication;
- significant extracranial injuries;
- continuing uncertainty about the diagnosis after first assessment;
- age greater than or equal to 65.

If the DP is to remain in custody, treat wounds as previously documented. Instruct the custody staff or HCP clearly both verbally and in writing on the level of observations needed. These would normally be for an assessment every 30 minutes to include rousing and speaking to the DP (seeking a sensible response and/or GCS for those suitably trained). It is important to remember that other conditions – hypoglycaemia, uraemia, meningitis, stroke – may create

confusion. If the level of consciousness appears to be worsening or the DP develops further symptoms such as increasingly severe
headache, blurred or double vision, vomiting,
has a seizure or develops any unusual or
strange behaviour you should be contacted
urgently or the DP transferred to hospital by
ambulance. On release he may be given a
standard head injury warning card, and
advised to stay with a responsible adult for
the next 48 hours (also can be given the
carer's advice card).

After significant head injury a full mental
health assessment is necessary to inform the
decision regarding fitness for interview and, in
particular, consideration should be given to
tests of memory and recall.

Police restraint injuries

The police use verbal warnings to control difficult
situations, but they are also able to employ a wide
variety of techniques, implements and weapons
to control and restrain subjects. Police dogs may
also be deployed and can cause a variety of typical bite injuries. There is a potential to cause
injury, and their use may result in transient or
longer-lasting complications; some techniques
have the capability to cause serious or life-
threatening injury. You are frequently asked to
assess and document injuries and give guidance
on management. Hospital referral may be needed
for further evaluation and treatment and you,
acting as an independent examiner, have a duty
to organize transfer when appropriate as medical
needs hold priority over police procedure. Take a
clear and detailed history from the DP and
arresting officers. You should also notify the duty
inspector if you are concerned about the possible
use of excessive force at arrest, but it is not within
your remit to judge whether inappropriate force
has been used: you are not in full possession of
the facts relating to the risks present at the time
of arrest.

Unarmed restraint

Familiarize yourself with the hierarchy of police
techniques taught to match different levels of
threat, such as open-handed moves, pressure point
application and holds and knee and elbow strikes
so that you can interpret any alleged injuries. Neck
restraints are not taught, as serious injury or even
deaths could ensue. When a DP alleges such a hold
examine for signs suggesting asphyxia such as
petechial bruising to eyes, mouth and head and
neck. In scuffles, clothing may be grabbed around
neck areas and cause ill-defined lines of redness or
bruising.

Restraint asphyxia is a life-threatening situation
and fatalities have been reported. It happens when
someone is unable to maintain adequate respiratory movement. Risk is increased in obesity, lying
prone, restraint face down especially with pressure
applied and when there is respiratory muscle
fatigue such as after a pursuit. Cardinal signs of
asphyxia – congestion, cyanosis and petechiae –
may be found in these cases.

Rigid handcuffs

The fixed connecting bar between rigid handcuffs
can be used to apply controlled force across the
wrist. Once applied, simple pressure allows them
to close with a ratchet mechanism; they normally
sit at the narrowest part of the wrist just distal to the
radial and ulnar styloid processes. They may be
applied with the arms to the front or behind the
person in the 'stack' position. Once in place, they
are checked for tightness, then locked to prevent
further tightening, although this may not be possible with violent or struggling prisoners. Further
tightening may cause increasing pain, disrupt skin
and even produce circulatory or neurological
damage. Intoxication with drugs, alcohol or both
may dull awareness of pain and increase the likelihood of injury.

Soft tissue injuries such as erythema, abrasions
and bruising, and less frequently lacerations, are
caused by excessive tightness or by movement

Table 6.2. Nerve damage secondary to handcuff injury

	Motor function (test against resistance)	Sensory function (loss of temperature, pain and touch)
Median nerve	Weakness of thumb abduction at right angles to palm and of thumb opposition (tested palm up)	Palmar aspect of lateral 3½ digits and nail beds
Ulnar nerve	Weakness of abduction of little finger and flexion at MCP joint with IP joints held extended (tested palm up) Weakness of abduction of index finger (tested palm down)	Palmar and dorsal aspect of medial 1½ digits
Radial nerve	No motor loss with lesions at wrist	Dorsal aspect of lateral 3½ digits and extending down to wrist but not nail beds.

Notes:
MCP, metacarpophalangeal; IP, interphalangeal.

within the handcuff; these may normally be managed with simple wound care. Numbness or hyperaesthesia affecting the cutaneous nerves distal to cuff application can occur, but the DP should be reassured that all these injuries normally heal in just a few days; if any problems persist they should seek further medical advice.

The median, ulnar and most commonly radial nerves may be injured from direct compression: single or multiple nerves can be affected. A table of clinical tests to guide examiners for damage to these nerves is given in Table 6.2.

Carefully document any damage detected to motor or sensory nerve function, preferably on body diagrams. The DP can be advised that full recovery will usually occur in a few weeks, but if problems persist he should seek further medical advice and may need nerve conduction studies.

Wrist fractures secondary to the use of handcuffs are rare, but may occur to the styloid processes of the radius and ulna and scaphoid. Loss of movement, extensive bruising and swelling with extreme tenderness all indicate the need for X-ray.

Batons

These can be made of different materials and are available in various sizes. They may be used for defensive purposes, and also for offensive jabs, strikes or held at both ends to push a person

backwards. Police are trained to target areas defined as low (limbs), medium (limb joints and clavicle) or high risk of injury (head, neck, loin and abdomen) commensurate with the level of risk perceived.

Injuries normally consist of bruising that may be non-specific, circular from jabbing or typical 'tram-line', that is two parallel lines of bruising with central pallor. Tracking of bruising away from the site of the blow can also occur, and other injuries described can be associated with lacerations especially if a strike has been over a bony site.

If a fracture is suspected transfer to hospital for X-ray is mandatory. This also applies in suspected injury to internal organs such as spleen, kidney, or heart as there is a risk of fatality. Caution is needed when assessing those who are intoxicated.

Baton rounds

These may be used in public order or as an alternative to firearms against individuals with a bladed weapon. They are normally deployed at 20–40 metres unless used as an alternative to firearms when a closer range is permissible. They are aimed at the belt area and injuries are normally confined to torso and lower limbs. Bruising, abrasions and occasionally lacerations may occur. Serious internal injury might occur on impact to the chest, face or neck area when hospital referral could be needed.

CS and PAVA incapacitant spray

Since the introduction of these agents injuries from the application of direct force during arrest have decreased. The active ingredient of CS spray, o-chlorobenzylidine malonitrile, is solid at room temperature but, dissolved in a solvent (methyl isobutyl ketone) with nitrogen as the propellant, is used as a liquid aerosol. The spray is aimed at the face to affect the mucous membranes of eyes, nose and mouth. The solvent rapidly evaporates, leaving the CS particles to irritate; they fail to affect 10% of subjects, particularly those intoxicated with drugs or alcohol.

Effects normally subside in 30–60 minutes with adequate ventilation, but more problems may be seen after exposure to high concentrations in confined spaces or in those with medical susceptibilities. Never use water to remove residue as it will cause the CS to redissolve and exacerbate effects. Contaminated clothing should be removed when possible.

Some forces now use PAVA (pelargonic acid vanillyamide) incapacitant spray in a solvent (ethanol and water) with a nitrogen propellant. This is the synthetic equivalent of capsaicin (active ingredient of natural pepper). It is directed to the eyes where it causes extreme discomfort and closure. Management should be the same as following CS exposure.

Clinical effects to the eyes can include lachrymation, pain, blepharospasm, conjunctival reddening, blurred vision, photophobia, periorbital oedema, iritis and corneal abrasions due to rubbing the eyes. Contact lenses should be removed if worn. Thereafter, ventilation normally affords relief or a fan may assist in blowing air into the eyes. If symptoms persist for longer than one hour, irrigate with sterile normal saline. If eye symptoms persist after a few hours or a corneal abrasion is found refer for ophthalmic advice.

Effects to the mouth, nose and respiratory system can cause stinging, burning, sneezing, rhinorrhoea, coughing, tracheitis, shortness of breath and bronchospasm. Pulmonary oedema can rarely develop 12–24 hours after exposure. Detained persons with pre-existing respiratory conditions are at greater risk, needing a full and thorough assessment with consideration for the need for bronchodilators and medical review. Pre-existing cardiac conditions including hypertension could potentially be worsened, and GTN may need to be used for angina, with hospital referral if the pain does not subside. Those with cardiac dysrrythmias exacerbated or induced should also be transferred to hospital.

Skin effects include burning, erythema, chemical burns with blistering and allergic contact dermatitis [18] but these normally settle rapidly. Delayed skin irritation from the solvent may be found 8–16 hours post-exposure, taking up to a week to subside. General management involves removal from exposure and placing the subject in a well-ventilated area. Medical personnel should wear gloves, and contaminated clothing (preferably dry) should be removed and placed in sealed (double) plastic bags. The skin, especially skin folds, should be washed with copious soap and water if symptoms persist more than 2 hours post-exposure. Treat any burns in the same manner as thermal burns. Topical steroids may be considered for contact dermatitis.

Taser (Thomas A Swift's electronic rifle)

The Advanced Taser M26 was introduced on trial for a year from April 2003 in five forces in the UK to bridge the gap in use of force hierarchy when baton or police dog had been deemed ineffective and the next option was to deploy a firearm. It is a small hand-held, battery-powered device delivering repetitive low current, high voltage impulse shocks to incapacitate a person. It contains a ballistic cartridge comprising a small explosive and a compressed nitrogen cylinder that is punctured on detonation, projecting two barbs at high speed. The two barbs (8 mm in length with a 1-mm barb about 3 mm from the tip) are attached to the weapon by wires (up to 6 metres) and become lodged in either the clothing or the skin of the subject, so completing the electrical circuit to allow the passage of 50 000-volt pulses. All arrested persons subjected to the discharge of a Taser must be examined by the FP.

The neuromuscular stimulation caused by the current is both painful and fatiguing. The barbs may penetrate the skin up to 6 mm and should normally be easily removed by the FP supporting the skin around the barb and applying a little traction.

Difficulty in removal or a sensitive site, such as around the eyes or genitals, indicates the need for hospital referral. Examination may reveal small circular burns on areas of skin where current has entered from barbs retained in clothing. Puncture of superficial blood vessels may also occur, as well as secondary injuries from falling. If the fall is uncontrolled or from a height there is a potential for severe injury, so a clear history is vital.

Other theoretical adverse effects include ventricular fibrillation that may be precipitated by metabolic acidosis [19], other cardiac arrythmias, BP changes, nerve or muscle injury (including incontinence due to loss of smooth muscle control), spontaneous abortion or seizures. There is also the potential for interference to an implanted device such as a pacemaker.

Although fatalities have been reported following Taser, no established direct links between cause of death and Taser deployment have been found. Cases of death most commonly involve those using phencyclidine, amphetamine or cocaine. Other cases involve those with underlying cardiac disease or secondary serious injury. There appears to be a delay of up to 30 minutes between Taser use and collapse, but if examination reveals the DP to be agitated or unwell, to have used stimulant drugs or have underlying cardiac disease hospital admission might be advisable.

Despite these concerns Taser carries a lower rate of injury to officers and those they arrest than physical skills, CS spray and batons. In addition it carries a lower injury rate to subjects than use of police dogs [20].

REFERENCES

1. General Medical Council (2006) booklets. *Good Medical Practice; Management for Doctors; Seeking Patients' Consent* and *Confidentiality*. London: GMC.
2. British Medical Association Ethics Committee and Association of Police Surgeons (2004) *Health Care of Detainees in Police Stations*. London: BMA.
3. Bennett T, Holloway K (2004) *Drug Use and Offending: Summary Results of the First Two Years of the NEW-ADAM Programme*. Findings 179. A Research, Development and Statistics Directorate Report. London: HMSO.
4. British Medical Association Health Policy and Economic Research Unit (2003) *Violence at Work: the Experience of UK Doctors*. London: BMA.
5. Hawton K, James A (2005) Suicide and deliberate self-harm in young people. *BMJ* **330**: 891–4.
6. *British Medical Association, Scotland, survey* (August 2006).
7. http:fflm.ac.uk/library/.
8. Norfolk GA (1997) 'Fitness to be interviewed'– a proposed definition and scheme of examination. *Medicine Science and the Law* **37**: 228–34.
9. Mohan G, Harrison BD, Badminton RM, Mildenhall S, Wareham NJ (1996) A confidential enquiry into deaths caused by asthma in an English health region: implications for general practice. *British Journal of General Practice* **46**: 529–32.
10. British Thoracic Society and Scottish Intercollegiate Guidelines Network BTS/SIGN (2003 and update 2004). *British Guideline on the Management of Asthma*. London, Edinburgh: British Thoracic Society and Scottish Intercollegiate Guidelines Network.
11. Levy D (1996) Management of diabetes in clinical forensic practice. *Journal of Clinical Forensic Medicine* **3**: 31–6.
12. National Institute for Clinical Excellence (2002) *Management of Diabetes*. Available at www.nice.org.uk
13. Stark M, Rogers D, Norfolk G (eds.) (2006) *Good Practice Guidelines for Forensic Medical Examiners*, 2nd edn. Association of Forensic Physicians.
14. Syed F, Beeching N (2005) Lower-limb deep-vein thrombosis in a general hospital: risk factors, outcomes and the contribution of intravenous drug use. *Quarterly Journal of Medicine* **98**(2): 139–45.
15. Wells PS, Anderson DR, Bormanis J, *et al.* (1997) Value of assessment of pretest probability of deep vein

thrombosis in clinical management. *Lancet* **350**: 1795–8.

16. Cummings P (1994) Antibiotics to prevent infection in patients with dog bite wounds: a meta-analysis of randomized trials. *Annals of Emergency Medicine* **23**(3): 535–40.

17. National Collaborating Centre for Acute Care (2003) Head Injury: *Triage, Assessment, Investigation and Early Management of Head Injury in Infants, Children and Adults.* Available at www.rcseng.ac.uk

18. Ro Y, Lee C (1991) Tear gas dermatitis. Allergic contact sensitization due to CS. *International Journal of Dermatology* **30**(8): 576–7.

19. Fish R, Geddes L (2001) Effects of stun guns and Tasers. *Lancet* **358**: 687–9.

20. Jenkinson E, Neeson C, Bleetman A (2006) The relative risk of police use of force options: Evaluating the potential for deployment of electronic weaponry. *Journal of Clinical Forensic Medicine* **13**: 229–41.

FURTHER READING

Codes of Practice C 9.5–9.14 and H 9.6–9.16 for England and Wales, July 2006. London: HMSO.

7

Custody medicine: mental illness and psychological conditions

Victoria Evans and Gavin Reid

Introduction

While certain conditions may be over represented in those in police custody the range of conditions is no different from those present in the general population. Clinical assessment of the detainee should, therefore, be of the same standard and afford the same respect and dignity to that detainee as if it had been carried out elsewhere in a typical clinical setting. The range of options thereafter and the recommendations which can be made differ from practice in the community. Criminal justice and public safety considerations need to be taken into account, although patient care remains of primary importance.

As in other areas of clinical forensic medicine, it cannot be overemphasized how important it is to keep clear, comprehensive, legible contemporaneous notes.

Clinical assessment includes a consultation and an examination of the mental state, supported by gathering background information. The circumstances of the arrest may include details of clinical relevance, and previous convictions may also be helpful in showing a pattern of deteriorating social functioning or a previous psychiatric disposal. The family, friends or local community services may be useful informants. Physical examination is required if there is any suspicion of an organic cause of an abnormal mental state.

A police station is not an easy place in which to make a clear diagnosis. When assessing a detainee, the task is not to make a definitive diagnosis, but rather to determine those cases where expert assessment is indicated, particularly if the use of mental health legislation may be required. Alternatively, the task may be to advise that a detainee is not fit for interview or advise that an appropriate adult is required. Forensic physicians should be familiar with local arrangements for psychiatric assessment and any schemes for diversion from custody.

An abnormal mental state may be due to a mental disorder, intoxication or withdrawal from alcohol or illicit substances. It is also important to consider causes of an acute confusional state such as seizures, head injury, organic brain disease or an abnormal metabolic state such as hypoglycaemia. The individual's presentation may be due to a reaction to the custody environment combined with intoxication. The effects of illicit substances and alcohol are dealt with in Chapters 8 and 9. Whenever possible, mental health assessment should be undertaken after the effect of any intoxicant has ceased.

The forensic physician should be alert to the unusual or less obvious presentation of mental disorder, such as the elderly person with dementia found wandering along the motorway.

Most mental state assessments carried out by a forensic physician will not be a request for specific assessment under the provisions of mental health legislation, but as an integral part of the routine assessment of fitness to detain or interview. Whenever mental illness or learning disability is diagnosed or suspected, this should be drawn to the attention of the custody officer, so that this can be given due consideration.

Examination of the mental state

This is the core component of any assessment: information from other sources supplements the mental state examination.

In examining the mental state, the person's behaviour and physical appearance should be considered as indicators of possible mental disorder. The more consistent the clinician is in style and approach, the easier it is to identify abnormalities. The clinician's own reaction towards the detainee, whatever that might be, should also be viewed objectively.

The general arrangements for the consultation should be as clinical as possible. The detainee and the doctor should both be seated. It is important to balance confidentiality and safety. Careful consideration should be given in each case as to whether a chaperone should be present in the examination room, but in any case it is prudent to ask an officer to wait outside the door.

A professional and clinical approach is often very effective in calming an agitated, fearful or aggressive detainee. In all circumstances, the consultation should begin with an introduction by the doctor and a brief explanation as to what will happen and why. Thereafter, personal details should be checked, and an account of recent circumstances obtained. Details concerning previous treatment, including medication, admissions to hospital and whether or not this involved the use of mental health legislation are required. A history of alcohol or substance misuse, a past medical history, previous offending and anything else of relevance should be noted. The underlying purpose is to gain an overview of the individual. During the course of

this structured interview, which may be brief, the doctor will simultaneously be observing the appearance, speech and mood of the detainee, together with evidence of any abnormal thinking. Some initial impression of intelligence will also have been gained from the use of vocabulary and capacity for self-expression. Specific questions can be asked about perceptual abnormalities, orientation, intellectual level or literacy if needed. Functional illiteracy is more common than learning disability and is often concealed by detainees through shame or embarrassment. By the end of the examination, the doctor should have formed a view as to whether or not a mental disorder is present, its general nature and its severity.

Clinical syndromes

The most common and important mental disorders encountered in detainees include schizophrenia, bipolar affective disorder, personality disorder and psychotic depression. Symptoms of psychosis may be either positive or negative.

Positive psychotic symptoms include hallucinations, delusional beliefs and a lack of insight. Hallucinatory experiences may be auditory, visual, tactile, olfactory or somatic. One or more of these positive symptoms of psychosis may be present in a particular detainee. During assessment, questions should always be sufficiently open to allow the detainee to describe his/her own experience.

The negative symptoms are the various forms of deficit which may be particularly evident in schizophrenia. These include loss of drive or energy together with blunting or coarsening of personality. The individual may present as shallow, facile and empty or may seem dour, unresponsive and inaccessible.

The pattern of mental illness may be reflected in a person's life-history. The educational and work history may show evidence of decline in keeping with the development of the disorder. While many patients with mental illness use a diagnostic term about themselves and may use clinical terms to describe their symptoms, others never gain insight nor use such terminology. Such lack of insight may result in non-compliance with treatment and precede presentation in a custodial setting.

Schizophrenia usually develops in early adult life and many patients are left with chronic deficits despite treatment with antipsychotic medication. Low grade residual positive symptoms may be present in addition to the negative features such as lack of volition, apathy and blunted affect. Schizophrenia is typically a lifelong disorder which may well have periods of acute relapse with marked hallucinatory or delusional symptoms. There may be ideas of reference in that a patient may believe that the radio or television is referring directly to them.

Manic depressive illness or bipolar affective disorder, is characterized by recurrent episodes of illness with a predominant abnormality of mood, either elation (hypomania) or depression. A mixed affective state can also occur.

Dual diagnosis, for example the coexistence of mental disorder and substance misuse, is common, especially in detainees in police custody. It is a risk factor for death in custody and can make assessment of the detainee's mental state more complex.

Drugs can cause, exacerbate or mask psychotic symptomatology. Patients with mental illness may 'self-medicate' with illicit drugs or alcohol in an attempt to gain relief from distressing symptoms or as a part of a deteriorating lifestyle. A careful history may help to distinguish the contributions of mental illness and substance abuse to an individual's presentation.

There should be an awareness of malingering, where a detainee is simulating the symptoms of mental illness. This is much less common than is sometimes believed. Individuals with mental disorder, including personality disorder, who behave in an abusive or offensive manner may be considered to be 'faking' symptoms. As in other branches of medicine, the manner in which an ill person behaves is a product not just of the illness itself but also of the individual's underlying personality, past experiences and environment. Corroborative information from other sources

can be invaluable in determining if a patient is malingering.

It is in disposal that criminal justice factors must be considered. Mental illness on its own does not necessarily require admission to hospital, diversion from the criminal justice system or that an individual is not fit to interview: each case must be considered on its merits. If a hospital bed is required and the detainee is facing serious charges, the bed must be in a hospital which offers adequate security. Every forensic physician should have a working knowledge of the range of services in his own area and how these may be accessed.

Fitness for interview

Great care should be exercised in determining whether or not a person who is mentally ill or who has learning disability can be interviewed by the police and/or is fit to be charged. The Police and Criminal Evidence Act 1984 (PACE) Codes of Practice (Annexe G) provide detailed guidance on good practice when assessing whether a detainee is fit for interview. In particular, the guidance emphasizes that both the effect of the mental disorder on the detainee's functional ability to give reliable answers and the effect of the nature and purpose of the interview on the detainee's physical and mental state must be taken into account. A detainee with a major mental disorder may still be fit for interview. The custody officer should be informed of the presence of any mental disorder so that the attendance of an appropriate adult may be secured if this has not already been done. Failure to do so may result in a court deciding subsequently that the content of any interview is unreliable. It is important to understand that fitness for interview may change as withdrawal symptoms resolve or mental illness responds to treatment.

Appropriate adult

There should be an awareness of any local Appropriate Adult Scheme. As mental disorder can disadvantage a detainee during police interview it may be appropriate for a psychiatrist or forensic physician to advise that an appropriate adult is required. The role of the Appropriate Adult is to support the interviewee. Guidance relating to who should be an appropriate adult varies and local guidelines should be consulted.

Assessment of suicide risk

This is a crucial part of the forensic physician's task. There will always be some successful suicides in police custody which could not be predicted. However, consideration of the factors below in every case should alert the examining doctor to the possibility of an increased risk of suicide and hence the need for extra vigilance on the part of the custody staff or, possibly, admission to hospital. In the event of a detainee being transferred to prison any relevant information regarding suicide risk must be passed on to the mental health services in the prison.

Risk factors include: a history of mental illness; alcohol or drug abuse; experience of sexual or child abuse; recent bereavement or relationship break up; financial problems; previous suicidal behaviour; history of suicide in the family; family pressures; social isolation; and access to lethal means. Special additional factors which arise out of detention in police custody include: the nature of the offence – in particular, offences involving violence, sex, arson or in a domestic setting; feelings of guilt; first time in custody; worries about children or other family concerns; and withdrawal from drugs or alcohol.

The Mental Health Act 1983 (MHA 1983)

This legislation currently applies in England and Wales whether the process is civil or criminal. All forensic physicians should have access to a copy of this Act and be familiar with the context of the latest Code of Practice, as published by the Department of Health and the Welsh Office.

It is important to remember that the Act specifically excludes promiscuity or other immoral conduct, sexual deviancy or dependence on alcohol or drugs alone as reasons for compulsory admission under the Act. Where 'mental disorder' as defined in the Act is also present, the provisions of the Act are applicable.

The sections of the Act most frequently encountered by forensic physicians are:

Section 2 (MHA 1983): Compulsory admission to hospital for assessment

Grounds: that the patient
  (a) is suffering from a mental disorder of such a nature or degree which warrants the detention of the patient in a hospital for assessment (or for assessment followed by medical treatment) for at least a limited period; and,
  (b) ought to be so detained in the interest of his own health or safety or with a view to the protection of other persons.

Recommendations: two medical recommendations – ideally one doctor to be s12 approved (see below) and to have had previous acquaintance with the patient.

Application: approved social worker (ASW) or nearest relative. Duration: not more than 28 days.

Note: the most commonly used section of the Act.

Section 3 (MHA 1983): Compulsory admission to hospital for treatment

Grounds: that the patient
  (a) is suffering from mental illness, severe mental impairment, psychotic disorder or mental impairment, and his mental disorder is of a nature or degree which makes it appropriate for him to receive medical treatment in a hospital; and,
  (b) in the case of psychopathic disorder or mental impairment, such treatment is likely to alleviate or prevent a deterioration; and,
  (c) it is necessary for the health or safety of the patient or for the protection of other

persons that he should receive such treatment and it cannot be provided unless he is detained under this section.

Recommendations: two medical recommendations – ideally at least one doctor to be s12 approved (see below) and one doctor to have had previous acquaintance with the patient. Usually one of the doctors will be the consultant psychiatrist under whose care the patient is to be admitted.

Application: ASW or nearest relative. If the nearest relative objects, the application cannot proceed unless there are grounds to make an application to displace the nearest relative.

Duration: a period not exceeding six months in the first instance.

Note: this section of the MHA 1983 is more rarely used by forensic physicians. Usually the patient will have been in hospital and a firm diagnosis made: subsequent non-compliance with treatment has then led to relapse.

Section 4 (MHA 1983): Compulsory admission for assessment in an emergency

Grounds:
  (a) as for Section 2; and,
  (b) the matter is of urgent necessity and there is not enough time to get a second medical recommendation.

To be satisfied that an emergency has arisen there must be evidence of the existence of a significant risk of mental or physical harm to the patient or others; and/or the danger of serious harm to property; and/or the need for physical restraint of the patient.

Recommendations: one medical recommendation.

Application: ASW

Duration: Up to 72 hours

Note: this should hardly, if ever, be used, and never for 'administrative convenience'.

Section 136 (MHA 1983): Police power to remove to a place of safety

Grounds: the person whom the constable removes must be in a place to which the public have access

and must appear to the constable to be suffering from mental disorder and to be in immediate need of care and control.

Purpose: to enable a mental health assessment as soon as practicable by a doctor and an ASW. Once the assessment is complete, unless the outcome is to arrange compulsory admission under the appropriate section of the MHA 1983, the detainee must be released.

Duration: up to 72 hours.

Note: the extent to which this power is used varies throughout the country. The involvement of the forensic physician in assessments under the provisions of this section largely depends on whether or not the usual place of safety is the police station.

Section 135 (MHA 1983)

This gives a police constable authority to enter and search premises as specified on a warrant issued by a Justice of the Peace subsequent to information laid on oath by an ASW, in order to remove to a place of safety for assessment where there is reasonable cause to suspect that a person suffering from a mental disorder

(a) has been, or is being, ill-treated, neglected, or kept otherwise than under proper control; or,
(b) being unable to care for himself, is living alone in any such place. Such entry is usually undertaken in the presence of an ASW and a registered medical practitioner.

Duration: maximum 72 hours.

Other provisions of the Act

Forensic physician involvement may be sought from time to time – referral to the Act itself and to the Code of Practice is to be recommended in such instances.

Part III of the Act refers to patients concerned in criminal proceedings or under sentence. Powers under these sections of the Act are usually exercised by the courts or within the prison system and therefore forensic physicians will not normally be involved.

Section 12 approval refers to s12(2) of the Act, by which a practitioner may be approved by the Secretary of State as 'having special experience in the diagnosis or treatment of mental disorder'. At present only some forensic physicians are so approved. However, those with the requisite experience are recommended to apply for approval, as in most areas the majority of acute mental health assessments involve forensic physicians. The Scottish equivalent is referred to as Section 22 approval (relating to the Scottish legislation).

Summary of options following mental health assessment

These are not mutually exclusive:

1. Where the problem is a social one, refer to social services.
2. If organic pathology is expected, take appropriate remedial action. Consider referral to local district hospital.
3. Voluntary admission to psychiatric facilities.
4. Compulsory admission to hospital under the appropriate section of the MHA 1983. This must never be undertaken lightly as it may be that the length of detention in hospital is a greater deprivation of liberty than a court would or could impose for the misdemeanour that has brought the offender to police attention.
5. Release of the detainee back into the community either after assessment under s136 of the MHA 1983 or on police bail with referral to the Mentally Disordered Offenders Panel (or local equivalent). In all cases due consideration must be given to and, where appropriate, arrangements made for continuity of care in the community setting whether medical, social or both.
6. Where a detainee is considered fit to detain and fit for interview, and there is a history of mental disorder, which might give rise to vulnerability during interview, or mental disorder is present or suspected, involvement of an Appropriate Adult should be advised in writing.
7. Where a serious offence has been committed, or the local psychiatric facility has refused the patient admission because of a diagnosis of personality disorder or psychopathy, consideration should be given to the following:
   (a) Is the patient's psychiatric state so bad that it puts him/her or others at risk and he/she cannot be managed in police custody? If the answer is yes, then admission to a Regional Secure Unit should be considered. This is usually a lengthy business and will involve initial assessment as for s2 of the MHA 1983, involving the district psychiatric team, before an emergency request is made for assessment by the duty forensic psychiatrist and their team.
   (b) Can the patient be safely managed in police custody and is he/she fit to go before the court? If the answer is yes, the best course is to let the court make an appropriate disposal. It may be helpful to the court in their deliberations to have a short handwritten report from the doctor stating his opinion.

The new mental health legislation in England and Wales

After eight years of debate and controversy, the terms of a new Mental Health Act 2007 have finally been agreed. The new Act will amend the MHA 1983 and the Mental Capacity Act. It is not known when this will become effective. The major changes to the 1983 Act include the following:

(a) *Definition of mental disorder:* a single definition will apply throughout the 1983 Act, abolishing references to categories of disorder.
(b) *Criteria for detention:* a new test is introduced as to whether a person's ability to make decisions about medical treatment is significantly impaired because of mental disorder. Unless this test is met, an individual may not be detained under Part 2 of the 1983 Act. It also applies to the 'treatability' test more widely than at present, with the effect that no one may be detained for medical treatment under the 1983 Act unless such treatment is likely to alleviate or prevent deterioration in their condition.

(c) *Professional roles:* the groups of practitioners who can take on the role of the ASW and responsible medical officer (RMO) have been broadened.

(d) *Nearest relative (NR):* it gives to patients the right to make an application to displace their NR and enable county courts to displace a NR where there are reasonable grounds for doing so. The provisions for determining the NR will be amended to include civil partners.

(e) *Supervised community treatment:* this is introduced for patients following a period of detention in hospital. It will allow a small number of patients with mental disorder to live in the community whilst subject to certain conditions under the 1983 Act to ensure that they continue with the medical treatment that they need. Before such an order can be imposed, the clinician must have regard to a patient's history and risk of deterioration.

Several other changes include a right to advocacy for detained patients, safeguards over the use of electroconvulsive therapy, changes in the timing of referral to a mental health review tribunal and abolition of finite restriction orders.

Mental health legislation in Scotland

The Mental Health (Care and Treatment) (Scotland) Act 2003 gained royal assent in April 2003 and came into force in October 2005, replacing the previous 1984 Act. The new Act has some key differences including the introduction of the Mental Health Tribunal for Scotland and an emphasis on the role of service users and carers. The Act is based on a set of ethical principles including: least restrictive alternative; benefit; child welfare; respect for carers; participation; informal care; reciprocity; respect for diversity; equality and non-discrimination. These principles must be considered when applying the Act. The 2003 Act clarified and enhanced the role of the Mental Welfare Commission for Scotland. This body has specific duties ensuring patients subject to mental health legislation receive appropriate

care. The Criminal Procedure (Scotland) Act 1995 has been amended in light of the 2003 Act.

The most frequently encountered sections are as follows:

Short-term detention: s44 of the Mental Health (Care and Treatment) (Scotland) Act 2003

This allows a patient to be detained in hospital for 28 days. The use of this section is preferred over an emergency detention in both the legislation and Code of Practice to the Act. It can follow on from an emergency certificate. This section requires an approved medical practitioner (AMP) (a psychiatrist approved by the Health Board under s22), to examine the patient. If the AMP believes the grounds are met, he/she must sign the certificate within three days of the examination. The AMP must consider that it is likely that the patient has a mental disorder, and it is likely that the ability to make decisions about medical treatment is significantly impaired as a result of that disorder. It must be necessary to detain the patient in hospital for the purpose of determining what medical treatment is required or to give such treatment. There must be a significant risk to the health, safety or welfare of the patient or to the safety of any other person. The granting of a short-term detention certificate must be necessary.

The AMP must consult with and gain consent from a mental health officer (MHO) (an appropriately trained and qualified social worker). The MHO must interview the patient and, if practicable, consult with their named person if one exists.

The section may be cancelled by the RMO (typically the patient's consultant), the Mental Welfare Commission or by a tribunal. The patient or their named person may ask the tribunal to review the case.

Emergency detention: s36 of the Mental Health (Care and Treatment) (Scotland) 2003

This allows a patient to be detained in hospital for 72 hours and for the removal of the patient to hospital within 72 hours beginning when the certificate is granted. This certificate can be used if an AMP and MHO are unavailable. Any registered medical practitioner may complete an emergency detention certificate once they have examined the patient and believe the criteria to be met. The medical practitioner must consider it likely that the patient has a mental disorder and it is likely that the patient has significantly impaired decision-making ability with respect to medical treatment for mental disorder. It must be necessary as a matter of urgency to detain the patient in hospital for the purpose of determining what medical treatment is required, and, if the patient was not detained in hospital, there would be a significant risk to their health, safety or welfare, or to the safety of any other person. There must also be an undesirable delay in making arrangements for a short-term detention certificate.

A medical practitioner must sign the certificate on the day of the examination or within four hours if the examination ends after 20.00 hours. The medical practitioner must consult with an MHO unless it is not practicable to do so. The MHO can give consent by telephone if they know the patient well and have seen them recently. If the MHO refuses consent, the opinion of a second MHO may be sought in exceptional circumstances.

An emergency certificate cannot be granted if immediately prior to the medical examination the patient was subject to:

an emergency certificate; a short-term detention certificate or an extension of this certificate; a compulsory treatment order; or an interim compulsory treatment order. Separate certificates exist to deal with a patient living in the community who is subject to a compulsory treatment order or compulsion order and defaults from treatment or who requires compulsory admission.

Assessment order and treatment order: s52 of the Criminal Procedure (Scotland) Act 2003

An assessment order requires written or oral evidence from one fully registered medical practitioner. This order may therefore be used by a forensic physician. In practice, this is likely to be unusual. The patient must appear to have a mental disorder, the category of which does not require to be specified. It must be likely that detention in hospital is required to meet the criteria specified for a treatment order. These include there being reasonable grounds for believing the patient has a mental disorder and that medical treatment is available which would be likely to prevent the mental disorder worsening or alleviate any of the symptoms, or effects, of the disorder. In addition, if the person were not provided with such medical treatment, there must be a significant risk to the health, safety or welfare of the person or to the safety of others.

It must also be likely that there would be a significant risk to the person's health, safety or welfare, or to the safety of any other person, if the assessment order was not made. A suitable hospital bed must be available within seven days and consideration should be given to any alternative to allow assessment without the use of the assessment order. The assessment order allows detention in hospital for 28 days which may be extended for a further seven days.

A treatment order requires written or oral evidence from two medical practitioners, one of which must be an AMP. The main differences are that this order permits treatment under the Act and it can be in effect until a disposal is given.

Compulsory treatment order or compulsion order

This replaces s18 of the Mental Health (Scotland) Act 1984. This requires two recommendations, one by an AMP, and consent from a MHO. This is granted for six months in the first instance and can be renewed by the tribunal upon application. A compulsion order has equivalent powers but is imposed by the court as a disposal.

Restricted status

This can result from a restriction order made in conjunction with a compulsion order; by virtue of being a transferred prisoner; from an assessment or treatment order. Such patients require permission from Scottish Ministers with regard to such areas as transfer between hospital, discharge and time out-with hospital. There are also statutory reporting requirements.

Section 200 of the Criminal Procedure (Scotland) Act 1995

This allows a court to remand a person in custody or on bail for assessment of physical or mental condition. It allows remand to hospital for assessment of a person's mental condition. Use of this section requires the person to have been convicted of an offence punishable by imprisonment, and it must appear to the court that enquiries should be made into the mental and physical condition. Detention in hospital requires evidence from one medical practitioner that the person appears to be suffering from a mental disorder and a suitable hospital bed is available. Typically, an assessment order, described above, is favoured over this section.

Place of safety

Under s297 of the Mental Health (Care and Treatment) (Scotland) 2003, a police constable who reasonably suspects a person of suffering a mental disorder and that person is in immediate need of care or treatment, may remove that person from a public place to a place of safety. The constable must consider that it is in the interest of that person, or necessary for the protection of any other person for this to be done. The person may be detained at a place of safety for a period of up to 24 hours and, in the event of absconding, the constable may take that person into custody and return him to a place of safety. The period of detention is to allow a medical examination to take place. The agreed place of safety is a matter for the local authorities and may be a hospital, a care home service or any other suitable place. An exception is that a police constable may, where no place of safety is immediately available, remove the person to a police station.

Separate powers exist where a patient subject to the powers of the Act is not in a public place to allow access and removal of the patient to a place of safety. This requires the authority of a sheriff or a Justice of the Peace.

FURTHER READING

Code of Practice: Mental Health Act 1983 (1993) London: HMSO, and the Act itself.

Code of Practice: Mental Health (Care and Treatment) (Scotland) 2003 (2005) Scottish Executive, and the Act itself.

Codes of Practice: Police and Criminal Evidence Act 1984 (1995) London: HMSO.

McManus JJ, Thomson LDG (2005) *Mental Health and Scots Law in Practice*. Edinburgh: W Green & Son Ltd. ISBN 9780414014756.

8

Substance misuse

Margaret M. Stark and Guy A. Norfolk

Introduction

Substance misuse is a major and growing problem often resulting in drug-related criminal activity. Forensic physicians are seeing an increasing number of substance misusers in the setting of a police station [1]. These misusers may be intoxicated, withdrawing or dependent on alcohol or drugs. The police may request a medical assessment of substance misusing detainees in order to: assess their fitness for detention and fitness to be interviewed; conduct a mental state examination; undertake a comprehensive examination of their fitness to drive a motor vehicle; and perform an intimate search for drugs.

Some substance misusers will, for a variety of reasons, attempt to hide their misuse from the authorities on arrest. Therefore, it is most important that examining forensic physicians make a conscious effort to look for any indication of substance misuse or dependence. A sympathetic approach from the doctor is more likely to result in disclosure and a reliable history from the detainee, who should be reassured that effective treatment will be given where necessary and that the overriding consideration of the doctor is their clinical safety and wellbeing.

Criminality and drug use

The relationship between crime and drug use is very complex and takes a number of forms, with much of the crime committed reflecting the lifestyle and circumstances of the drug users themselves. Drug-related crime encompasses any criminal activity which is committed either to fund the purchase of drugs or as a consequence of drug misuse. Examples include acquisitive crimes, such as shop-lifting or burglary; offences under the various acts established to control the possession, distribution and consumption of drugs, primarily the Misuse of Drugs Act 1971; and criminal acts carried out by persons in an abnormal mental state due to drug intoxication or withdrawal, such as assault or damage to property. However, it should be noted that crime and addiction do not inevitably go together and that effective treatment programmes result in substantial reductions in criminal activity amongst drug users [2].

Drug laws

Two main statutes regulate the availability of drugs in the UK: the Misuse of Drugs Act 1971 and the Medicines Act 1968. The Medicines Act 1968 governs the manufacture and supply of medicinal products and divides drugs into prescription only medicines (POM), which must be prescribed by a doctor, a dentist or in exceptional circumstances another healthcare professional; pharmacy medicines (PM), sold under the supervision of a pharmacist from a pharmacy; and general sale list medicines (GSL),

Clinical Forensic Medicine, third edition ed. W. D. S. McLay. Published by Cambridge University Press. © Cambridge University Press 2009.

Table 8.1. Misuse of Drugs Act 1971

Penalty purposes

Class A	Major natural and synthetic opiates
	MDMA
	LSD
	Cocaine
	Injectable amphetamines
	Fungi containing psilocin or esters of psilocin ('magic mushrooms')
Class B	Dihydrocodeine
	Codeine
	Oral amphetamines
Class C	Cannabis
	Anabolic steroids
	Benzodiazepines
	Gamma-hydroxybutyrate
	Ketamine

Notes:
MDMA, 3,4, methylene-dioxymethamphetamine (ecstasy); LSD, d-lysergic acid diethylamide.

which can be sold from any premises without supervision or advice from a doctor or pharmacist.

The Misuse of Drugs Act 1971 aims to prevent the unauthorized use of drugs which are likely to be misused and are capable of having harmful effects sufficient to constitute a social problem. It is also the way the UK fulfils its obligation to control drugs in accordance with international agreements. The drugs are divided into various classes for penalty purposes (see Table 8.1). Regulations made under the Act divide controlled drugs into schedules that take account of the needs of medical practice (see Table 8.2).

Table 8.2. Misuse of Drugs Regulations 1985

Control purposes

Schedule 1	Prohibited drugs except with a Home Office licence (no medical uses), e.g. cannabis, LSD, MDMA
Schedule 2	Only available as prescription medicines with full controlled drug requirements in relation to prescribing and safe custody, keeping of registers, e.g. most opiates and cocaine
Schedule 3	Only available on prescription, e.g. some barbiturates and two benzodiazepines – temazepam and flunitrazepam
Schedule 4	Other benzodiazepines, anabolic steroids, ketamine
Schedule 5	Available without prescription – preparations containing small amount of controlled drugs

Another important piece of drug legislation is the Drugs Act 2005. One of the aims of the Act is to increase the effectiveness of the Drug Interventions Programme by getting more offenders into treatment. Under this legislation the police now have the power to test offenders for heroin, crack and cocaine on arrest for certain trigger offences, such as robbery or burglary, and to require a person with a positive test to undergo an assessment by a drugs worker. When forensic physicians are aware that detainees have undergone drug testing, they may like to ask about the results as these could inform their examination and management decisions.

Definitions

A *drug* is 'any substance, other than those required for the maintenance of normal health, that, when taken into the living organism may modify one or more of its functions' (World Health Organization (WHO) definition).

Drug misuse has been defined as 'any taking of a drug which harms or threatens to harm the physical and mental health or social well-being of an individual, of other individuals, or of society at large, or which is illegal' [3]. Drug misuse can occur in the absence of *dependence*, which is defined as 'a state, psychic and sometimes also physical, resulting from the interaction between a living organism and a drug, characterised by behavioural and other responses that always include a compulsion to take the drug on a continuous or periodic basis in order to experience its psychic effects and sometimes to avoid discomfort of its absence. Tolerance may or may not be present' (WHO definition). Drug dependence can occur without drug misuse but it is more common for both to occur together. It is important to note that for drug dependence to exist psychological dependence must be present but that physical dependence may not necessarily occur.

Tolerance occurs when increased doses of a drug are required to produce the same effect and will only be maintained if the drug is taken regularly and in sufficient doses.

Co-morbidity is the simultaneous presence of two or more disorders, often referring to combinations of severe mental illness, substance misuse, learning disability and personality disorder, whereas *dual diagnosis* is a more specific term used to describe people with a combination of substance misuse (including alcohol) and mental illness. Dual diagnosis is a particularly common problem amongst those with a history of offending and involvement in the criminal justice system. Therefore, forensic physicians should be diligent in enquiring about a history of substance misuse in all those detainees with a mental disorder and vice versa.

General principles

A careful and well-documented history and examination are required to look for objective signs of intoxication, dependence or withdrawal. Often more than one drug is misused; this may be a combination of prescribed and illicit substances as well as alcohol. The prescribed dose of a drug may not necessarily indicate accurately the true amount taken per day; some may be sold and perhaps other drugs taken as well. For each drug an estimate of the average quantity taken each day, the frequency of use, time of the last dose, amount used in the past 24 hours as well as the route of administration should be noted. The effect of a particular drug on an individual varies and the

severity of withdrawal, for example, is influenced by psychological factors. On-site urine analysis can be regarded as an adjunct to the history and examination in confirming substance misuse [4].

Specific drugs (classified by their most characteristic pharmacological effect)

Drugs that stimulate the nervous system

These drugs, which include amphetamine, methamphetamine, khat and cocaine, result in euphoria, increased energy and alertness with loss of appetite. Aggressive behaviour and confused thinking may also occur leading to exhaustion and sleep. The heart rate, blood pressure and respiratory rate may be increased and associated with dry mouth, sweating, dilated pupils and hyperactive reflexes. Hallucinations, delusions and paranoia may occur as well as fits, coma and death.

Stimulants such as amphetamines, methamphetamine, cocaine and ecstasy can cause psychological dependence but do not produce a major physical withdrawal syndrome. However, there may be insomnia and a severe depression which will require that the detainee is closely supervised whilst in custody and may need pharmacological treatment.

Amphetamine is the most popular stimulant and may be taken intravenously, orally or sniffed (snorted). The clinical effects come on quickly and can last several hours. A mixture of amphetamine and heroin is known as a speedball.

Methamphetamine (MA) is commonly used recreationally but individuals may binge. There is limited information on the prevalence of MA usage in the UK so far, although there is some evidence that it is increasing. It can be found as tablets, powder, 'base' or crystal MA 'ice'. The effects are sympathomimetic and instantaneous when the drug is smoked or injected, producing a 'rush' and euphoria that can last 4–12 hours. With the oral or snorting route there is no 'rush'; effects from oral ingestion occur in around 30 minutes and via snorting 3–5 minutes. Effects may continue for up to 24 hours; the half-life of the drug is 12 hours.

Khat (catha edulis) is chewed for its stimulant effect or maybe taken as an infusion; the main component is cathinone, so the effects produced are similar to those seen with amphetamine. Effects commence within 15 minutes and may last for a couple of hours.

Cocaine hydrochloride is a white powder that can be snorted, taken orally or injected. Crack cocaine, produced by treating cocaine with an alkaline solution resulting in small lumps or 'rocks', may be smoked in a pipe, inhaled as vapour after heating on foil, or injected. The onset of action, half-life and duration of effects depend on the route of administration. Snorting results in a peak effect within 30–120 minutes; with smoking or intravenous routes peak effects occur within 5 minutes.

The euphoric effects wear off very quickly and therefore have to be quickly repeated. Larger doses or a 'binge' may result in anxiety and panic leading to paranoia. A combination of cocaine and heroin taken by injection is a 'snowball'.

Ecstasy (3,4, methylene-dioxymethamphetamine – MDMA) is a stimulant with hallucinogenic properties. A moderate dose of 75–100 mg produces effects within 20–60 minutes that last for 4–6 hours. In addition to the general effects of stimulants described above, trismus (spasm of the muscles of mastication) and bruxism (grinding of teeth) may be noted. Other effects reported include catatonic stupor and hyponatraemia, pneumomediastinum, paranoid psychosis, liver and renal problems, hyperpyrexia, disseminated intravascular coagulation, rhabdomyolysis and death.

Anabolic steroids may be used by athletes or body-builders and taken orally or by injection. Effects include mood swings with an increase in aggressive behaviour, psychiatric problems such as depression and paranoia, and rarely hepatitis and liver tumours and human immunodeficiency virus (HIV) from sharing injecting equipment.

Nitrites ('poppers'), such as amyl nitrite, are used as euphoric relaxants and to enhance sexual performance. The effects of inhalation of the vapour, which are almost instantaneous and last only minutes, include headache, dizziness and flushing. Excessive use may result in methaemoglobinaemia.

Drugs that alter perceptual function

LSD (d-lysergic acid diethylamide) is usually taken orally with sympathomimetic effects within 5–10 minutes and psychological effects within 30–60 minutes (both dose-related); duration of effects is 8–12 hours and there is a recovery period of 10–12 hours. The effects depend very much on the individual and the situation they are in, with the same user having a bad or good 'trip' on different occasions or even within the same trip, so friendly reassurance can help until the drug has worn off. Visual effects such as intensified colours and distorted shapes occur but true visual hallucinations are rare; there may be distortions of hearing. In the recovery stage of an LSD experience there may also be apprehension and distraction that is not immediately obvious to onlookers and therefore a detainee's fitness to be interviewed may be affected. The forensic physician should advise the police accordingly.

Cannabis is the most widely consumed illegal substance in the UK. When smoked, effects occur within a few minutes and last up to one hour with low doses, 2–3 hours with higher doses. If it is ingested it may take an hour or more to have an effect which can last 12 hours or more. The effects include drowsiness, giggling, euphoria, poor concentration and memory, tachycardia, increase in blood pressure, red eyes, loss of co-ordination and an ataxic gait.

Hallucinogenic mushrooms or 'magic mushrooms' contain psilocybin and psilocin and are taken orally raw or cooked to enhance potency.

Drugs that depress the nervous system

Depression of the nervous system leads to sedation and relief of anxiety but, because of disinhibition, may initially result in euphoria, excitation and risk-taking.

Physical effects include disorientation, drowsiness, slurred speech, nystagmus, loss of co-ordination, ataxia, coma and death. At high doses cerebral depression may occur, so these drugs are more dangerous when taken with other cerebral depressants such as alcohol.

Volatile substance misuse is the deliberate inhalation of a volatile substance to achieve a change in mental state. There are many substances which can be misused including fuel gases, such as butane; petrol; aerosol propellants; glues and adhesives containing toluene; and cleaning agents such as trichlorethylene. These substances can result in a mixture of sedative, anaesthetic and hallucinogenic effects.

Death can occur from a variety of mechanisms including direct effects, such as anoxia, vagal inhibition (if the larynx is stimulated directly), respiratory depression and cardiac dysrhythmias, and secondarily following trauma. In addition, unexplained sudden death has been reported either during exposure or in the hours after. These substances should be discontinued abruptly. There is no physical withdrawal syndrome.

Ketamine is an anaesthetic agent which can be taken intranasally, orally or by injection. Effects start within 30 seconds or so after intravenous use, 2–4 minutes if used intramuscularly and 10–20 minutes if taken orally. The duration of action depends on the route of administration and varies from 10 minutes to one hour. Users can experience a cocaine-like 'rush' with psychological dissociation.

Gamma-hydroxybutyrate (GHB or GBH) is an anaesthetic with primarily sedative properties. Clinical effects start within 10–15 minutes but the duration of action is unpredictable.

Benzodiazepines are often misused with other drugs such as heroin and cocaine. Effects of intoxication are similar to those seen with alcohol. The withdrawal syndrome from benzodiazepines includes the major complications of fits and psychosis. In addition anxiety symptoms, such as sweating, insomnia, headache, tremor, nausea and disordered perceptions, such as feelings of unreality, abnormal bodily sensations and hypersensitivity to stimuli, may be seen. Treatment of benzodiazepine withdrawal should be with a long-acting drug such as diazepam to prevent the medical complications of withdrawal.

Barbiturates are particularly dangerous drugs when taken in overdose and cause a physical and psychological dependence. They have limited therapeutic uses now, having been largely replaced by the benzodiazepines, but may still occasionally be encountered in forensic practice.

Opiates

Opiate intoxication results in a feeling of wellbeing. There may be euphoria or the misuser may seem distant and drowsy with an inability to concentrate. The pupils will be small or pin point. Severe intoxication can result in respiratory depression and death. Tolerance develops to the analgesic and respiratory depressive actions of opiates but not the action on the pupil or the bowel so that a dependent individual usually displays a typically constricted pupil and suffers from constipation.

The start of the abstinence syndrome will depend on the opioid used. For example, heroin withdrawal will usually start within 8 hours, progress to a peak and then gradually improve over 48–72 hours, whereas withdrawal from methadone may lead to a longer abstinence syndrome. The misuser may experience sweating, lachrymation, rhinorrhoea, yawning, a feeling of going hot and cold, anorexia, abdominal cramps, nausea, vomiting, diarrhoea, tremor, restlessness, insomnia and generalized aches and weakness. On examination there may be dilated pupils, gooseflesh, an increase of pulse rate and blood pressure, and hyperactive bowel sounds.

Treatment of opiate withdrawal

Symptomatic treatment may be helpful for a number of detainees but it should be remembered that symptomatic treatment is not as effective as substitution treatment. Paracetamol and the non-steroidal anti-inflammatory drugs, such as ibuprofen, may be useful for generalized aches and pains. Other drugs may be used for specific problems: loperamide (Imodium®) for abdominal cramps and diarrhoea; promethazine, which has antiemetic and sedative properties, or metoclopramide for nausea and vomiting. Benzodiazepines are useful for the treatment of anxiety and insomnia but should not be used in naïve users who may need to be interviewed as the drugs will affect cognition and memory. Failure to produce symptom relief may indicate tolerance due to dependence on benzodiazepines or alcohol.

If the detainee is taking prescribed lofexidine this should be continued in police custody.

Substitution treatment includes methadone, buprenorphine or dihydrocodeine. Methadone and buprenorphine have a long duration of action (24–36 hours) and, therefore, can be given once a day. Dihydrocodeine may be suitable for those less severely dependent on opiates not controlled with symptomatic medication. If the detainee is receiving opiates as part of a detoxification programme this prescription should be continued once the presence of intoxication by other drugs has been excluded. The detainee may be carrying prescribed and accurately labelled medication on arrest or the details may be verified with the local clinic or chemist. If there is concern about the dose, for example a very large dose (methadone 100 mg), the dose can easily be split and the detainee reviewed at each stage. Otherwise, treatment should be given after a full assessment of the detainee. It may be necessary to review the detainee after a period of time to establish whether there are signs of withdrawal. Both methadone and buprenorphine should be self-administered under supervision by the authorizing doctor.

Sudden cessation of opioid use in a dependent pregnant woman may be life-threatening to the fetus and special care should be taken to ensure that a pregnant woman continues any prescribed medication and that treatment is instigated promptly to alleviate withdrawal.

The assessment of fitness to interview is of the utmost importance; mild opiate withdrawal may not affect a detainee's fitness with respect to an interview, but in more severe cases the detainee may require treatment prior to being interviewed. Continuing in police custody any substitution therapy or treatment that the detainee has been receiving in the community is unlikely to influence fitness for interview. However, when substitution therapy is initiated in custody, or when symptomatic treatment of withdrawal symptoms alone is provided, the doctor may well need to assess the impact of the treatment before the interview takes place (see Fig. 8.1).

Overdose

Naloxone is an opioid antagonist used to reverse the effects of intoxication. If naloxone is used, observation in hospital is required as most misused opioids have a longer half-life than naloxone. Furthermore, administration of naloxone to a polydrug misuser has the risk of precipitating cardiac arrhythmias (particularly in cocaine misuse). Whenever possible, naloxone should be given by intravenous injection. The intramuscular route can be used when it is difficult to establish intravenous access but this has the disadvantage of a slower onset of action.

Harm minimization

Harm minimization aims to reduce the damage from drug misuse. Many substance misusers have little or no contact with doctors and the attendance of a forensic physician provides an opportunity to provide advice about minimizing the harm from continued substance misuse. For example, advice can be given on safer injecting behaviour; general awareness of blood-borne viruses and the availability of hepatitis B vaccination; education on the risks of overdose; and information about the local agencies involved in counselling and treatment. Treatment may be needed for the medical

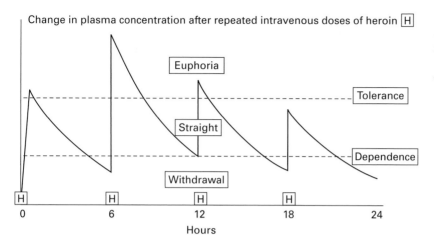

Change in plasma concentration after repeated intravenous doses of heroin [H]

Fig. 8.1 Schematic diagram of heroin and methadone use. (Reproduced from Ghodse [5].)

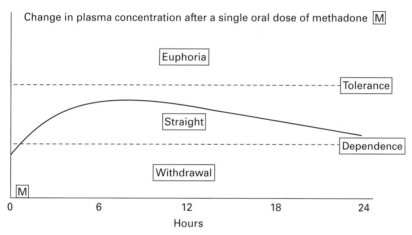

Change in plasma concentration after a single oral dose of methadone [M]

complications of substance misuse (see Table 8.3). All detainees should be seen as a potential infectious risk, but the police should not be informed of a detainee's HIV status as this would be a breach of patient confidentiality.

Mental Health Act

Drug misuse and dependence are explicitly excluded as grounds for compulsory admission under the Mental Health Act 1983. However, the mental state of a detainee may occasionally be such as to require assessment in hospital in the interests of their own health or for the safety of others. Chronic misuse of stimulants or cannabis may precipitate a psychotic illness. In the absence of mental disorder, substance misuse in itself is not an indication for an appropriate adult (see page 77) to be called. For changes under MHA 2007, see book website. www.cambridge.org/9780521705684.

Concealment

There are two distinct groups of individuals who swallow packets containing illicit drugs in an attempt to avoid detection by law enforcement

Table 8.3. Medical complications of drug misuse

Self-neglect, malnutrition, dental decay

Complication of injection
- intra-arterial may cause vascular damage resulting in gangrene
- intravenous may cause superficial thrombophlebitis, deep vein thrombosis, pulmonary embolism; post thrombotic complications such as limb swelling and ulcers

Inhalation of certain drugs may precipitate asthma or bronchitis; pneumothorax, pneumomediastinum, vomiting with inhalation and asphyxiation

Infection
- at the injection site may result in cellulitis and abscess formation
- septicaemia and infective endocarditis
- increased risk of tuberculosis
- hepatitis and HIV

Acute and chronic liver disease

Kidney problems and amyloidosis

Psychiatric complications

Overdose and death

agencies. 'Body-packers' are international smugglers who ingest packages of drugs in order to transport and subsequently retrieve them in a foreign country. 'Body-stuffers' or 'contact precipitated concealers' are individuals who ingest drugs at or around the time of their arrest in order to 'swallow the evidence'. Whereas body-packers take great care to package the drugs in such a way as to ensure their safe transit through the gastrointestinal tract without rupture, body-stuffers take no such elaborate precautions as they swallow packages in an unplanned attempt to conceal evidence. The drugs concerned have usually been prepared for street sale or carried for personal use and may be loosely wrapped in cellophane, plastic bags, paper or aluminium foil. These containers carry with them the obvious risk of leakage; subsequent absorption of the drugs contained therein may lead to toxic complications and possible death. The speed of onset of toxic effects depends on the integrity of the packaging and there may be significant delay [6].

Forensic physicians may be asked to undertake intimate searches to look for drugs concealed in the ears, mouth, nose, vagina or rectum of detainees.

An intimate search consists of the physical examination of a person's body orifices other than the mouth. In England and Wales, intimate searches are governed by s65 Police and Criminal Evidence Act 1984 (PACE) as amended by s59(1) of the Criminal Justice and Public Order Act 1994 and the Drugs Act 2005. In Scotland, in the absence of informed consent, an application in the interests of justice and to obtain evidence may be made to a sheriff for a warrant to conduct an intimate search. Intimate searches for drugs should take place in a properly equipped medical room, not a police station, by a registered medical practitioner or registered nurse [7]. Occasionally concealed packages may be at risk of rupture and full resuscitation facilities must be available.

The search must be authorized by an officer of inspector rank or above and can only take place after the detainee has given the appropriate consent in writing to the police. Forensic physicians should satisfy themselves that the consent is fully informed. Intimate searches for drugs only apply to persons who are believed to have Class A drugs concealed on them. Class A drugs include major natural and synthetic opiates (heroin and methadone), LSD, cocaine, ecstasy and injectable amphetamines but not cannabis, a commonly concealed substance. If a detainee refuses to be searched the forensic physician may have to arrange admission and observation in hospital.

Drug treatment monitoring systems

The National Drug Treatment Monitoring System (NDTMS) is the process by which information is collected, collated and analysed from and for those involved in the drug treatment sector in England and Wales. The NDTMS is a development of the Regional Drug Misuse Databases, which had been in place since the late 1980s. Responsibility for the NDTMS in England lies with the National

Treatment Agency. The data are collected by the treatment provider (soon to be by electronic data transfer) and there is no need for forensic physicians to submit data.

REFERENCES

1. Payne-James JJ, Wall IJ, Bailey C (2005) Patterns of illicit drug use of prisoners in police custody in London, UK. *Journal of Clinical Forensic Medicine* **12**:196–8.
2. Gossop M (2005). *Drug Misuse Treatment and Reductions in Crime: Findings From the National Treatment Outcome Research Study (NTORS)*. London: National Treatment Agency for Substance Misuse. www.nta.nhs.uk/publications/documents/nta_drug_treatment_crime_reduction_ntors_findings_2005_rb8.pdf (accessed August 2007).
3. Royal College of Psychiatrists (1987) *Drug Scenes. A Report on Drugs and Drug Dependence*. London: Royal College of Psychiatrists.
4. Stark MM, Norfolk GA, Rogers DJ, Payne-James JJ (2002) The validity of self-reported substance misuse amongst detained persons in police custody. *Journal of Clinical Forensic Medicine* **9**: 25–6.
5. Ghodse H (2002) *Drugs and Addictive Behaviour – A Guide to Treatment*, 3rd edn. Cambridge: Cambridge University Press.
6. Norfolk GA (2007) The fatal case of a cocaine body-stuffer and a literature review – towards evidence based management. *Journal of Forensic and Legal Medicine* **14**: 49–52.
7. British Medical Association and Faculty of Forensic and Legal Medicine (2007). *Guidelines for Doctors Asked to Perform Intimate Body Searches*. London: British Medical Association (also available at www.fflm.ac.uk).

FURTHER READING

Department of Health (England) and the devolved administrations (2007) *Drug Misuse and Dependence: UK Guidelines on Clinical Management*. London: Department of Health (England) the Scottish Government, Welsh Assembly and Northern Ireland Executive.

Association of Forensic Physicians/Royal College of Psychiatrists (2006) *Substance Misuse Detainees in Police Custody – Guidelines for Clinical Management*, 3rd edn. Report of a Medical Working Group. Council Report CR132. London: Royal College of Psychiatrists.

Karch SB (2002) *Karch's Pathology of Drug Abuse*, 3rd edn. Boca Raton: CRC Press.

Karch SB (2007) *Drug Abuse Handbook*, 2nd edn. Boca Raton: CRC Press.

Stark MM, Gregory M (2005) The clinical management of substance misusers in police custody – a survey of current practice. *Journal of Clinical Forensic Medicine* **12**: 199–204.

9

Alcohol, drugs and driving

Ian F. Wall

The substance

Of the many types of alcohols, this chapter will discuss only one – ethanol. Ethanol (or ethyl alcohol) is one of a number of alcohols containing a hydroxyl group attached to a carbon atom.

Ethanol is a water-soluble molecule usually produced by the fermentation of fruits and grains by yeast. The process generally stops when the alcohol level reaches about 15% by volume (per cent v/v) because the yeast dies. This produces drinks such as cider, beer and wine. The alcohol content can then be increased by distillation to produce spirits such as whisky, rum or brandy with alcohol contents often between 35% and 45%. The 'fortified' wines such as sherry and port have alcohol added to give them strengths between 14% and 22%. One hundred millilitres of a drink with a strength of 10% alcohol will contain 10 ml of alcohol or approximately 10 g (as alcohol is slightly lighter than water the actual weight will be slightly less). In the United States, alcohol strengths are measured in terms of percentage proof with US proof spirit containing 50% of alcohol by volume.

A UK unit of alcohol is 10 ml or 8 g of pure alcohol and is equivalent to half a pint of 3.5% beer, a small (125 ml) glass of wine or a 25 ml pub measure of 40% spirit. In view of the increasing social problems of alcohol excess, alcohol manufacturers are now required to state the number of units of alcohol on the bottle or can.

Metabolism

As with most other drugs, alcohol is absorbed in the small intestine, the absorption being fastest in the duodenum, but some absorption occurs in the stomach. Peak blood alcohol concentrations generally occur 30–60 minutes after ingestion, but the time to peak levels is influenced by many factors. As soon as alcohol enters the bloodstream elimination begins. The overall elimination rate is fairly constant (though there is significant variation from person to person) giving rise to the classic blood alcohol curve (Fig. 9.1).

Many factors affect the absorption and elimination of alcohol; these include:

Sex and weight: as alcohol is highly water soluble, once absorbed it enters the systemic circulation and is evenly distributed throughout the total body water. Therefore, generally, if two people of the same sex drink the same volume of alcohol, the lighter person will have a higher peak concentration because of the smaller volume of distribution. Furthermore, as women have more body fat and fewer muscle cells than men, and fat contains very little water, but muscle contains substantial

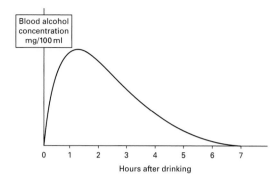

Fig. 9.1 Blood alcohol curve.

quantities of water, higher peak alcohol levels are reached in women than men of the same weight. The weight of body fluid expressed as a percentage of a person's total weight is known as the Widmark factor. A quick way of calculating the theoretical maximum alcohol level is to apply a formula devised by Widmark:

$$C = \frac{A \times 100}{D \times W}$$

where C is the peak alcohol concentration in blood in milligrams per 100 ml of blood, A is the amount of alcohol consumed in grams, D is the weight of the drinker in kilograms and W is the Widmark Factor (0.68 for men and 0.55 for women). In practice, the maximum concentration will never be reached as by the time all the alcohol is absorbed, elimination is beginning to take place.

Effect of food: the consumption of food during or before ingestion has a significant effect on absorption, with carbohydrate-rich foods tending to have a larger effect than fatty meals; the reduced blood alcohol concentration is due to a combination of delayed and reduced absorption of alcohol.

Type of drink: alcohol of 10–20% volume is maximally absorbed, with drinks of lesser strength being absorbed more slowly and stronger strength drinks irritating the stomach and delaying gastric emptying, thus slowing absorption.

Duration of drinking: if alcohol is drunk more slowly it may be eliminated almost as quickly as it is being absorbed, leading to a flattening of the blood alcohol curve.

Other factors: many other factors can also affect alcohol absorption. Gastric surgery may lead to a more rapid absorption. Some drugs slow gastric emptying, for instance chlorpromazine, tricyclic antidepressants, amphetamines and opiates. Other drugs may hasten gastric emptying, examples being metoclopramide and erythromycin. Alcohol is broken down by the enzyme alcohol dehydrogenase; some studies have shown less enzyme activity in the stomach of women, which may explain why they have higher peak alcohol levels than men.

Rate of elimination: once absorbed, almost 90% of alcohol is oxidized in the liver by alcohol dehydrogenase to form acetaldehyde, and further metabolized to acetic acid. The remainder is excreted unchanged, mainly in the urine but also in sweat and breath. Experimental studies have shown that rates of elimination of alcohol can vary from person to person. Dubowski [1] found a mean elimination rate of 14.94 mg/100 ml of blood per hour, other surveys showed a mean rate of 18.6 mg/100 ml per hour. The range can be anything from 10 to 25 mg, with chronic alcoholics having well-developed liver enzyme systems often achieving these high levels of elimination. Most scientists work on an average rate of 18 mg/100 ml per hour but will give a range using 10–25 mg/100 ml per hour.

Effects of alcohol

Ethanol is a central nervous system (CNS) depressant, but is now known to affect a number of excitatory and inhibitory amino acid transmitters as well as dopamine and 5-hydroxytryptamine (serotonin). This partly explains the apparent initial stimulatory effect of alcohol, because it acts first on higher centres of the brain which control inhibition, but

Table 9.1. Effects of alcohol

Blood alcohol mg/100 ml	Stage of influence	Effects
Under 50	Sobriety	No obvious effect but subject may be more talkative with a sense of wellbeing
50–100	Euphoria	Slurred speech, bravado, some loss of concentration and sensory perception
100–150	Excitement	Emotional instability
		Marked loss of concentration
		Poor sensory perception
150–200	Drunkenness	Disorientation, mental confusion and dizziness
		Decreased pain sense, impaired balance and slurred speech
200–300	Stupor	General inertia, approaching paralysis
		Marked lack of response to stimuli
		Vomiting, incontinence of urine and faeces
300–450	Coma	Coma and anaesthesia
		Depressed or abolished reflexes
Over 450	Death	Probable death from respiratory paralysis

then in larger doses, depresses medullary processes. There is a marked variation in the susceptibility of drinkers to the effects of alcohol.

Alcohol initially produces a sense of euphoria with disinhibition and increased self-confidence, the latter resulting in gregarious behaviour. Increased self-confidence can be manifest by aggression and loud and outrageous behaviour. Mood changes are not always predictable: some may be disinhibited, others become sleepy, introverted or depressed. In addition, the CNS effects become more marked with stupor leading to coma and death, as illustrated in Table 9.1.

The diagnostic criteria [2] for alcohol intoxication are:

• Recent ingestion of alcohol
• Clinically significant maladaptive behavioural or psychological changes (e.g. inappropriate sexual or aggressive behaviour, mood lability, impaired judgement, impaired social or occupational functioning) that developed during or shortly after alcohol ingestion
• One or more of the following signs, developing during, or shortly after, alcohol use:
  • Slurred speech
  • Unsteady gait
  • Inco-ordination
  • Nystagmus
  • Impairment in attention or memory
  • Stupor or coma
• The symptoms are not due to a general medical condition and are not better accounted for by another mental disorder.

In assessing persons for alcohol intoxication you must exclude other medical conditions: head injuries, metabolic disorders, effects of other drugs, neurological problems, psychiatric disorders, febrile illnesses and carbon monoxide poisoning. Do not overlook acute hypoglycaemia, an occasional complication of severe intoxication [3].

Alcohol has a moderate to high abuse potential with up to 10% of users becoming dependent and developing into alcoholics. Chronic alcohol consumers develop tolerance to the effects of alcohol; when alcohol intake is abruptly stopped, symptoms and signs of withdrawal develop, the severity depending mainly on the duration and amount of alcohol consumed. Alcohol withdrawal symptoms [4] can develop six to eight hours after the last alcohol consumption and can occur well before the alcohol level reaches zero in dependent individuals. Symptoms and signs include anxiety, irritability, tremor and insomnia leading to sweating, raised pulse and blood pressure, hallucinations, delirium tremens and, ultimately, alcohol withdrawal seizures.

In the custodial setting, withdrawal from alcohol can have serious consequences and you should assess the degree of dependence, then initiate treatment to prevent the serious, potentially fatal, complications of delirium tremens and convulsions. Benzodiazepines are the drugs of choice, the starting dose depending on the severity of the withdrawal, for example either chlordiazepoxide 20 mg or diazepam 10 mg, given three or four times per day [5]. However, admission to hospital may be necessary if symptoms are severe.

Alcohol and driving

Even at low doses, there is clear evidence that alcohol impairs driving performance. The classic study on the relationship between accident risk and blood alcohol concentration (BAC) was the Grand Rapids study [6] in 1964 where data were collected on 5895 drivers involved in accidents and on 7590 drivers not involved in accidents. Comparison of the two groups showed that accident risk was statistically more likely at BAC levels greater than 80 mg/100 ml of blood with the risk rising exponentially (see Box 9.1).

Box 9.1 The relationship of accident occurrence to blood alcohol

Blood alcohol (BAC)

mg/100 ml	Accident occurrence
50–100	1.5 times as frequently
100–150	4 times as frequently
Over 150	18 times as frequently

This relationship between BAC and accident risk, illustrated in Fig. 9.2, led to the introduction of the legal limit in 1967. More recent research [7] showed a significant increase in crash risk at BAC levels of 40 mg/100 ml.

Accident risk is also related to driver inexperience, with a sharp increase at much lower alcohol levels.

This has resulted in several countries having lower legal limits for young or inexperienced drivers.

Road traffic legislation

The Road Safety Act 1967 set a legal driving limit of 80 mg/100 ml blood (or 35 μg/100 ml of breath or 107 mg/100 ml of urine) and allowed for mandatory roadside screening tests and the provision of blood or urine tests at police stations. The legislation was updated by the Transport Act 1981 which allowed the use of evidential breath testing machines as the sole evidence of drink driving. These provisions were revised by the Road Traffic Acts (RTA) of 1988 and 1991. The main legislation in the UK is as follows:

Section 3A – causing death by careless driving while under the influence of drink or drugs

Section 4 – driving, being in charge of or attempting to drive a motor vehicle while unfit through drink or drugs

Section 5 – driving, being in charge of or attempting to drive a motor vehicle while over the prescribed limit

Section 6 – relating to the provision of specimens of breath for analysis

Section 7 – relating to the provision of specimens of blood or urine for analysis

The Police Reform Act 2002 and the Criminal Justice (Northern Ireland) Order 2005 permit the taking of blood from incapacitated drivers for future consensual testing. The Railways and Transport Safety Act 2003 introduced Preliminary Impairment Tests (PITs) by police officers.

Legal limits

In the United Kingdom, the current legal limits are:

Blood – 80 mg per 100 ml of blood

Breath – 35 μg per 100 ml of breath

Urine – 107 mg per 100 ml of urine.

Most other European countries now have lower legal limits, though the penalties for drink driving

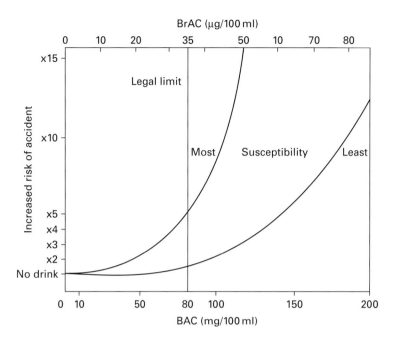

Fig. 9.2 Risk of road traffic accidents related to levels of alcohol in the blood (BAC) and breath (BrAC).

differ. Lowering the legal limit from 50 to 20 mg/100 ml in blood in Sweden resulted in a fall in casualties [8]; cost–benefit analyses [9] have shown that reducing the legal limit to 50 mg/100 ml in the UK would save 50 lives, prevent 250 serious injuries and save £75 million per year.

Road Traffic Act procedures

Police procedure

A police officer in uniform may require a person driving, attempting to drive or being in charge of a motor vehicle on a road or other public place to take a breath test if he suspects that the person:
- has been drinking or
- has committed a moving traffic offence.

Where an accident has occurred, a police officer in uniform may require any person whom he has reasonable cause to believe was drinking or attempting to drive or was in charge of the vehicle at the time of the accident to take a screening breath test. Several makes of screening breath testing devices are available, some of which give digital readings. Furthermore, appropriately trained police officers can now require, under the Railways and Transport Safety Act, a person to undertake a PIT at the roadside. A person who:
- is unfit to drive or
- has provided a positive breath test or
- has refused/failed to take a breath test or PIT

will be arrested and taken to a police station where the driver will be required to provide an evidential breath test.

Police officers use a series of standardized Police Manual of Guidance forms for the various procedures. These are:
- Form MG DD/A – Drink/Drugs Station Procedure – General
- Form MG DD/B – Drink/Drugs Station Procedure – Specimens/Impairment Supplement
- Form MG DD/C – Hospital Procedure
- Form MG DD/D – Alcohol Technical Defence Form

- Form MG DD/E – Drug Sample Information Form
- Form MG DD/F – Preliminary Impairment Test.

The Faculty of Forensic and Legal Medicine have produced a s4 Road Traffic Act Assessment Form which is a useful aide-memoire for doctors. It can be downloaded from the Faculty website [10].

Police station procedure

The police officer will commence the procedure using form MG DD/A. The three current evidential breath testing machines in the UK – Intoximeter EC/IR, Camic and Lion Intoxilyzer 6000 – all measure alcohol levels using an infrared spectrophotometer. The person is required to produce two samples of breath in a timed cycle.

If the breath alcohol level is 39 μg/100 ml or less, no action is taken unless it is suspected the person is impaired; if the level is between 40 and 50 μg/100 ml inclusive, the person has the statutory option to replace the sample with a specimen of blood or urine; if the level is 51 μg/100 ml or more an automatic prosecution will result.

If

- no reliable breath testing machine is available *or*
- no trained machine operator is available *or*
- the machine is operating unreliably *or*
- the person has a statutory option *or*
- the police officer believes that for medical reasons a specimen of breath cannot be provided,

the police officer will proceed to a blood/urine option and continue with form MG DD/B. It is for the police officer to decide whether to request a blood or urine specimen. If the police officer chooses a blood sample, a forensic physician or healthcare professional (HCP) will be called. If the police opt for urine, the sample will be taken by the police officer.

It is very important for the doctor or HCP to use the standard kits provided (which have special safety devices to try to reduce the risk of needlestick injury) and to have a standard routine for the procedure because many technical defences have arisen. Obtain witnessed informed consent to take the sample, and establish any medical reasons why

a sample of blood cannot be taken. It is for you to decide where the sample should be taken from and, once taken, to divide the sample equally between two bottles and shake to disperse the preservative. Label both bottles, placing them in secure containers and then tamper-proof bags. The driver is allowed to retain one sample for independent analysis and given a list of approved analysts. The time the sample is taken, the time the specimens are sealed and the time one is offered to the driver should be noted. In addition, it is good practice to make a brief assessment of fitness to detain and release.

If the police officer decides to request a specimen of urine, the person is required to provide two samples of urine within one hour; the first sample is discarded and the second sample is used for analysis (having been split into two samples similar to the blood option procedure). It should be noted that there is no statutory provision for moving on from a urine sample to a blood sample.

When a juvenile is involved, the procedure should not be unduly delayed while the attendance of an appropriate adult is secured since this is not an interview under the Police and Criminal Evidence Act 1984 (PACE). However, without the agreement of a parent or guardian, a juvenile cannot consent to the provision of blood and, where necessary, the requirement to provide a sample of urine is recommended.

Hospital procedure

If a driver is taken to a hospital, the police officer needs to establish first if the person can give valid consent, then obtain permission from the hospital doctor to permit an examination by a forensic physician, or permit the taking of a specimen of breath, blood or urine, or to undertake a PIT. It is important not to compromise any medical care of the driver.

Under current legislation, if the person is able to give consent and the police officer elects for a blood sample, this can only be taken by a doctor. In the future, it is possible that legislation may be changed to permit the sample to be taken by a HCP.

If the police officer decides that the person is unable to give valid consent for medical reasons, the Police Reform Act 2002 legislation can be used. A blood sample may be taken for future testing for alcohol or drugs from a person who has been involved in an accident and is unable to give consent where

- the forensic physician taking the specimen is satisfied that the person is not able to give valid consent *and*
- the doctor in immediate charge of the patient is satisfied that the taking of the specimen would not be prejudicial to the proper care and treatment of the patient *and*
- the person does not object to or resist the specimen being taken and has not refused consent to the sample being taken before losing competence.

The specimen is not tested until the person regains competence and gives valid consent for analysis. The British Medical Association and the Faculty of Forensic and Legal Medicine have produced a joint guidance document [11] which gives excellent advice about the ethical and practical issues involved in this procedure. Again, currently, the sample of blood can only be taken by a doctor, and it is not permissible to take a specimen of urine instead.

Complex defences

Numerous technical defences have arisen over the years and it is important to be aware of the most common ones. Unless with reasonable excuse, failure to provide a sample of breath, blood or urine is an offence (s7 RTA).

Failure to provide a sample of breath

Examples of medically acceptable reasons include mouth, lip or facial injury, tracheostomy, chest wall injury and some neurological problems. Many cases have been challenged on the basis that the person has respiratory problems.

The evidential breath machines are designed to measure the alcohol levels in deep lung air. The Home Office requirement for the machines is that the subject must exhale a minimum of 1.2 litres of air and, once this has been satisfied, to continue blowing until deep lung breath has been detected, which is achieved by monitoring the rise in alcohol level with increasing exhaled volume, until at the end of the breath, the alcohol level no longer rises and a plateau is reached. The volume of air that has to be exhaled by the person in order to reach deep lung air will therefore depend on the size of the person's lungs. Research [12] showed that, of 30 patients with respiratory problems, nine were unable to provide a sample of breath on the Lion Intoxilyzer 6000 and, although the machine requires a minimum volume of 1.2 litres, eight of the nine subjects had forced vital capacities (FVCs) of more than 1.5 litres. Although most of these patients had respiratory problems at the severe end of the spectrum, it was often not possible for subjects with lung diseases (particularly COPD) to complete the required number of attempts because of the long periods needed for exhalation and recovery.

The responsibility to decide whether there is a reasonable excuse for failing to provide a breath sample rests with the police officer, but forensic physicians are sometimes asked to examine a detained person to assess if a reasonable excuse exists. If there is doubt, give the person the benefit of that doubt and recommend a blood/urine option.

Failure to provide a sample of blood

Medical reasons for failing to provide a blood sample include poor venous access, failure of the forensic physician to take the sample and needle phobia.

It is for the doctor to decide where the sample should be taken from, and it is generally accepted that up to three attempts are likely to be considered reasonable. A minimum of 2 ml of blood is required for analysis (the laboratory requires 1 ml) but if sufficient blood is not obtained at the first attempt, do not add the blood from one attempt to blood from another, as the legislation states that the blood has to have been taken from one continuous sample. If you are unable to obtain an adequate sample after three attempts, abandon the procedure and advise the police officer that a medical reason for failing to provide exists. The police officer should then opt for a urine sample.

Needle phobia appears an increasing problem. If this is alleged, take a full history with specific attention to immunizations, body piercing, dental procedures, tattoos and current and past psychiatric history. Note when the problem started and whether it is due to fear of needles or blood products. A standard approach [13] using diagnostic guidelines is very important. Rix [14] also gives some practical advice in distinguishing 'repugnance' from 'phobia' and 'unwillingness' from 'inability'.

If you are unsure that needle phobia exists, it is best to act with caution and recommend a urine sample. The best way to get a successful prosecution is to obtain a sample, any sample, for analysis.

Failure to provide a sample of urine

Although this is technically a police procedure, it is important to be aware of some of the potential reasons why persons fail to provide a sample of urine:

- Drugs acting on the bladder, e.g. tolterodine, methadone
- Neurological problems affecting the bladder
- Embarrassment – case law has determined that the officer present should be of the same sex as the detained person. In order to pass urine, it is necessary to relax the bladder sphincter muscles; anxiety causes muscle tension and difficulty in micturition. Self-conscious feelings elicited when others are present may possibly interfere with the ability to relax the bladder sphincters. This is known as avoidance paruresis [15], sometimes

called shy bladder, bashful bladder or bladder shyness.

Drugs and driving

There is increasing evidence [16] that drugs driving, including prescribed, over-the-counter and illicit drugs, is an increasing problem. The relevant legislation is s4 RTA; being unfit is defined thus: a person shall be taken to be unfit to drive if his ability to drive properly is for the time being impaired.

It is for the court to decide if the person was unfit to drive and this will usually comprise three elements (though it is not necessary for all three to be present):

- witness observations of the manner of driving
- the results of a medical assessment
- toxicological analysis.

Once suspicion is directed to a drug other than alcohol as responsible for the accused's condition, the police have no legal right to require the provision of specimens of blood or urine at a police station unless a doctor has advised that the subject's condition might be due to some drug other than alcohol. In drug cases, where a choice exists, blood is generally a better medium for analysis than urine.

Following arrest, the police officer will continue using form MG DD/B and will request the doctor to undertake an examination to ascertain if there is a condition present that might be due to a drug. However, the doctor's role is more wide ranging than this and includes:

- assessment of fitness for detention;
- excluding a condition that may mimic intoxication;
- determining whether a person's ability to drive is impaired;
- determining whether there is a condition present that might be due to a drug.

The police can require a specimen for analysis providing the doctor has advised them that there is a condition present that might be due to a drug – the doctor does not have to establish impairment for a sample to be legally required.

It is helpful to ascertain the circumstances from the arresting officer, whether impairment tests have been carried out and what findings the custody officer noted. There is no formal definition of a 'condition' or 'impairment' but useful advice [17] has indicated that in deciding what a condition is, a doctor can use information relating to events which occurred before the examination of the suspect. For example, the suspect might say that he had taken drugs or was in possession of drugs at the time of arrest. However, this is a controversial issue and it would be helpful if case law clarified the position.

Establish informed consent for the examination and explain that the information will not be treated confidentially. Take a full medical history including details of any current medical problems and details of recent events, particularly about any road traffic accident that led to the event. Note past medical history (with specific reference to diabetes, epilepsy, asthma and visual and hearing problems), past psychiatric history and alcohol and drug consumption (prescribed, over the counter and illicit). Perform a physical examination to include general observations of demeanour and behaviour, any injuries, speech, hiccoughs and any smell of alcohol on the breath. Examine the cardiovascular system noting pulse, blood pressure and temperature. Examine the eyes, noting the state of the sclera, size of the pupils and the presence of nystagmus.

Carry out a series of standardized field impairment tests (FITs). These consist of a Romberg test, Walk and Turn test, One Leg Stand test and a Finger Nose test. Precise details of how these should be carried out are available on the pro forma (see www.fflm.ac.uk/library) produced by the Faculty of Forensic and Legal Medicine. In Scotland, forensic physicians use the form F97. If the driver does not consent to an examination, you should still make observations.

The importance of a comprehensive examination cannot be overemphasized as many conditions mimic intoxication including:

- head injury
- metabolic disorders, e.g. hypo- or hyperglycaemia, uraemia, hepatic coma
- neurological disorders, e.g. multiple sclerosis, epilepsy, vertigo, cerebral tumour, stroke, Parkinson's disease
- psychiatric disorders, e.g. hypomania
- fatigue
- pyrexia.

At the end of the examination, decide whether there is a condition present that may result from some drug. In the case of short-acting drugs, the observations of the police officer and particularly their results from an earlier PIT may be crucial. Inform the police officer whether there is a condition present that might be due to a drug (and what that condition is). Armed with this information, the police officer will then continue with the blood/urine option procedure. It should be noted that currently, for s4 cases, a specimen of blood or urine can only be required if the police officer has been advised by a medical practitioner, never a HCP, that the person has a condition that might be due to some drug.

The standardized impairment tests remain controversial. Recent research [18] has shown that the forensic medical examiner supported the police officer's assessment of impairment using the test in 77% of cases. However, it was not possible to obtain biological samples from the 23% of cases where the forensic medical examiner did not corroborate the findings of the police officer; although it was only possible to obtain a small number of specimens from persons whom the police officer considered to be unimpaired, a significant number of these were drug positive (71%). It was concluded that, although useable in its current form, further development of the tests and procedure is required to improve performance.

The Railways and Transport Safety Act 2003 not only introduced legislation concerning PITs by police officers, but also enacted the requirement for a person to undergo a Preliminary Drug Test. Thus, if the police officer considered that the motorist had failed a PIT, the person could be arrested and required to have a sample of sweat or saliva tested for drugs. The implication is that a positive test allows the police officer to proceed to a blood/urine option without the requirement for a medical examination (which, as indicated above, is partly for the detained person's medical welfare and safety). Though the legislation is in place, the type approval for the necessary drug testing equipment has not yet been established. Other research projects in progress from the Home Office Police Scientific Development Branch involve the use of hand-held devices to detect impairment.

Under certain circumstances, for example the person does not have a primary care physician and is believed to be driving under the influence of drugs, you may need to follow the General Medical Council's code and inform the Driver and Vehicle Licensing Agency about the driver's condition.

REFERENCES

1. Dubowski RK (1985) Absorption, distribution and elimination of alcohol: highway safety aspects. *Journal of Studies on Alcohol* Suppl 10: 98–108.
2. DSM-IV. *Diagnostic and Statistical Manual of Mental Disorders* (2000) 4th edn. Washington DC: American Psychiatric Association.
3. Stark MM, Rogers DJ (1998) Hypoglycaemia: a hidden danger. *Journal of Clinical Forensic Medicine* 5(4): 211–2.
4. Association of Forensic Physicians/Royal College of Psychiatrists (2006) *Substance Misuse Detainees in Police Custody Guidelines for Clinical Management. Report of a Working Party.* May 2006.
5. Naik P, Lawton J (1996) Assessment and management of individuals under the influence of alcohol in police custody. *Journal of Clinical Forensic Medicine* 3: 37–44.
6. Borkenstein RF, Dale A (1964) *The Role of the Drinking Driver in Traffic Accidents (the Grand Rapids Study).* Indiana University, Bloomington: Department of Police Administration.
7. Compton RP, Blomberg RD, Moskowitz H, *et al.* (2002) Crash risk of alcohol impaired driving. *T2002 Proceedings of the 16th International Conference on Alcohol, Drugs and Traffic Safety.* 4–9 August 2002. Montreal, Canada, pp. 39–44.
8. Aberg L, Utzelmann HD, Berghaus G (1992) Behaviour and opinions of Swedish drivers before and after the 0.02% legal BAC limit in 1990. *T9 Proceedings of the 12th International Conference on Alcohol, Drugs and Traffic Safety.* Cologne, Germany.
9. Department of the Environment, Transport and the Regions (1998) *Combating Drink-driving – Next Steps. A Consultation Document.* London: DETR.
10. Wall IF (2007) *Section 4 RTA Assessment Form.* [Online] Available at http://fflm.ac.uk/library/ [7 June 2007].
11. British Medical Association and the Faculty of Forensic and Legal Medicine (2007) *Taking Blood Specimens from Incapacitated Drivers – Guidance for Doctors.* [Online] Available at http://fflm.ac.uk/library/ [7 June 2007].
12. Honeybourne D, Moore AJ, Butterfield AK, Azzan L (2000) A study to investigate the ability of subjects with chronic lung diseases to provide evidential breath samples using the Lion Intoxilyzer 6000 UK breath alcohol testing device. *Respiratory Medicine* 94: 684–8.
13. Stark MM, Brenner N (2000) Needle phobia. *Journal of Clinical Forensic Medicine* 7: 35–8.
14. Rix K (1996) Blood or needle phobia as a defence under the Road Traffic Act of 1988. *Journal of Clinical Forensic Medicine* 3: 173–7.
15. International Paruresis Association (2007) *About Avoidance Paruresis.* [Online] Available at www.paruresis.org/ [7 June 2007].
16. Tunbridge RJ, Keigan M, James FJ (2001) *The Incidence of Drugs in Road Accident Fatalities.* TRL Report 495. Crowthorne, UK: TRL Ltd.
17. Stark MM, O'Keefe V, Rowe D (2000) Interpretation of Section 7(3)(c) of the Road Traffic Act 1988 (Letter to the Editor). *Journal of Clinical Forensic Medicine* 7: 59.
18. Oliver JS, Seymour A, Wylie FM, Torrance H, Anderson RA (2006) *Monitoring the Effectiveness of UK Field Impairment Tests.* Road Safety Research Report No 63. London: Department for Transport.

10

Injury

Jack Crane

The accurate description and interpretation of injuries is one of the most important functions of the forensic physician. Marks of violence may be found on the victim of an assault, either physical or sexual, on a child suspected of having been abused, on a police officer arresting a violent suspect, on a prisoner alleging ill-treatment whilst in custody, or on a body found dead in suspicious circumstances. The doctor asked to carry out an examination in such cases must be able to record injuries accurately, be aware of their medico-legal significance and be able to give a useful opinion on how they may have been caused.

Describing wounds

The examination should preferably be made in good light; in practice however, conditions may be less than ideal, for example, when called out at night, in the rain, to examine a dead body in a dark entry. Under such circumstances a powerful torch or floodlighting of the scene may be required. A few basic items of equipment are also essential: a hand-lens (or better still, an illuminated magnifier), a ruler with clear metric markings, a tape measure and a pair of calipers. Body charts (examples are available on the Faculty of Forensic and Legal Medicine website (www.fflm.ac.uk)) are invaluable for recording injuries. A portable ultra violet torch

may help to highlight faint bruises. In cases of serious assault or when injuries have distinctive characteristics of patterning, wounds must be professionally photographed with a suitable scale included beside the wound. Self-adhesive tape, incorporating both imperial and metric graduations, is readily available for this purpose.

The important points to consider in describing a wound are the nature of the injury, its age, its size and shape and its location. When examining the living, injured areas need to be palpated to discern swelling and tenderness.

Nature of the injury

Under the Offences Against the Person Act 1861 a 'wound' required the integrity of the body surface to be breached, however superficially or minutely. As this obviously excludes bruising and internal injury, it is unrealistic in a medical sense. In legal terms, however, there is the definition of 'causing serious bodily harm' to cover any injury to any tissue or organ. Local reaction to injury also includes erythema and oedema that, on occasions, may be the only indication of the application of violence. Thermal damage also occurs locally as a response to chemical and electrical burns and due to the application of dry heat. Scalds are due to the application of moist heat. In spite of the confusing assortment of names used by doctors and others, it

Editorially revised for this third edition.
Clinical Forensic Medicine, third edition ed. W. D. S. McLay. Published by Cambridge University Press. © Cambridge University Press 2009.

is essential that for medico-legal purposes, forensic physicians, like forensic pathologists, use a standardized nomenclature when describing wounds. The classification that should be used is:

1. Bruises – (a term familiar to all) or contusions
2. Abrasions – familiar as scratches or grazes
3. Lacerations – irregular cuts or tears
4. Incisions – to be differentiated from lacerations (see below)
5. Stab or penetrating wounds

Of course, a variety of types of wound may coexist following a single traumatic incident. Furthermore, a single wound may show characteristics of different types, for example a bruised abrasion or an abrasion within which is a laceration.

Age

Injuries inflicted just before examination or indeed shortly before death show no sign of healing; this process (and eventual resolution) provides some guidance as to the age of the wound, but the many variables – such as site, force applied, amount of tissue damage, infection, treatment – all make judgements difficult. Bruises often become more prominent some hours or even days after infliction because of diffusion of blood closer to the skin surface. Bruises resolve over a variable period, ranging from days to weeks. The larger the bruise the longer it will take to disappear. Reddish-blue, blue or purplish-black bruises are almost certainly recent. As the extravasated red cells are destroyed, the ageing bruise goes through variable colour changes of bluish-green, greenish-yellow and brown [1, 2]. Estimating the age of non-recent bruises is one of the most contentious areas of forensic medicine. It must be clearly understood that it is impossible to age a bruise precisely; if you are asked to do so in court as a medical witness, you would be prudent simply to state that a bruise undergoing these colour changes is obviously not recent.

During life, an abrasion remains moist until it forms a scab, which consists of hardened exudate. The time taken for this process varies mainly with its depth, but also with any disturbance to which the surface is subjected, for instance, across a joint. The scab organizes over a period of days up to a couple of weeks, before detaching, leaving a pink, usually intact surface. The colour gradually fades, unless the lesion is extensive, develops keloid or becomes very scarred. After death, an unscabbed abrasion dries and has a parchment-like brown colour. Abrasions caused after death tend to have a hard, yellow, translucent appearance and are devoid of any colour change at the periphery.

A laceration, or any wound healing by secondary intention, is associated with scab formation and eventual scarring, both taking days or weeks to develop. An incision, the edges of which are apposed, heals within a few days. The wound's colour, as with a bruise, may help in assessing the age of the lesion.

Size and shape

Size is determined with the aid of a ruler or a pair of calipers and must be measured on the metric scale. Since measurements given in imperial units may still be easier for a jury to understand, it is acceptable for you to include the equivalent size in inches after that given in millimetres or centimetres. You should also note the shape of the wound, using simple terms such as circular, triangular, V-shaped, crescentic, and outline them on the appropriate body chart. Wounds also have depth, but it is often not possible to estimate this clinically, nor to see the base. This may have significance, as in distinguishing lacerations or incised wounds of the scalp, and in identifying and recovering foreign (trace) material.

Position

First, the general location should be noted – for example, on the right upper limb, face or scalp. Then the precise location should be determined using fixed anatomical landmarks, such as 'on the scalp, 3 cm above and 1 cm behind the outer opening of the left ear' or 'on the inner aspect of the right upper arm, 5 cm above the medial epicondyle of the humerus'. On the neck, use landmarks such as the prominence of the thyroid cartilage and the sterno cleidomastoid muscles; on the trunk, the nipples, umbilicus and bony prominence of the pelvis can be points of reference. In females, the position of the nipples will vary with posture and the bulk of the breast. Technical anatomical terms are useful in reports for putting the site of the injury beyond doubt, but explain these in language suitable for a lay audience when giving oral evidence or a written statement.

Types of injury

Transient lesions

Friction and irritants applied to the skin often cause transient erythema, sometimes accompanied by swelling. The skin over a weal may or may not be reddened. In susceptible individuals, a light touch causes a histamine reaction, seen as dermatographia. On the face, neck, upper chest and arms and behind the ears, patchy reddening, which persists for a time varying from minutes to several hours, may be seen in some sensitive individuals, as a response to fear or embarrassment. It diminishes on digital pressure and must not be confused with bruising. Simple pressure from tight clothing may also cause erythema.

Red marks outlining an apparent injury, for example the mark of a hand on a slapped face or the buttock of a child, should be photographed without delay, as such images may fade within an hour or so after infliction.

Reddening on the genital area, for example within the vulva, cannot be attributed to trauma with any certainty. These problems of interpretation are considered further in Chapters 11–13.

Bruises

A bruise is due to the application of blunt force. The blow ruptures small blood vessels beneath the intact skin surface and blood escapes to infiltrate the surrounding tissues under the pumping action of the heart (see Fig. 10.1). It follows that established bruising is only produced during life; post-mortem wounds are not associated with any significant bruising as there is no internal pressure in the small vessels that have been ruptured.

Pinhead-sized haemorrhages within the skin, usually termed petechiae, may be produced by mechanical trauma as in reproducing the texture of clothing (see below), but may also be produced by sucking (as in love bites) and are often seen on the serous membranes and conjunctivae as well as the skin as a result of congestion, possibly associated with mechanical asphyxia. Purpura is seen in those with a haemorrhagic tendency; in the elderly, lesions tend to be larger and less regular in outline. Larger blotchy areas of haemorrhage within the skin are often referred to as ecchymoses, but take care in the use of the term lest you become embroiled in problems of definition in the witness box. When blood collects within a mass beneath the skin, rather than being diffused within the tissues, it forms a haematoma. Do not confuse bruising with naevi or Campbell de Morgan spots. Innocent striae running transversely across the lower back of adolescents have been mistaken for injuries caused by beating. Cyanosis is also a cause of blue discoloration in the skin, which may be a source of confusion as is hypostasis, particularly in early stages of its development.

The initial site of a bruise corresponds with the point of impact but, if the victim lives, its boundaries are likely to exceed the original area of contact. Thus, one cannot state that a bruise, 6 cm diameter, was caused by an object of similar dimensions.

The extension of bruising can also mislead as to the actual site of the injury. Since a bruise is a simple mechanical permeation of the tissue spaces by fluid blood, its extension may be affected by gravity. Bruising of the thigh could result from a blow on the hip and facial bruising from an injury to the scalp. Difficulty arises when a bruise, as it extends, tracks along tissue planes from an invisible to a visible situation. Bruising of this kind may not

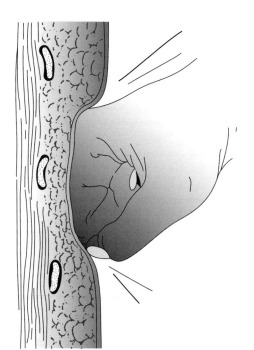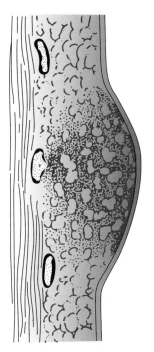

Fig. 10.1 Bruising.

become apparent externally for some time and then at a point well removed from the site of the original injury. This delay in the appearance of bruising is of considerable significance since lack of positive findings at an initial examination is not inconsistent with positive findings at an examination 24 or 48 hours later. Therefore, in many cases of assault, it may be essential to conduct a further examination a day or so later.

The size of a bruise is not necessarily related to the severity of the blow. In the living, a small bruise usually indicates no more than a slight blow, whereas a small bruise on a dead body may result from a violent blow if death occurred soon after the injury was inflicted. In contradistinction, a minor knock may produce a large bruise in the very young, the elderly, alcoholics or those with a compromised peripheral circulation. Bruising which seems inconsistent with the violence inflicted should lead one to exclude the possibility of a bleeding diathesis. Much depends on the general health of the individual and the condition and

resilience of the skin, factors to be taken into account when recording findings made on general examination.

Some areas of the body bruise more readily than others, and this depends, among other things, on their blood supply and the density of the supporting tissues. Where there is an underlying bony surface and the tissues are lax, such as the facial area, a relatively light blow may produce considerable puffy bruising, particularly around the eyes. The scalp is a tissue that bruises more readily than it appears to; bruising there is easily detected at postmortem examination when the scalp is reflected, but in the living, scalp bruising frequently goes undetected.

Sometimes a bruise has a pattern that may indicate the agent responsible. This is particularly so when death occurs soon after the injury is sustained, the pattern remaining sufficiently clear for diagnosis. In the living, this may become obscured as the area of bruising tends to extend and merge with others. Despite this, it may still be possible to

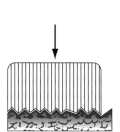 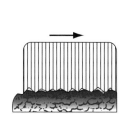 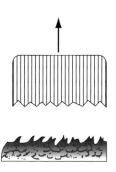

Fig. 10.2 Abrasion.

make out such features as the links of a dog chain or the ridges on the patterned sole of a shoe. Beating with a rod often leaves a patterned bruise consisting of an area of central pallor outlined by two narrow parallel bands of bruising ('tramline bruising'). Perhaps the commoner pattern of bruising is that composed of petechial haemorrhages reproducing the texture of clothing. This may occur if a person is struck a violent blow on a clothed area of the body or if the clothing is grabbed and twisted over the skin. Another type of patterning occasionally seen is the streaky linear purple bruising on the neck, wrists or ankles caused by the application of a ligature.

Other bruises of particular medico-legal significance are the small circular or oval bruises, usually about 1–2 cm in diameter, characteristic of fingertip pressure from either grabbing with the hand or prodding with the fingers. They are often seen on the limbs in cases of child abuse when the child is forcibly gripped by the arms or legs and shaken, or on the abdomen when the victim is poked and prodded. Similar bruises from the fingertips may be seen on the neck in manual strangulation and are then usually associated with other signs of asphyxia.

When sexual assault is alleged, the presence of bruising on the victim may help to corroborate the complaint and give some indication as to how much violence was used. Moreover, bruising found elsewhere than about the genitalia gives some indication of how the attack was conducted, for example bruising on the back could be in keeping with the complainant having been pinned to the ground. Grip marks or 'defence' injuries may be present on the upper arms and forearms, while bruising on the thighs and inner sides of the knees may occur as the victim's legs are forcibly pulled apart. Bruising of the mouth and lips is frequently caused when the assailant places a hand over the face to keep the victim quiet. Also in cases of sexual assault, discrete areas of bruising – 'love bites' – may be found on the neck, breasts and other parts of the body.

Abrasions

An abrasion is an injury often involving only the outer layers of the skin; that is, it does not penetrate the full thickness of the epidermis. From a clinical standpoint it is of little importance but to the pathologist or forensic physician, an abrasion is valuable in that, unlike a bruise, it always indicates the precise point of impact. In theory the abrasion does not bleed as blood vessels are confined to the dermis. Nevertheless, because of the corrugations of the dermal papillae, many abrasions do extend into the corium and thus bleeding will occur.

The abrasion may have a linear arrangement and close examination may show ruffling of the superficial epidermis to one end, indicating the direction of travel of the opposing surface (see Fig. 10.2). Thus a tangential blow could be shown to have been horizontal or vertical, or it may be possible to infer that a body had been dragged over a rough

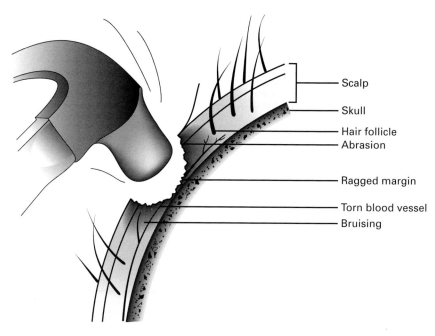

Fig. 10.3 Laceration.

Scalp

Skull

Hair follicle
Abrasion

Ragged margin

Torn blood vessel
Bruising

surface. Trace material will often adhere to abraded skin and should be preserved. Multiple scratches running in different places may corroborate a history of being pulled through bushes, and trace vegetation may provide further confirmation.

The patterning of abrasions is clearer than that of bruises because abrasions, once inflicted, do not extend or gravitate. In manual strangulation small, crescentic marks caused by fingernails, although causing little in terms of injury, may be the only external feature by which one can prove that a hand has gripped the neck. Similarly a victim of strangulation, whether manual or by a ligature, may attempt to tear away the assailant's fingers or the ligature and leave linear vertical abrasions on the skin. A victim resisting a sexual or other attack may rake her nails down the assailant's face leaving linear parallel abrasions on the cheeks. Biting may also abrade the skin in a way that not only clearly demonstrates the mechanism but may also assist in the identification of the assailant (see Chapter 17).

Lacerations

Whenever blunt force splits the full thickness of the skin the wound is called a laceration. These wounds are often inflicted during assaults when the victim is struck with a stick, bottle, stone, hammer or pistol butt. They can also be sustained in falls and road traffic accidents.

Lacerations have characteristic features (see Fig. 10.3). They are ragged wounds with irregular division of the tissue planes. They tend to gape because of the pull of elastic and muscular tissues. Their margins are often bruised and abraded; these are important diagnostic features that must be looked for with a hand-lens if necessary. Blood vessels, nerves and delicate tissue bridges may be exposed in the depth of the wound soiled by, for instance, grit, dirt or particles of glass. Occasionally, the margins are shelved or flaps of skin are produced by a shearing blow, the direction of which can then be deduced. Laceration of skin overlying bone may split the skin so cleanly as to simulate an

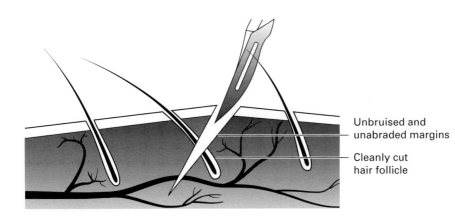

Fig. 10.4 Incision.

Unbruised and
unabraded margins

Cleanly cut
hair follicle

incision; this is particularly so on the scalp, face or shin, but close examination of the wound together with the history of how the injury came to be sustained should clarify the situation.

The shape of a laceration may indicate the agent responsible. For example, blows to the scalp inflicted with the circular head of a hammer or the spherical knob of a poker could cause crescentic lacerations; when the face of the weapon is square or rectangular, as the butt of an axe, its corners will produce a three-legged laceration. Lacerations may be inflicted after death but the distinction from antemortem wounds is usually not difficult because of the absence of antemortem abrasions or bruising of the margins.

Lacerations are rarely self-inflicted because they cause pain. The suicide or attempted suicide victim is more likely to inflict incised wounds.

Incisions

These wounds are caused by sharp cutting instruments, and their infliction in criminal circumstances implies intent. They are frequently caused in slashing movements by bladed weapons such as knives and razors, but sharp slivers of glass, the sharp edges of tin cans and sharp tools are examples of objects that may be used accidentally or criminally. Axes, hatchets and the like, though capable of cutting, usually produce lacerations when they are blunt or wielded so that a glancing blow is struck. Glass is another material often responsible for irregular lacerated wounds.

An incision is usually longer than its depth (see Fig. 10.4). The margins tend to be straight, unbruised and without abrasion. The deeper tissues are cut in the same plane, blood vessels and nerves are cleanly divided and bleeding is often profuse. When they cross Langer's cleavage lines of the skin, the wounds tend to gape as elastic tissue contracts, and when caused by a slash with a blade, are deeper at their origin and shallower at the end from which the blade is withdrawn. These wounds are rarely soiled. When the skin is lax, as on the wrist and neck, it may crease as the blade is drawn over it, causing notching of the wound. A blunt weapon can cause a similar appearance.

When incised wounds are inflicted in an attack, the usual target is the victim's head and neck. When the attacker has a sexual motive, injury and mutilation of the breasts and genitalia may be seen (particularly in homicidal cases). Incisions to the fingers and forearms may be as a result of a defensive gesture by the victim as described below.

Incised wounds, found in suicide or attempted suicide, are often multiple and parallel, most of them being tentative and superficial and are usually located on the front of the forearm or wrist or on the front and sides of the neck.

Stab wounds

The typical feature of these penetrating wounds is a depth greater than their width or length. The list of instruments is endless, including knives, scissors, screwdrivers and pokers. Stabbing can cause serious penetrating injuries to deeper structures leading to rapid death, usually from haemorrhage or occasionally air embolism. Delayed deaths from infection, pulmonary embolism or other complications may also occur. Occasionally, a stab wound track perforates a limb, and the blade of the weapon extends to injure another structure.

Some stab wounds are accidental, as occur from time to time in butchers' shops, some are suicidal (although this is not common) but in most cases infliction is deliberate by another person, and in such circumstances may be associated with the presence of defence injuries to the arms and hands.

The appearance of the wound in the skin will vary depending on the weapon responsible. The double-edged blade of a dagger tends to produce an elliptical wound with sharp edges and clean-cut ends, whereas a stab wound from a single-edged blade such as a kitchen knife may cause squaring-off or fish-tailing of one extremity of the wound caused by the non-cutting back of the blade (see Fig. 10.5). When blunt weapons are used, for example a pair of scissors, the wound will be more rounded with bruising surrounding its margins. Wounds caused by scissors can also sometimes have a cross shape caused by the blade screws or rivets. The blade of a weapon, which is partially withdrawn and then reintroduced at a slightly different angle, may give the stab wound a notched appearance.

Remember that the external dimensions of a stab wound are a poor guide to the width of the knife blade. The skin tends to retract after the blade of the weapon is withdrawn, causing the length of the wound to shorten while its width increases. Moreover, the blade of the weapon may not have been

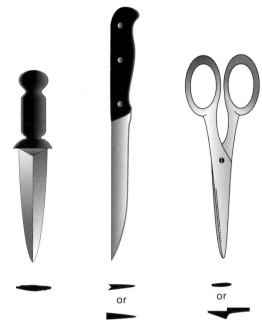

Fig. 10.5 Stab wounds.

introduced and withdrawn perpendicular to the skin surface and, as a result, the wound may be considerably longer than the actual width of the blade.

Defence wounds

The natural response to attack by an assailant, with or without a weapon, is to shield oneself with raised arms. In consequence, deflected blows are received usually on the extensor and ulnar surfaces of the forearms and hands. These may take the form of bruises, abrasions or lacerations. In the course of an assault there is a great deal of movement, and defence injuries should be sought in less familiar sites. A victim lying on the ground curls up to protect the face and the front of the trunk from kicking feet, so that other surfaces of the limbs are liable to defensive bruising.

If the assailant is armed with a sharp instrument, such as a knife or razor, bruises and lacerations are replaced by incised wounds. In a struggle, the victim will often try to wrest the weapon from the assailant, sustaining injuries in the process. If the blade of the weapon is grasped in the hand, expect incisions on the palm and the palmar surfaces of the fingers and between the fingers.

Self-mutilation

Self-inflicted injuries are seen in a variety of circumstances, but they tend to fall into three broad categories. First, there are those individuals attempting to commit suicide or who, in desperation, are making a cry for help. Injuries in this group are often multiple, parallel, superficial linear incisions, mostly of a tentative nature. The preferred sites are the forearms (both flexor and extensor aspects), the front surfaces of the wrists and occasionally on the neck. Old linear scars in these areas suggest previous similar attempts. Inexpertly executed tattoos are a not uncommon form of self-mutilation, carrying the dangers of infection, especially when the needles used are contaminated with hepatitis B or C virus or human immunodeficiency virus (HIV).

The second group comprises individuals who allege that they have been assaulted by someone else; the motive is often malicious, directed against an individual, but may be for financial gain. An example of the former is a young woman, jilted by her boyfriend, who concocts a story that she has been sexually assaulted and deliberately injures herself to give support to her story. Such wounds are of a trivial nature, consisting for the most part of linear abrasions and superficial incisions. Common characteristics are that such wounds tend to be found in groups, with roughly parallel orientation and with each wound having much the same depth throughout its length. There is usually no significant bruising and the wounds tend to be located on those areas of the body easily accessible to the victim: on the face, on the front of the trunk, on the arms and on the fronts of the legs. The clothing is often deliberately and

extensively torn, soiled or disarranged. The whole picture is incompatible with a real struggle, where a more random infliction is to be expected in type, site and severity of injury. When confronted, the complainant often admits how he/she came by the wounds.

In the third situation, encountered by the forensic physician, a prisoner intentionally injures him/herself, and then alleges that he/she has been assaulted by the police while in custody. A thorough and meticulous examination in these cases is essential since the medical evidence may go a long way in corroborating or refuting the allegations. As already discussed, the injuries are commonly multiple abrasions and occasionally incisions but the determined prisoner will inflict serious damage on him/herself, including bruises and head injuries, by using items and materials within his cell. The prudent doctor should examine the cell for agents that could have been used as weapons. In one case, a prisoner with multiple linear abrasions on his legs made an allegation that he had been assaulted by the police. The wounds were deliberately self-inflicted, and were found to have been made by the bristles of a toilet brush. Infliction of injuries on a willing 'victim' by others, for example a cell-mate, has been known in an attempt to throw suspicion on the police.

Cigarette burns may also be self-inflicted but are less common since the subject anticipates that they will be painful. Bruising, which is also painful to sustain, is infrequently seen and, therefore, if present, should raise suspicions that the prisoner's allegations might not be without foundation. Psychotic patients are capable of inflicting bizarre and painful injuries upon themselves, which do not conform to the patterns outlined. Any injuries, self-inflicted or otherwise, found on a prisoner must be carefully documented and preferably also photographed. Suspected terrorists and those with a previous history of complaints against the police should be examined on detention, before and after interview and before release from custody.

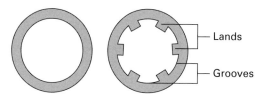

Fig. 10.6 Smooth bore (left) and rifled (right) gun barrels in cross-section.

Firearm wounds

Some basic knowledge of ballistics is essential for a proper understanding of wounds caused by firearms. There are essentially two types of weapon, smooth bore and rifled (see Fig. 10.6)

Smooth bore weapons

Shotguns are the commonest type of smooth bore (that is, the barrel lining is smooth) weapons. They are commonly used in agricultural activities and by sportsmen. They may be either single- or double-barrelled. The usual barrel is from 66 to 81 cm (26 to 32 in.) in length, but criminals frequently shorten this ('sawn-off shotgun') to aid concealment and give a wider spread of shot. In double-barrelled weapons, the right barrel is usually a true cylinder but the diameter of the left barrel narrows towards the muzzle: this is called 'the choke'. Choking of the barrel helps to keep the shot together over a longer distance. The bore or gauge of a shotgun is determined by the number of solid balls of lead, each with the diameter of the barrel, that can be prepared from one pound of lead. Thus if 12 balls can be made from one pound of lead, the weapon is of 12-bore. In the 12-bore shotgun the diameter of the unchoked barrel is 19 mm (0.73 in.).

Shotgun ammunition consists of a cardboard or plastic cartridge case with a brass base containing primer. Inside the main part of the cartridge are a layer of powder, one or more felt or card wads and a mass of pellets (lead shot of variable size).

Rifled weapons

These are characterized by a number of parallel but spiral lands (projecting ridges) and grooves (depressed spaces between the lands) on the interior of the barrel from the breech to the muzzle. This rifling causes the bullet to spin, thus imparting gyroscopic steadiness to its flight. The rifling also leaves characteristic scratches, rifling marks, unique to that weapon, on the bullet.

There are three common types of rifled weapons: the rifle, revolver and pistol. The rifle is a long-barrelled shoulder weapon capable of firing bullets with muzzle velocities of 450–1500 m/s. Examples include the Armalite, the Kalashnikov and the SA80 military rifle. Most military weapons are 'automatic', which means that the weapon will continue to fire while the trigger is depressed until the magazine is empty. It is thus capable of discharging many rounds within seconds. The revolver, which has a low muzzle velocity of the order of 150 m/s, is a short-barrelled rifled weapon with its ammunition held in a metal drum that rotates each time the trigger is released. The spent cartridge case is retained within the cylinder after firing. The self-loading pistol, often called 'semi-automatic' or erroneously 'automatic', has its ammunition held in a metal clip-type magazine under the breech. Each time the trigger is pulled the bullet in the breech is fired and the spent cartridge automatically ejected. At the same time, a spring mechanism pushes the next live cartridge into the breech ready to be fired. The muzzle velocity of pistols may be between 300 and 360 m/s.

Shotgun wounds

When a shotgun is discharged, the lead pellets emerge together en masse, gradually diverging in a cone-shape as the distance from the weapon increases. The pellets are accompanied by particles of unburnt powder, flame, smoke, gases, wads and cards. A number of different factors affect the appearance of the entrance wound on the body but probably the most important of these is the range of fire. Both the estimated range of fire and the site of the wound are crucial factors in determining whether the wound was self-inflicted or not.

Contact wounds are caused when the muzzle of the weapon is held against the skin. This usually leaves a circular or oval entrance wound, depending on whether the muzzle was perpendicular or not to the skin surface. The margins of the wound are usually clean-cut although they may be bruised or abraded due to so-called 'recoil' impact of the muzzle. In the case of a double-barrelled weapon the circular abraded imprint of the non-firing muzzle may be clearly seen adjacent to the contact wound. The wound margins and the tissues within the base of the wound are usually blackened by smoke and there may even be charring of the wound margins or singeing of the skin hairs by flame. Because the shot and gases are contained within the wound there is often severe disruption of the underlying tissues and the gas forced into the wound may cause the tissues along its track to turn pink from carbon monoxide. The severity of the injuries associated with these contact wounds is dramatically demonstrated in wounds to the head where there is often gross mutilation with bursting ruptures of the scalp and face, multiple explosive fractures of the skull and extrusion or partial extrusion of the underlying brain. Most contact wounds of the head are suicidal in nature with the temple regions, the mouth and under the chin being the common sites. In these types of head wounds, fragments of scalp, skull and brain tissue may be dispersed over a wide area. The pellets and wads may or may not be retained within the fragmented skull.

At close range, with the muzzle up to 15 cm (6 in.) from the body, the entrance wound is still usually round or oval with fairly clean-cut margins. The clothing or skin may show slight burning from the flame and there may be blackening by smoke and unburnt powder. Blackening due to smoke is rarely seen beyond about 20–40 cm while punctate abrasions or 'tattooing' from unburnt powder usually only extends to about a metre or so. The wads and

cards travel a relatively short distance, rarely being found beyond 2 m.

Up to about a metre, the pellets tend to travel as a compact mass and thus usually cause a single circular hole, although at the upper end of this range the edges of the wound will be crenated and scalloped. With increasing range of fire, from about 1 to 3 m, the pellets start to scatter and cause variable numbers of satellite pellet holes surrounding a larger central hole. Longer distances reveal a greater scatter of pellets. At long ranges, over about 8–10 m, there is no main entrance wound, only 'peppering' of the skin from individual pellets (see Fig. 10.7).

As a rough rule of thumb, which is often incorrect, burning and singeing occur over the first 15 cm (6 in.), soot staining can be seen for the first 40 cm (15 in.) and a single large hole persists for at least 1 m (3 ft).

Rifled weapon wounds

Entrance bullet wounds tend to be neat round holes ranging from about 3 to 10 mm diameter. The wound margin is usually fairly smooth and bordered by an even zone of creamy-pink abrasion. This collar of abrasion will be eccentric and the entrance hole more oval if the bullet strikes the skin at an angle (see Fig. 10.8). If there is thick bone immediately subjacent to the skin, particularly with close range wounds to the head, the entrance wound may appear atypical with irregular ragged margins. This is because the underlying bone resists the entry of gases which accumulate under the skin and blow back causing subsidiary tears in the wound margins and giving it a stellate or irregular lacerated appearance. Careful examination of such wounds should reveal evidence of burning of the wound margins, blackening in the base of the wound and possibly the imprint of the muzzle on the skin surface (see Fig. 10.9). Atypical entrance wounds are also found when bullets have ricocheted, struck an intermediate target, or have fragmented before striking the skin.

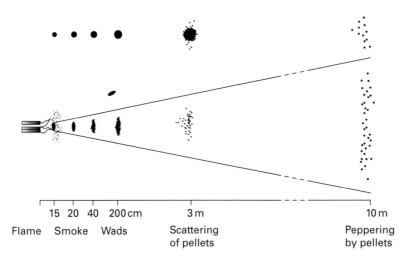

Fig. 10.7 Dispersal of shot from a shotgun.

| 15 | 20 | 40 | 200 cm | | 3 m | | 10 m |
| Flame | Smoke | Wads | | | Scattering of pellets | | Peppering by pellets |

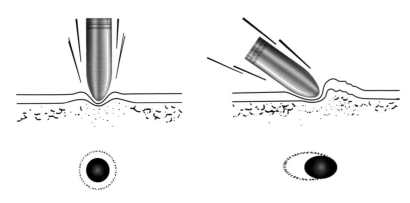

Fig. 10.8 Perpendicular (left) and angled (right) bullet penetration.

In contact wounds, the entrance hole may be bordered by the imprint of the muzzle. The margin may be charred and parchmented by flame and the surrounding skin may be pink in colour due to the effects of carbon monoxide in the underlying tissues. Punctate discharge abrasion and soot soiling are usually absent but the subcutaneous tissues within the depth of the wound are commonly soiled. In close range wounds, singeing due to flame is rarely seen beyond about 15 cm (6 in.) with sooty soiling extending to about 30 cm (12 in.). Punctate discharge abrasion, which may be particularly heavy with revolver ammunition, is often present with ranges up to about 60 cm (24 in.).

Exit bullet wounds tend to be larger than the corresponding entrance wounds and usually consist of irregular lacerations or lacerated holes with everted, unbruised and unabraded margins. There are exceptions, however, and one must not be too dogmatic in the interpretation of bullet injuries particularly when there are multiple wounds on the body. Remember that close range wounds may not show the typical features associated with flame, smoke and discharge particles if clothing or other material is interposed between the skin surface and

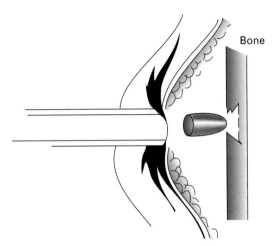

Fig. 10.9 Stellate close-range bullet wound due to underlying bone.

the muzzle of the weapon. Care must also be taken when cleaning bullet wounds to remove blood and debris, as smoke soiling of the wound margins or surrounding skin can easily be wiped away.

It is inadvisable to express an opinion on the calibre of a bullet based on the size of the entrance wound, nor is it possible to state confidently, from the appearance of an entrance wound, whether the bullet was fired from a rifle or a pistol. The differentiation between high and low velocity wounds is best determined by an assessment of the internal damage, although, as a rule of thumb, a large ragged exit wound is more consistent with the high velocity of a rifle bullet than that of a pistol or revolver.

Torture

Abuse of human rights is so widespread throughout the world that reference must be made to it in this book. As far as the forensic physician is concerned, torture is seen in two main contexts: first, that perpetrated by criminal and terrorist groups and second, that carried out, or allegedly carried out, by the police or other security force personnel during the detention and interrogation of prisoners and suspects.

The Northern Ireland experience was of torture as a sinister and abhorrent weapon used by terrorist groups to instil fear and division in the community. The victims were usually members of their own organization suspected of giving information to the police or to a rival group, members of rival organizations and occasionally captured members of the security forces. Often, the torture occurred during interrogation and usually ended with the victim being shot. The victim was usually bound, with the wrists and ankles bearing the pale streaky bruises and abrasions caused by ligatures. 'Beating up' was fairly standard, with extensive bruises and abrasions to the face and body. The typical picture included black eyes, fractures of the nose and jaws and displacement of the teeth. Burning with a cigarette causes discrete circular, yellow (in the dead, parchmented) burns while more severe burns may be caused by branding with a hot poker. Patterned injuries due to being struck with the butt of a rifle or pistol may be seen while incisions and stab wounds are inflicted by knives. It is not uncommon for a finger or the lobule of the ear to be amputated. Finally, the victim may have been hooded and taken to a deserted spot, made to kneel on the ground and then shot, at close range, through the back of the head, possibly with a *coup de grace* on the face. In some instances, the beating had been so severe that death by shooting must have come as a merciful relief.

Doctors with access to prisoners in custody have an onerous responsibility to ensure that they are properly treated during detention and interrogation. The Tokyo Declaration of 1975 defines torture as 'the deliberate, systematic or wanton infliction of physical or mental suffering by one or more persons acting alone or on the orders of any authority, to force another person to yield information, to make a confession, or for any other reason'. The Declaration also lays down guidelines for doctors when faced with cases or suspected cases of torture. The methods employed during interrogation range from apparent physical abuse to the more subtle use of threats and intimidation. Sexual humiliation and 'waterboarding' or simulated drowning are notorious techniques associated with the conflict in Iraq. Hooding, prolonged standing, and the use of continuous high-pitched sound have all been used and subsequently condemned, as have attempts to disorientate the prisoner by offering food at erratic times, frequently waking the person up after short intervals of sleep and by burning a light in the cell 24 hours per day. A doctor, charged with the responsibility of caring for prisoners, particularly in interrogation units, must satisfy himself that such methods are not employed.

Actual physical abuse can be curbed by regular medical examinations of prisoners. However, methods of physical assault may be employed which, on casual examination, leave no apparent marks of violence. These include vigorous hair pulling (detected by scalp tenderness and areas of recent balding), face slapping (detected by redness, tenderness and swelling) and blows to the side of the head such as by the arm of the interrogator. Both vigorous face slapping and blows to the head may result in perforation of the eardrum and, therefore, it is imperative to examine the ears carefully during routine examination. Blows to the abdomen may not leave any apparent mark, but just occasionally the faint petechial impression of the clothing may be seen on the skin of the abdominal wall. Pinching, squeezing and blows to the testes have been employed, so the scrotal skin must be carefully examined for bruising or other marks. The underlying testes may be swollen and tender. Doctors do not normally inspect the soles of the feet, but it has been known for prisoners to be repeatedly struck here with a baton. In all cases of suspected or alleged ill-treatment of prisoners it is essential that you carry out a methodical and detailed 'head-to-toe' examination. You should accurately record all injuries and marks, ensure that they are photographed and that the appropriate authorities are informed immediately.

Investigation of suspicious death

The forensic medical examiner is often one of the first experts to attend the scene of a suspicious death. Your preliminary function is to confirm the fact of death, then to ensure, as far as possible, that no further disturbance of the scene takes place until the other appropriate investigators (see Chapter 15) have arrived. Calls to scenes frequently occur at unusual hours, and you must ensure that you have appropriate equipment and clothing ready to hand; often the items required may not be easy to locate at 3 o'clock in the morning. The wearing of protective disposable overalls and overshoes is mandatory at all scenes, and it goes without saying that such garments must be changed if you are subsequently asked to examine a suspect in the case. Ideally, a colleague should perform this function.

Do not try to take 'control' of the scene nor undertake procedures best left to the pathologist, for example the taking of liver temperatures. The scene is the responsibility of the investigating police officer, and you must be prepared to accept his instructions regarding the approach to the body and how much or how little you are expected to do. Avoid the unnecessary touching of objects, particularly possible weapons. Disturb the body and clothing as little as possible, even though this may mean that some injuries, for example those on the back of the body, are not seen. A more detailed examination of the body will be undertaken by the pathologist at a later stage, and the full extent of the injuries can then be assessed.

In summary, the main functions of the forensic medical examiner are to observe the scene, to confirm that death has taken place, to ensure that trace evidence is not removed or destroyed from the body or its surroundings, to offer an opinion as to the possible nature, as opposed to the cause, of death and, where necessary, to assist and supervise the removal of the body from the scene. In addition, the taking of detailed contemporaneous notes, possibly complemented by clear line diagrams, will ensure that the doctor subsequently required to make a statement or attend court about the case has sufficient documentation to refresh the memory.

REFERENCES

1. Langlois NEI, Gresham GA (1991) The ageing of bruises: a review and study of the color changes with time. *Forensic Science International* **50**: 227–38.
2. Munang LA, Leonard PA, Mok JYQ (2002) Lack of agreement on colour description between clinicians examining childhood bruising. *Journal of Clinical Forensic Medicine* **9**: 171–4.

FURTHER READING

Knight B (1991) *Forensic Pathology* (London: Edward Arnold) provides a detailed description of wounds and their interpretation.

Mason JK (ed.) (1993) *Forensic Medicine – An Illustrated Reference* (London: Chapman and Hall Medical) and Gresham GA (1986) *Colour Atlas of Wounds and Wounding* (Boston: MTP Press Ltd) both illustrate the appearances of the various types of injuries encountered in forensic medical practice.

Payne-James JJ (2007) Restraint injuries and crowd control agents. In: Rogers DJ, Stark MM, Norfolk GA, ed. *Good Practice Guidelines for FMEs*. London: Metropolitan Police Service.

Payne-James JJ, Crane J, Hinchliffe J (2005) Injury assessment, documentation and interpretation. In: Stark MM, ed. *Clinical Forensic Medicine. A Physician's Guide*, 2nd edn. Totowa, NJ: Humana Press pp. 127–58.

Various sections in Payne-James JJ, Byard RW, Corey T, Henderson C (eds.) (2005) *Encyclopedia of Forensic and Legal Medicine* (London: Elsevier/Academic Press) particularly volume 1 pp. 151–7 (asphyxia); volume 2 pp. 153–8 (deliberate self-harm); volume 3 pp. 119–29 (sharp and cutting edge wounds); volume 4 pp. 87–91 (sexual offences: injuries and findings after sexual contact).

11

Child abuse: physical

Robert Sunderland

Violence towards the vulnerable may be part of the human condition, and vulnerability increases the younger the victim. In recent wars more lives were lost at home from domestic violence than from injuries on the battlefield. Child abuse is common and has been throughout history. Although it has frequently gone unrecognized, increasing awareness and changing definitions have sometimes led to over-diagnosis.

Child abuse is both emotive and emotional. Doctors, lawyers and journalists are not immune. Some doctors have admitted fabricating evidence to support children's allegations [1], a position that has ill-served the profession, justice or children. The forensic examination must be impartial, independent and objective if miscarriages of justice are to be prevented. Indeed, the interests of justice require us to consider the possibility that the allegations are false. The courts place the child's needs paramount; it is the doctor's duty to remain impartial and assist the court in understanding medical information. The doctor must remain within their area of expertise. It is the lawyer's not the doctor's duty to act as advocate.

It is essential to be aware of precise definitions in law, understand the forensic principles, different types of injury and their causation as well as the natural history of healing and changes in appearance with time.

The severity of an injury does not indicate intent or mechanism. Accurately assessing the significance of an injury may be vital for the future of the child and family; relatively minor injuries can be more difficult to evaluate than gross injuries. An unappreciated non-accidental minor injury leaves the child at risk; a misinterpreted accidental injury renders the child and family vulnerable to the consequences of a wrongful diagnosis of abuse.

A complete investigation of alleged abusive injuries will include the child's background and past history, together with a full and careful physical, social and psychological assessment. Where there are concerns or history to suggest coagulation or bony problems the blood is screened for clotting defects and a full skeletal survey done. Formal haematology or radiology opinions by paediatric experts may be required.

Non-accidental injury (NAI)

It may be helpful to analyse alleged injuries into the three components of the NAI label:

1. Is there an *injury*? Is it a malformation, or consequence of disease?
2. If it is an injury, is it consistent with an *accidental injury*? Is it consistent with offered accidental scenarios or are alternative accidental explanations plausible?

Clinical Forensic Medicine, third edition ed. W. D. S. McLay. Published by Cambridge University Press. © Cambridge University Press 2009.

3. If the injury is consistent with a *non-accidental* aetiology, is it consistent with the offered cause? Was there chastisement? The determination that NAI was abusive is the responsibility of social services and the courts.

The risk factors for non-accidental injury include unwanted pregnancy (and refused abortion), social isolation, scapegoating, handicapped child, drug and alcohol abuse, previous domestic violence, injured pets and past problems with anger management.

Features that should raise suspicion when an injured child presents include:

(a) Is the history consistent with the injury? Carefully consider the offered mechanism of the injury and make a commonsense judgement on the credibility of the explanation given. The development of the child must be considered – would it be capable of the actions or movements described?

(b) Multiple injuries of differing ages. Healing occurs, fractures knit and bruises resolve. Dating injuries from their appearance is an imprecise art that can mislead. However, bruises of different colour and fractures with different stages of callus formation are unlikely to have been caused at the same time from the same accident.

(c) Discrepancies in varying and changing explanations. Fabricated stories are more difficult to keep consistent than describing a witnessed event. The story may be changed if the abuser thinks that the original is doubted.

(d) Delay in reporting, sometimes of hours and sometimes of days. A concerned parent is more likely to seek medical advice soon after an accident, but be aware that parents may observe for a while rather than 'trouble the doctor'.

(e) The parents may seek help from different outlets or become afraid and withdraw. 'Doctor shopping' is seen in both the 'worried well' and in fabricated or imposed illness (FII). Some cases of FII may be better considered as hypochondria by proxy rather than Munchausen by proxy.

(f) Denial and collusion. The denial is invariably strong and is supported by both partners. A weak partner may collude with the abusing parent rather than recognize and confront the abuser's need for help. Sometimes an older child may collude with a parent, especially if there is gain for the child (such as school avoidance).

(g) The behaviour of the child may be significant. Does he show fear of one parent, being unwilling to make eye contact? Is there a wary, haunted look, the so called 'frozen watchfulness'? Although not always present, it is striking evidence of chronic abuse when seen. Excessive compliance during the examination is also a clue; an abused child may seek comfort and affection from comparative strangers.

The diagnosis of child abuse does not rest on medical evidence alone. Unilateral decisions should not be made. The results of all strands of the investigation are best co-ordinated through collaboration between all investigating agencies (usually police, social and health services) in a case conference. Medical evidence is often inconclusive. Although some advocates may wish clear definitive information, courts are not helped by over-confident opinion where evidence is lacking. Both justice and families are ill-served by certainty where there is uncertainty. It bears repetition that the examining doctor's duty is to remain impartial.

Types of injury

It is important to strip search the whole body in every case; marks may be hidden by long sleeves and high-necked jumpers. It is also helpful to view the whole picture rather than concentrate on individual injuries; for example, bruising on more than one side or plane of the body is significant. The examination should include the inside of the mouth and lips, behind the ears, the palms and soles and in-between fingers and toes. The object causing the injury – bruise or abrasion – may leave the pattern of its shape.

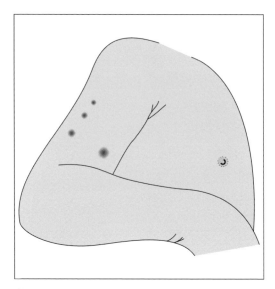

Fig. 11.1 Grip marks on right arm caused by squeezing with an adult right hand which has encircled the limb from its inner aspect.

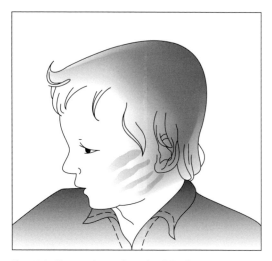

Fig. 11.2 Slap marks on the side of the face: an outline of individual fingers is often seen.

Spot bruises: caused by harsh fingertip pressure, 0.5–2.5 cm in size, sometimes in clusters corresponding to the fingers of the grasping hand. Look for the thumb-print on the opposite side (Fig. 11.1) or if the child is shaken, there may be thumb marks on the trunk in front and finger bruises on the back.

Slap marks: found often on the face (where they may involve the ear – look behind, at the other ear and check the eardrum for barotrauma) and on the trunk and buttocks. There may be clear lines of petechial haemorrhages (Fig. 11.2).

Knuckle punches: these show as rows of three or four roughly round bruises 0.5–1 cm; favoured sites being the head and back and particularly over the spine (Fig. 11.3). Where the skin covers bone, a rounded swelling may also be present, for example on the side of the head or over the facial bones.

Instruments: bruising from the use of belts, straps, canes, pieces of wood, hair brushes and electric flex (which wraps around limbs)

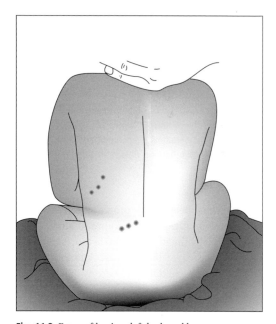

Fig. 11.3 Rows of bruises left by knuckles.

may all leave recognizable marks (Fig. 11.4). These are frequently to be seen on the buttocks and thighs, and may involve the genital area. Look for grip marks on the arms where the

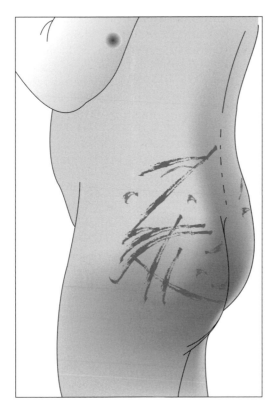

Fig. 11.4 Typical site of weals and bruises caused by canes, belts and other instruments. The loop of a doubled, flexible instrument such as a dog lead may leave rounded impressions, as seen here on the upper thigh.

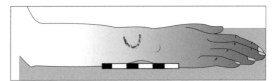

Fig. 11.5 Pattern of bruises caused by biting.

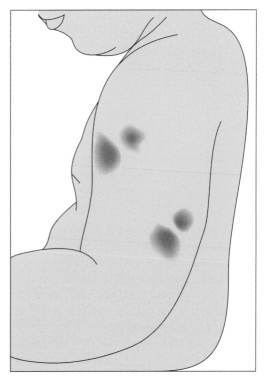

Fig. 11.6 Pinch marks (see text).

child has been held roughly, and also for defence injuries on the hands and arms.

Bite marks: human bite marks are distinctive, crescent-shaped lines of discoloration. A bite made by a child has a narrow arch and is smaller than one made by an adult, which often involves teeth behind the canines (Fig. 11.5). Animal bites are characterized by puncturing and tearing of the tissues, unlike the human whose bite compresses, so causing the distinctive bruises (see also Chapter 17).

Pinch marks: these may form a butterfly-shaped bruise with one wing (caused by the thumb) larger than the other (Fig. 11.6). If near the lip, the under surface of the nose may be scraped by the finger nail, or the frenulum torn. Finger nails leave thin linear paired bruises.

Some bruises are in themselves highly suggestive of abuse. Children rarely injure the eye or ear in 'rough and tumble', seeming instinctively to protect these sense organs. Other suggestive non-accidental injuries include black eye without clear history of an accident (Fig. 11.7), bruising on the inner side of the thighs, bruised face in pre-mobile babies and central spinal bruising.

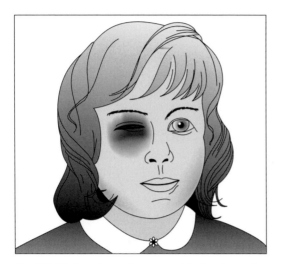

Fig. 11.7 Black eye (a much more graphic description than 'periorbital haematoma').

Other significant injuries to note include:

- torn frenulum in pre-mobile babies is commonly caused by blunt trauma; in the absence of history of a heavy fall, consider a glancing blow across the mouth or roughly forcing a feeding bottle into the mouth, which may also cause bruised lips and displaced teeth with bleeding gums;
- friction burns of prominent areas such as the chin and cheeks from dragging over carpets and furniture;
- hair pulling leaving bald patches;
- marks around the mouth and face indicative of gagging;
- encircling marks on the wrists and ankles where the child has been tied up, perhaps to a chair;
- pinch or ligature marks round the penis and scrotum.

Burns and scalds

Approximately 10% of abuse involves burning, but it can be very difficult to determine whether some burns were inflicted deliberately. The heat source may leave an unmistakable pattern on the skin, for example the outline of a flat-iron (Fig. 11.8). The degree of heat generation must be considered; the depth of the burn may indicate how long the contact must have been maintained to produce the marks. The burn may be in an accessible position, and the ability of the child to draw away from the heat source is an important factor. Other abuse injuries may be present.

Hot water is like acid to a baby's skin. Partial thickness burns may be caused by less than one second immersion into water at 60 °C, and full thickness burns can occur in the same time in water at 90 °C.

Dipping into hot water is seen especially on the hands when a 'tide' mark may be apparent, or a 'stocking' distribution from dipping the feet. Areas of scalding round the upper thighs with clear, unaffected areas on the buttocks arise when the child is forcibly sat in hot liquid (see Fig. 11.9).

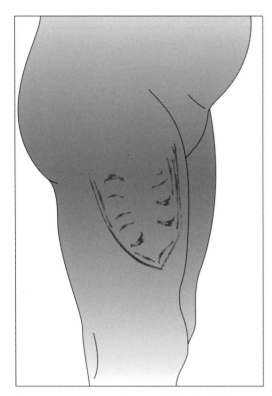

Fig. 11.8 Burns from an iron applied to the thigh.

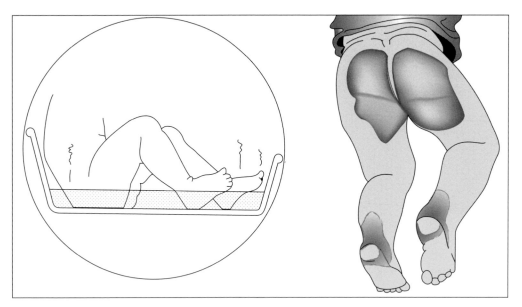

Fig. 11.9 Scalding.

Any child accidentally or intentionally immersed in hot water may struggle or splash; the absence of splash marks is not proof of abuse.

Cigarette burns give a round, punched out lesion of roughly 1 cm when applied at right angles to the skin (Fig. 11.10). Such circular injuries are caused when a lighted cigarette is deliberately held against the skin; when a child brushes against the cigarette or when the cigarette is dropped accidentally there may be an elliptical or irregular burn which often heals without scarring. Cigar and matchstick burns may also occur. They are often full thickness, and leave characteristic scars. Frequently found on the arms and legs, they may be seen in other situations such as the genital area or even between the toes.

Bone and joint injuries

Injury to the skeleton results from impact, whether intentional or not. The severity of injury may not indicate mechanism. The type of fracture as well as the age and development of the child should be considered in evaluating offered explanations: spiral fractures of long bones indicate a twisting force; metaphyseal fractures only occur in growing bones.

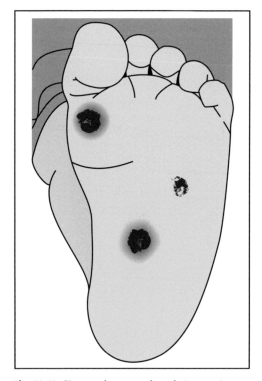

Fig. 11.10 Cigarette burns on the sole (see text).

Not all fractures are apparent on clinical examination, especially when they have begun to heal, whereas fresh fractures may be missed on initial X-ray but be apparent when callus forms. Some small children can have serious bone injuries without showing much external sign. Accidental rib fractures are rare in infants whereas, over the age of five years, abuse fractures are uncommon. A skeletal survey is advisable in suspicious cases, and may reveal old healing fractures in the seemingly straightforward case.

Spiral fractures in a pre-mobile child are highly suspicious of abuse unless there is a clear history of an accident where the child's limb was trapped and twisted.

Periosteal reaction without fracture is seen where there has been twisting of a long bone so that the periosteum shears. Bleeding under the periosteum provokes calcification, seen radiologically as an extra line of opacity running alongside the affected length of bone. Thin lines of periosteal calcification are seen in normal growing bones when it is usually symmetrical.

Metaphyseal fractures are seen as a disruption of the normal bony outline, sometimes with angulation and displacement. Found most commonly at the elbow, wrist, knee and ankle; they are of particular significance in babies as yet unable to walk. The possibility of rickets should be excluded.

A closely detailed history of the incident should be taken, and the X-rays examined by a specialist. The mechanism of the fracture should be worked out in consultation with the radiologist or orthopaedic surgeon. The age of the fractures is estimated from the amount of callus formed, although skull and metaphyseal fractures pose difficulty, as they heal differently, and may appear fresh after some weeks. If, as a forensic physician, you are assisting the paediatrician, careful notes of all accompanying lesser injuries may be important in any subsequent court proceedings.

Neurological injuries

A baby with unexplained encephalopathy requires specialist examination for intracranial and retinal haemorrhages as they may have an inflicted head injury. The opinion of a paediatrician, paediatric ophthalmologist, radiologist and neurologist or neurosurgeon will be necessary. Permanent neurological damage and loss of vision in such cases is possible. Accompanying the neurological signs, 'silent' visceral damage may be present and, here again, it is necessary to use any visible external mark to help understand the mechanism of injury.

Neurological damage may also be caused by blows, suffocation and poisoning (including household remedies, iron medicines and salt).

Mistaken diagnoses

Errors in diagnosis will distress parents innocent of any ill-treatment. Where an independent third party is present, abuse is unlikely. Bizarre mishaps can have serious repercussions, yet remain accidental. All the available evidence must be examined, and a case conference convened to review the whole matter. For example, in cases of FII where the perpetrator either inflicts injury (factitious/imposed illness) or fabricates medical history leading to inappropriate investigation or treatment (fictitious/fabricated illness) action to safeguard the child may only become possible after several apparently accidental occurrences.

Keep the following points in mind when examining any case of suspected physical abuse:
(a) Calcium deficiency, abnormalities in copper metabolism, rickets, scurvy, severe anaemia and haemophilia must all be excluded by appropriate investigation.
(b) Disorders of bone formation and 'brittle bones', although rare, must also be excluded routinely when the skeletal survey is performed [2].
(c) Pigment anomalies, Mongolian spots, birthmarks and skin disorders must be identified and dealt with accordingly.
(d) Blood extravasation seeping down tissue planes from lesser injury can simulate widespread bruising. An injury to the forehead may cause

blood to appear in the upper eyelids or inner corners of the eye, so simulating direct injury to the eye.

(e) Alopecia areata can be mistaken for hair pulling.

(f) Lesions of impetigo, chickenpox and, more rarely, shingles or chilblains may be mistaken for cigarette burns.

(g) Burns involving contact with hot radiators and other heaters need careful investigation as accidental contact is not uncommon.

(h) Accidental scalds from tipping pans or kettles usually produce a 'shield' injury including the shoulder of the dominant arm.

(i) In scalds received in the bath, sparing the soles of the feet occurs because of the thicker collagen in the soles and if the child was standing up especially in a metal bath (where the metal provides a cooler 'heat sink'). In pre-mobile babies, most scalds are accidents; most bruises aren't.

(j) Accidental fractures can have bizarre explanations: for instance, an impacted fracture of the upper end of the humerus is consistent with a fall on the point of the elbow.

(k) The possibility of self-inflicted injuries in older children should be borne in mind.

(l) In adolescents, horizontal striae running across the lumbar region have been mistaken for marks of beating [3].

The possible causes for the constellation of unexplained subdural and retinal haemorrhage (previously referred to as *shaken baby syndrome*) have been uncertain for years. Beginning in late 2007, an inquiry [4] has been sitting in Toronto under Justice Stephen Goudge into paediatric forensic pathology in Ontario, based on suspicion of wrongful convictions arising from a catalogue of faults within the provincial service. The inquiry is bringing into the public domain some of the controversies; transcripts of evidence are readily available.

The primary objective of child protection is to prevent and protect. This includes preventing an escalating pattern of injuries but also involves protecting families from erroneous allegations. In all but a few incidents, careful consideration of the history, thorough examination and the application of sound forensic principles will permit a firm opinion. The consensus of developmental experts is that a child is best reared in a loving home by their biological parents. Most parents in our communities endeavour to provide the best for their offspring. In a civilized society we should strive to provide these optimal conditions for growth to all.

REFERENCES

1. Dyer C (2002) Judge criticises paediatrician for 'overstating' sex abuse allegations. *BMJ* **325**: 235.

2. Bishop N, Sprigg A, Dalton A (2007) Unexplained fractures in infancy: looking for fragile bones. *Archives of Disease in Childhood* **92**: 251–6.

3. Davies H de la H (1985) Adolescent lumbar striae mistaken for non-accidental injury. *The Police Surgeon* **27**: 72–6.

4. www.goudgeinquiry.ca/index.html

12

Child abuse: sexual

Catherine White, with contribution from Cathy Cobley

In recent years two documents have had significant political influence on medical and social work practice related to child abuse. In his report on Victoria Climbié [1] Lord Laming (para 11.53) said: 'Investigation and management of a case of possible harm to a child must be approached in the same systematic and rigorous manner as would be appropriate to the investigation and management of any other possible fatal disease.' His inquiry was followed by the publication of *Working Together to Safeguard Children: a Guide to Inter-Agency Working to Safeguard and Promote the Welfare of Children* [2].

Definition of a child

According to the Children Acts 1989 and 2004, a child is anyone who has not yet reached his or her eighteenth birthday, but the term 'children' includes persons aged 18, 19 and 20 years who have been looked after by a local authority at any time after attaining the age of 16 years or who have a learning disability.

Definitions of abuse or neglect

Child abuse involves acts of commission or omission resulting in harm to the child. Harm takes various forms, but it is not uncommon for a child to suffer from more than one type of abuse. The definitions are taken from *Working Together to Safeguard Children* [2]. Emotional abuse and neglect do not usually come within the remit of forensic physicians and will not be considered in this chapter. It is imperative for the forensic physician to remember that one type of abuse rarely occurs in isolation, and a holistic approach to the child is required.

Physical abuse may involve hitting, shaking, throwing, poisoning, burning or scalding, drowning, suffocating, or otherwise causing physical harm to a child. Physical harm may also be caused when a parent or carer fabricates the symptoms of, or deliberately induces, illness in a child they are looking after. Physical abuse is considered in Chapter 11.

Emotional abuse is the persistent emotional ill-treatment of a child such as to cause severe and persistent adverse effects on the child's emotional development. It may involve conveying to children that they are worthless or unloved, inadequate, or valued only insofar as they meet the needs of another person. It may feature age or developmentally inappropriate expectations being imposed on children. These may include interactions that are beyond the child's developmental capability, as well as overprotection and limitation of exploration and learning or

The legal framework of child protection in England and Wales, contributed by Cathy Cobley, is to be found on pp. 134–5.
Clinical Forensic Medicine, third edition ed. W. D. S. McLay. Published by Cambridge University Press. © Cambridge University Press 2009.

preventing the child participating in normal social interaction. It may involve seeing or hearing the ill-treatment of another. It may involve causing children to feel frightened or in danger, or the exploitation or corruption of children. Some level of emotional abuse is involved in all types of ill-treatment of a child, although it may occur alone.

Neglect is the persistent failure to meet a child's basic physical and/or psychological needs, likely to result in the serious impairment of the child's health or development. Neglect may occur during pregnancy as a result of maternal substance abuse. It may involve a parent or carer failing to provide adequate food, shelter (that is, exclusion from home or abandonment) and clothing, failing to protect a child from physical harm or danger, failure to ensure adequate supervision (including the use of inadequate care-takers) or the failure to ensure access to appropriate medical care or treatment. It may also include neglect of, or unresponsiveness to, a child's basic emotional needs.

Sexual abuse involves forcing or enticing a child or young person to take part in sexual activities, including prostitution, whether or not the child is aware of what is happening. The activities may include physical contact, including penetrative (rape, buggery or oral sex) or non-penetrative acts. They may include non-contact activities, such as involving children in looking at, or in the production of, pornographic material or watching sexual activities, or encouraging children to behave in sexually inappropriate ways. This chapter is concerned with sexual abuse.

Confidentiality, consent, sharing of information

The examination of a child when abuse has been alleged or is suspected has two components, therapeutic and forensic. The examining doctor must take both into consideration when gaining consent (Fig. 12.1). As with any medical intervention, for the consent to be valid it must be fully informed (see also Chapter 4).

Although parental responsibility continues until the end of childhood at 18 years of age, a child acquires an increasing ability to influence matters that affect his/her welfare, so for the parent, it is 'a dwindling right which the courts will hesitate to enforce against the wishes of the child, the older he is. It starts with the right to control and ends with little more than advice.' (*Gillick* v. *West Norfolk and Wisbech Health Authority and Another* (1986) 1 FLR 224 – see Box 12.2).

If a Gillick competent child refuses an examination, that must be respected, but it is good practice to explore the reasons for refusal, and it may be possible to do a modified examination. Despite a refusal, if child protection concerns persist, you should still consider the sharing of information with other agencies, but the child should be informed of this. In obtaining consent from a parent or carer when the child is unable to consent for him- or herself, ensure that this person has legal parental responsibility.

Box 12.1

The doctor's primary duty is to act in the child's best interest . . . If there is conflict between doctor and parents or parents and child, then the child's needs are paramount.

Responsibilities of Doctors in Child Protection Cases with Regard to Confidentiality. Royal College of Paediatrics and Child Health February 2004, ISBN 1 900954 95 8 at page 9

Box 12.2 Gillick competency

A child is Gillick competent if he/she understands the nature, purpose and hazards of any proposed treatment, but he/she must also have an understanding of the consequences of

- the treatment
- failure of the treatment
- alternative courses of action
- inaction

Consent to Examination and Report

I, ... (parent/guardian of) ....
and / or I, ... (client) give consent for

a. full medical examination
b. collection of forensic specimens/clothing
c. taking of photographs for
    i.   record purposes and evidential purposes
    ii.   research and audit
    iii. teaching
d. use of the colposcope to make a DVD recording of the genital examination for:
    i.   record purposes and evidential purposes
    ii.   research and audit
    iii. teaching
e. anonymous use of records for teaching/research by the St. Mary's Centre

The purpose of the medical examination and report has been explained to me by
....
....

**I have been advised that I can strike out any of the above before I sign. It is
routine practice to share information with other agencies as part of child
protection procedures. It is routine that the medical records including pictures
are peer reviewed as part of quality assurance.**
**I understand that the information recorded on this form and any images taken
are for the purpose of providing evidence and may be required by a court.**

Signed.. Date ..../..../.......

Fig. 12.1 Consent form used at St Mary's Hospital, Manchester. The full version of the form can be found on the book website at www.cambridge.org/9780521705684.

Child sexual abuse

Research [3] for the National Society for the Prevention of Cruelty to Children showed that:

    1% experienced sexual abuse by a parent or carer;
    3% experienced sexual abuse by another relative;
    11% experienced sexual abuse by people known but unrelated to them;
    5% experienced sexual abuse by an adult stranger or someone they had just met.

The correct management of allegations of child sexual assault or abuse requires skill, sensitivity and good inter-agency communication and co-operation. Factors to be considered include:

- Why do an examination?
- Who should do the examination?
- Where should the examination be done?
- When should it be done?
- How should it be done?

Why do an examination?

The best interest of the child should be the foremost consideration. When you are elucidating what that is, consider the medical and psychological needs and any ongoing child protection concerns as well as any forensic issues. Good practice dictates that joint strategy discussion involving the police and social services should include input from health professionals in deciding what actions ought to take place. You may need to remind the other agencies that reassurance is a very important outcome of a medical examination for both child (and carers) even when the chances of obtaining forensic evidence are minimal, for example after considerable time delay between the alleged assault and disclosure. A strategy discussion may take place following a referral, or at any other time (for instance, if concerns about significant harm emerge in respect of a child receiving support under s17 Children Act 1989, Provision of care for children in need). The discussion should be used to

- share available information;
- agree the conduct and timing of any criminal investigation;
- decide whether a core assessment under s47 of the Children Act 1989 ('s47 enquiries') should be initiated, or continued if it has already begun;
- plan how the s47 enquiry should be undertaken (if one is to be initiated), including the need for medical treatment, and who will carry out what actions, by when and for what purpose;
- agree what action is required immediately to safeguard and promote the welfare of the child, and/or provide interim services and support; if the child is in hospital, decisions should also be made about how to secure the safe discharge of the child;
- determine what information from the strategy discussion will be shared with the family, unless such information sharing may place a child at increased risk of significant harm or jeopardize police investigations into any alleged offence(s);
- determine if legal action is required [2].

Who should conduct the examination?

These examinations require a high level of skill and knowledge; it is of the utmost importance that the examining clinician be correctly qualified. Joint Guidance [4] produced by the Faculty of Forensic and Legal Medicine with the Royal College of Paediatrics and Child Health (see Box 12.3) was last updated in April 2007.

The guidelines also stress that it is essential to obtain high quality photo documentation. If not obtained, you must document the reasons why.

> **Box 12.3** Single or joint examinations
>
> A single doctor examination may take place provided the doctor concerned has the necessary knowledge, skills and experience for the particular case. When a single doctor does not have all the necessary knowledge, skills and experience for a particular paediatric forensic examination two doctors with *complementary skills* should conduct a joint examination. Usually such examinations involve a paediatrician and a forensic physician (forensic medical examiner, police surgeon, forensic medical officer). However, it may be necessary to involve another medical professional such as a genito-urinary physician or family planning doctor, if the case demands it. If two professionals are involved they need to determine in advance of the assessment what skills they bring to the examination and who will undertake which component of the examination.

Skills required

These can be found in Palusci *et al.* [5] and include:
- an ability to communicate comfortably with children and their carers about sensitive issues;
- an understanding of and sensitivity to the child's developmental, social and emotional needs and his/her intellectual level;
- an understanding of consent and confidentiality as they relate to children and young people;
- competence to conduct a comprehensive general and genital examination of a child, and skill in the different techniques used to facilitate the genital examination (e.g. labial traction);
- an understanding, based on current research evidence, of the normal genital and anal anatomy, and its variants, for the age and gender of the child to be examined;
- an understanding, based on the current research evidence, of the diagnosis and differential diagnosis of physical signs associated with abuse;
- competence in the use of a colposcope and in obtaining photo documentation, ensuring that the latter properly reflects the clinical findings and documenting if it does not;

- an understanding of what forensic samples may be appropriate to the investigation and how these samples should be obtained and packaged;
- the ability to document comprehensively and precisely the clinical findings in contemporaneous notes;
- the competence to produce a detailed statement or report describing and interpreting the clinical findings;
- an understanding of the importance of communicating and co-operating with other agencies and professionals involved in the care of the child; this may include attending a case conference, referral to other healthcare professionals, e.g. paediatricians, psychiatrists, genito-urinary physicians;
- the ability to present the evidence, and be cross-examined, in subsequent civil or criminal proceedings;
- an understanding of the different types of post-coital contraception available, the indications and contraindications of the various methods, and the capacity to prescribe the hormonal types of contraception where appropriate (see Chapter 13);
- training in prophylaxis (including hepatitis B, human immunodeficiency virus (HIV)), screening and diagnosis of sexually transmitted infections (see Chapter 14).

Where should the examination take place?

There are minimum requirements [6] for the venue, of which the following is a brief summary. The surroundings should be age appropriate. This should take into consideration both chronological age and developmental age. There should be privacy. A busy accident and emergency (A&E) department or out patient clinic is unsuitable. It should be forensically sound in order to minimize the chances of cross-contamination of any forensic exhibits. There should be quick and easy access to other healthcare professionals. With this in mind, where better than a hospital base?

When should the examination be done?

This will depend upon
- medical needs (e.g. emergency contraception, post-exposure prophylaxis, injuries that need urgent attention)
- forensic considerations
  - time since last assault
  - nature of assault
  - actions of child since (e.g. washing, bowels open)
- age of child.

Bearing these considerations in mind, an examination for an historical allegation may be planned for a child-friendly time. However, when the allegation is of an acute assault, it is vital to see the child quickly to maximize the chances of
- identifying and documenting any injuries
- collecting trace evidence
- prescribing emergency contraception if appropriate
- prescribing post-exposure prophylaxis if appropriate.

It is well established that injuries with major forensic significance can quickly heal, leaving no or minimal residua. For example, grip mark bruises, erythema from bites, genital injuries such as oedema, bruises, abrasions, lacerations. Children examined soon after an assault are also more likely to have positive ano-genital findings [7].

Research into persistence data following sexual assault in children [7, 8] shows that the chances of obtaining positive swab results are reduced when the victim is a prepubertal child.

Taking all this into account, you may be better advised to discuss the case further with the investigating officer before planning an examination time. A benefit of delaying the examination is to give the police a chance to conduct a prior video interview with the child. Particularly with younger children, this increases the chances of having full disclosure of details of the assault, a help in directing the nature of the examination.

How should the examination be done?

These examinations are often lengthy. You need to allow for this. It is in everyone's interest to avoid interruptions.

History taking

Note keeping needs to be meticulous, precise and contemporaneous. It is a good idea to use a proforma developed for the task. A copy of the St Mary's proforma may be viewed on the book's website (www.cambridge.org/9780521705684).

Most of these cases will be police referrals rather than self-referrals. The initial history of the assault should be gained from the attending officer. Key points to note are:

- What has happened?
- When did it happen?
- When was last contact with alleged assailant?
- What actions have been taken since, e.g. changing clothes, washing, showering, bowels open, micturating, etc.?

Note the officer's name, rank and collar number. In the interests of your participation in later criminal justice proceedings, always record who gave what information and who else was present at the time.

You may wish to clarify the account with the child. Great caution is urged here, particularly with any child who has not yet been video interviewed, or young children. Any suggestion that a clinician has questioned a child about the details of the assault may make the child's evidence inadmissible, as it could be regarded as contaminated. If you feel that you have to ask questions about the assault, they must not be leading, that is to say suggesting the answer. They should be non-directional, open questions recorded verbatim in the notes, as should their subsequent answers.

Take a concise medical history. This will include details such as birth history, immunizations, development, previous and current medical problems, operations, social history, family history, drug history (including prescribed, over the counter, illegal). In adolescents, a menstrual and sexual history may be required. Depending on the nature of the alleged assault additional questions may need to be asked. For example, a history of anal assault necessitates a detailed bowel history. Tailor the history for each individual case, but be aware that further disclosure may occur after the examination. Remember that you are gathering evidence on behalf of the court, not trying to gather evidence to help support any allegations.

It is always a good idea at some point to get the child alone so that he/she can add bits he/she may have been reluctant to divulge in front of a carer. Particularly with sexual assault cases, it is important to give a young person some privacy, but still with the understanding that the information given may well be disclosed to the criminal justice system.

Communication problems

Where English is not the first language, interpreters must be used. It is not acceptable to use other family members as interpreters. If there are any other communication difficulties, the necessary professional help should be employed. Ideally, these should have child protection training.

The examination (see Table 12.1.)

Tailor the medical examination to the individual case, and carry it out with the greatest care and sensitivity. The young child who has been indecently touched by a family member, but not physically hurt, may well perceive an intrusive medical examination as more abusive than the alleged offence. At the same time, an examination that fails to reveal any evidence present is also detrimental to the welfare of the child. The child should feel in control of his/her body. It should not be necessary to restrain him/her physically, but very occasionally it may be necessary to examine a child under sedation. If your examination is incomplete, for instance because the child becomes distressed, record this in the notes. You must assess, on the facts of the case, what procedures to carry out, remembering that you may have to justify actions or omissions under cross-examination in court.

Your dual role is to act in a therapeutic capacity, assessing the general wellbeing of the child, and to gather any evidence that may help determine the veracity or otherwise of any allegations or suspicions of maltreatment. Although not obligatory, a proforma acts as an *aide-mémoire*, and facilitates the recording of information contemporaneously. Examination findings and opinion are separate entities, and should be clearly separated in any notes and subsequent reports or statements. It is of the utmost importance to document all negative, as well as positive, findings.

Assuming consent, the examination, no matter what the allegation, should be from head to toe. Explain the process to the child at a level commensurate with his/her maturity and understanding.

Note the rapport between child and carers, as well as his/her general behaviour. Take care how you use words to describe his/her demeanour; to describe a nervous teenager, giggling in her embarrassment at having to undergo her first ever gynaecological examination, as just 'giggling' may well paint a very different picture of her to a jury when read out by a defence barrister months afterwards.

Chaperones

It is good practice to have a chaperone present during the examination. The chaperone should be a trained member of staff, familiar with this type of examination. The chaperone's role is to help put the child and carer at ease, safeguard the child and the doctor and, in some cases, assist the doctor. For younger children it is often helpful to have their carer with them (assuming that this is not the alleged offender). It is better to ask older children whom they would like in the room other than the examining doctor and the chaperone. Again, document in the notes those present during the examination.

Height and weight

Check measurements on a Tanner growth chart (see book website) and record the percentiles. Failure to thrive and dips in normal growth pattern may be associated with abuse of all types.

Detail on the identification and documentation of injuries is found in Chapter 10, but readers are referred also to Chapter 11 (physical abuse of children).

The genital examination: female

In ideal conditions, the child is relaxed, the lighting excellent, with colposcope, camera and DVD available. Document how the examination was done and if any difficulties were encountered.

Use the frog leg position [8], with the girl supine on the examination couch, feet together, knees flexed and separated. If a young child will not allow this, have her sit on the carer's knee.

After carefully visualizing them, separate the labia and apply traction gently downwards and forwards, grasping them gently between thumbs and forefingers. A labelled line drawing is provided (Fig. 12.2).

If, in examining a young child in the frog leg position, you suspect any abnormality of the posterior hymen, re-examine her in the prone knee-chest position. Some so-called posterior hymenal abnormalities seen in the former posture may be purely positional, but the influence of gravity in the knee-chest position shows them to be normal. Examples, taken with permission from Heger *et al.* [9] are reproduced on the book website.

As well as photo documentation, notes should be made of the genital characteristics including Tanner staging (see book website), shape of hymen, amount of hymenal tissue (see Fig. 12.3), presence or absence of vaginal discharge. Take care to describe in words and on line drawings as well as photographs any abnormalities, injuries or lesions. Do this even if you are not sure of the significance or otherwise of what you are seeing. The face of a clock is often used to help locate position: with the child lying supine, 12 o'clock represents the

Table 12.1. Guide to the general examination

	General features	If history of acute assault
Clothing	Cleanliness, appropriateness e.g. for age, weather	Record if original clothing worn at time of assault. Damage, staining etc.
Skin	Cleanliness, infestation, track marks, chronic skin conditions	Bruises, abrasions, etc. or residua thereof; staining, e.g. from saliva, semen, etc.
Head	Hair cleanliness, infestation	Traumatic alopecia, debris or body fluids in hair. Fontanelle: swelling, bruising etc.
Eyes	Frozen watchfulness	Evidence of intoxication, petechial haemorrhages associated with asphyxia
Mouth	Dentition	Frenula, bruising inner aspects of lips from hand held over mouth. Petechial haemorrhages on roof of mouth after oral sex
Upper limbs		Nails – debris, length, bruising consistent with grip marks
Thorax	Heart and chest sounds. Breast development – Tanner staging	Injuries
Abdomen	Masses	Tenderness, swelling, pregnancy
Back	Spine	Bony tenderness, injuries
Lower limbs	Gait, mobility	Injuries
Genitalia	Tanner stage	Injuries

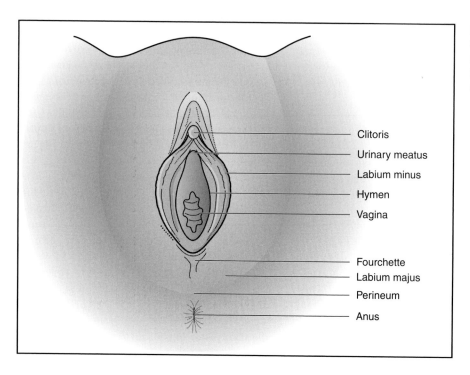

Fig. 12.2 General features of external genitalia in the female child.

- Clitoris
- Urinary meatus
- Labium minus
- Hymen
- Vagina
- Fourchette
- Labium majus
- Perineum
- Anus

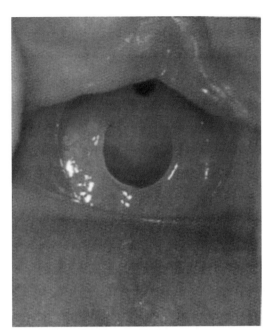

Fig. 12.3 An intact, broad crescentic hymen in a four-year-old child. Reproduced with permission from Heger, A *et al.* (2000) *Evaluation of the Sexually Abused Child, 2nd edn.* Oxford: Oxford University Press [9].

uppermost position, closest to the abdomen, 6 o'clock that nearest to the couch.

It may be difficult to see the edges of the hymen in some cases. Use the tip of a moistened cotton swab to unfold the edges gently and get a better view. A small amount of sterile water can be used to help 'float' the hymen.

In an older post-pubertal girl [8, 10], a urinary catheter (size 12 or 14 Foley) can be useful. Pass it into the vaginal canal, inflate the balloon, then slowly retract the catheter, displaying the edges of the hymen gently stretched over the balloon. Done carefully, this should not cause any discomfort. If your examination follows an acute assault it is most important to do this procedure *after* the forensic swabs have been taken in order not to contaminate them.

It is very rare to proceed to an internal vaginal examination in prepubertal girls [11]. In older girls,

where there has been an allegation of penetration, a full gynaecological examination, including insertion of a speculum, may be required. These decisions must be made on a case-by-case basis.

The genital examination: male

Genital injury in boys who have been indecently assaulted is rare, but inspect the penis and testicles carefully for signs of bruising, tears of the frenulum and 'love bites' or signs of sucking. Where the child's penis has been sucked saliva may persist on the skin for up to a week. Forensic swabs should therefore be taken (see Chapter 13, *Oral sexual acts*).

Anal examination

Inspect the anus in every case unless there has been an active decision not to do so. This may arise with a teenage girl, where the allegation is of vaginal penetration only and she declines this part of the examination. Disclosures of anal assault are sometimes withheld through embarrassment or in a sexually naïve child who may be unsure which orifice has been touched/penetrated, hence the need to examine this area. The child should be in the left lateral position or, if the knee-chest position has been employed during the hymenal examination, it may be done then. Separate the buttocks gently without using traction, and observe the perianal area and anal verge for signs of past and recent injury. The reader should consult Chapter 13 on perianal injury, and be familiar with the evidence-based content of *The Physical Signs of Child Sexual Abuse* [4].

Other features to be noted during the examination include soiling, general perianal skin condition, fissures (and note whether they are acute or chronic, show signs of healing, whether they extend to the anal verge or not), scars, bruising. Again, the face of a clock (see above) is useful to help locate position. Take care not to mistake venous pooling around the anal margin for bruising.

Significance of ano-genital finding

Over the years, greater knowledge of what is normal and abnormal in both abused and non-abused children has helped inform our understanding of the significance of examination findings. Nevertheless, gaps remain. Initial studies showed high injury rates in children examined following allegations of abuse. More recent work [7] has reversed these findings. The low injury rate has several explanations, including time delay from assault to examination and the tendency for most injuries to heal rapidly, leaving no residua; indeed, the assault may have caused no injury in the first instance. The chance of finding injuries depends upon such factors as

- time from assault to examination
- type of assault, e.g. penetration or not
- force used
- resistance of the child to the act
- use of lubrication
- size of penetrating object
- age of child

It is known that penile vaginal penetration can occur without causing any damage to a stretchy, oestrogenized hymen, [7, 10] casting doubt on the concept of the 'intact' hymen. A child may make an honest mistake and genuinely believe that full intercourse has occurred if a penis has been pushed against the vulval tissues. The prepubertal child experiences pain in these tissues when they are touched, as they are both delicate and sensitive. In preparing a report for court or giving feedback to the investigating officer following an examination, make these points clear, as non-medical people tend to assume that there would certainly have been physical signs had the allegation been true. Excessive claims are sometimes made for the value of medical evidence. Doctors must guard against trying to fit the evidence to the case, a fault that has all too frequently led to medical evidence being discredited in court. It can, however, be difficult to say to the investigating officer and social worker that one cannot find any medical evidence. You may feel that you are letting the child down by failing to find evidence, but it is very much worse for the child and does not assist the cause of justice if the medical evidence is later discredited.

Questions to be answered during the medical examination are:

- If you saw these findings in a child where there was no allegation or suspicion of abuse, would you consider abuse to be a likely cause?
- Do these findings occur in non-abused children?
- What is the mechanism of causation if the findings are due to abuse?

The differential diagnosis for apparent injury includes such diverse conditions as straddle injuries, lichen sclerosis et atrophicus, urethral prolapse, candidiasis, nappy rash and bubble bath dermatitis.

Findings of injury and any possible significance have been set out in guidance from the Royal College of Paediatrics and Child Health [4]. A link to the most recent (2007) revision can be found on the book website. Once again, it must be emphasized that no doctor should undertake examinations of children thought to have been sexually assaulted unless familiar with this text. Readers are referred to Chapter 16 for a description of current practice in taking swabs and other material for examination in clinical and forensic science laboratories.

Other considerations

These include the need to provide advice on emergency contraception and appropriate prescription; see Chapter 13.

Sexually transmitted infections (STIs)

Where the allegation suggests that transmission of STIs is a possibility, screening must be considered. This may be done at the time of the examination although, in acute cases where the incubation time has not elapsed, follow-up plans must be arranged. Working arrangements with local laboratories accepting the need for chain of evidence procedures should be in place.

Psychological support

The psychological impact of an assault upon a child depends upon many factors including those specific to the victim, the assault and the assailant. The child's response will also be influenced by the ability of the carers to support her/him. Response to assault changes with time, perhaps with a court case, so the ongoing needs of the child and carer should be assessed and reviewed appropriately. Not all will need professional help. For those who do, it should be tailored to their specific needs. These may be met by practical support from a support worker; these have been of great value in adult sexual assault cases. Here the support worker acts as a link figure, keeping the family informed of any criminal justice proceedings, liaising with witness support services and so on.

Medical follow-up and the sharing of information

The context of a child being examined for suspected abuse/assault will vary enormously from the child about whom there have been welfare concerns to a 'one-off sexual assault' by a stranger in a park. The duty of the doctor is to consider the holistic needs of that child, including school attendance, drug/alcohol abuse, family planning, failure to thrive. Suitable follow-up must be made as required, with systems in place to detect when appointments are not kept. If you are unsure of the clinical significance of findings, it may be necessary to review the child at a later stage.

Time and again, history has shown that without good inter-agency working, including the sharing of information, opportunities to help – even to save children – have been squandered. Lord Laming's report [1] made 108 recommendations, many of which focused on information sharing. As part of the initial consent process, both child and carer should be informed about the process of information sharing. The doctor must be familiar with local Child Protection Procedures. It may become apparent as you take the history that other children

(siblings, peers) are at risk from the assailant. Appropriate steps must be taken for their welfare to be assessed.

Photography

It is good practice to have high quality photo documentation of the ano-genital examination. Consent for obtaining these images has already been considered, but remember these are highly sensitive, so must be treated as such in terms of storage and access.

Storage/ownership of notes

The obligations on practitioners to ensure the security of what is highly sensitive material is dealt with in Chapter 4. Specific guidance relating to sexual assault examination findings can be seen on the book website.

Currently, there is no nationally agreed protocol for storage and disclosure of these images, but local protocols to ensure their confidentiality and safety must be in place (see Further reading, below). Their existence must be declared in any statement made for the courts. The defence may request that a medical expert acting on their behalf view them. It is good practice to do so together with the doctor who created the images. The images should not be disclosed to any non-medical persons except on the order of a judge. Images may be shared with other doctors as part of clinical governance/peer review/teaching as long as this was made clear at the time consent to take the images was obtained.

Peer review

Detection and prevention of child abuse is the responsibility of every healthcare professional, but some will come into contact with this type of work more than others. Regular, well-structured peer review allows a process of support and quality control as well as training. If cases involved in the criminal justice system are peer reviewed any dissenting views are disclosable to the courts. The local Crown Prosecution Service ought to assist in processes to accommodate this.

THE LEGAL FRAMEWORK OF CHILD PROTECTION IN ENGLAND AND WALES

Justifying state intervention: the concept of significant harm

The Children Act 1989 introduced the concept of 'significant harm' as the uniform threshold criterion below which state intervention in a child's life is not justified. Wherever the concept of significant harm is used, harm is defined to mean ill-treatment or the impairment of health or development (ss31(9) and 105). This definition was extended by the Adoption and Children Act 2002 to include, for example, impairment suffered from seeing or hearing the ill-treatment of another. 'Health' is defined to mean physical or mental health and 'development' is defined to mean physical, intellectual, emotional, social or behavioural development. 'Ill-treatment' is not defined exhaustively, the Act merely stating that it includes sexual abuse and forms of ill-treatment which are not physical. Although not expressly stated, it seems clear that this includes physical abuse and presumably also extends to cover emotional abuse, even if no physical harm results. There is, therefore, potential overlap between ill-treatment and the impairment of health or development.

The harm must be 'significant'. The Act does not define 'significant', but does provide that, where the question of whether harm suffered by a child is significant turns on the child's health or development, his/her health or development shall be compared with that which could reasonably be expected of a similar child (ss31(10) and 105). This requires a comparison to be made with a hypothetical 'reasonable' child. It seems that the appropriate standard for any individual child will not necessarily be the best that could possibly be achieved, but only what is reasonable for that particular child. Clearly some children have specific characteristics

which mean they cannot be expected to be as healthy or well developed as other children, therefore the hypothetical child must be attributed with similar characteristics. But whether or not the same would apply to a child's background, as opposed to physical or intellectual characteristics, is doubtful.

Identifying and reporting abuse

Guidance on inter-agency working issued by the Department for Education and Skills provides that: 'If someone believes that a child may be suffering, or may be at risk of suffering significant harm, then they should always refer their concerns to the local authority children's social care' (*Working Together to Safeguard Children*, 2006, para 5.16 [2]). Prior to the implementation of the relevant provisions of the Children Act 2004, if a practitioner had concerns about a child, it was common practice to enquire if the child was registered on the Child Protection Register, which provided a record of children in the area who were the subject of an inter-agency protection plan. As part of the Government's 'Every Child Matters' programme following the death of Victoria Climbié and the resulting inquiry by Lord Laming, the 2004 Act made provision for the setting up of information-sharing databases to contain information on every child in England and Wales, including any child protection concerns. The ContactPoint database, which will be operational in England from 2008, will allow authorized practitioners to see who else is working with the child, so that information can be shared and co-ordinated support delivered where necessary.

As soon as the local authority is made aware of the concerns, they have a statutory duty to make such enquiries as they consider necessary to enable them to decide whether they should take any action to safeguard or promote the child's welfare (s47 Children Act 1989). The resulting investigation will frequently be conducted in conjunction with the police, who will be concerned to gather evidence of any criminal offences committed with a view to prosecuting the abuser.

Emergency protection of children

If it is considered necessary to take emergency action to protect the child, an application can be made to a court for an emergency protection order (s44 Children Act 1989) which enables a child to be made safe when he/she might otherwise be likely to suffer significant harm. This may involve not only removing a child from home but also keeping a child in hospital against the wishes of the carers. The order lasts for a maximum of 15 days. The applicant (usually the local authority) gains parental responsibility for the child for the duration of the order and can thus give consent for medical examination.

In more urgent cases, a child may be taken into police protection (s46 Children Act 1989) for no more than 72 hours. No parental responsibility is acquired and so, if consent for medical examination is required, the local authority will need to apply for an emergency protection order.

In some cases the nature of the harm suspected is long term and cumulative, rather than acute and severe. For example, the child may be failing to thrive, or there may be suspicions as to neglect or sexual abuse which give cause for concern but which do not place the child at serious immediate risk. If the carers are not willing to agree to an assessment of the child, the local authority may apply to the court for a child assessment order (s43 Children Act 1989), under which the court can direct that an examination or assessment of the child (which may take a variety of forms) should take place. However, if the child has sufficient understanding to make an informed decision, he/she may refuse to submit to the examination or assessment. Furthermore, the child may only be kept away from home if this is specified in the order and if it is necessary to do so for the purpose of the assessment. The court is unlikely to allow a child to be kept away from home overnight solely for the convenience of those carrying out the order, but on occasions this may be necessary if the child is to be properly assessed. In view of the fact that the order only extends for a maximum of seven days, arrangements for carrying out the assessment should usually be made in advance of the application being made to a court, thus ensuring that once intervention is authorized, delay is kept to a minimum.

REFERENCES

1. *The Victoria Climbié Inquiry 2003: Report of an Inquiry by Lord Laming* (2003) London: HMSO.
2. Department for Education and Skills (2006) *Working Together to Safeguard Children: a Guide to Inter-Agency Working to Safeguard and Promote the Welfare of Children.* London: HMSO.
3. Cawson P, Wattam C, Booker S, Kelly G (2000) *Child Maltreatment in the UK. A Study of Prevalence of Child Abuse and Neglect.* London: NSPCC.
4. Royal College of Paediatrics and Child Health (2007) *The Physical Signs of Child Sexual Abuse: an Evidence-based Review and Guidance for Best Practice.* London: RCPCH.
5. Palusci V, Cox E, Shatz E, Schultze, J (2006) Urgent medical assessment after child sexual abuse. *Child Abuse and Neglect* **30**: 367–80.
6. Department of Health Working Draft (May 2007). *Guide for Services for Children Provided by Sexual Assault Referral Centres (SARCs).*
7. Heger A, Ticson L, Velasquez O, Bernier R (2002) Children referred for possible sexual abuse: medical findings in 2384 children. *Child Abuse and Neglect* **26**: 645–59.
8. Kellogg N, Menard S, Santos A (2004) Genital anatomy in pregnant adolescents: 'normal' does not mean 'nothing happened'. *Pediatrics* **113**(1): 67–9.
9. Heger A, Emans SJ, Muram D (2000) *Evaluation of the Sexually Abused Child*, 2nd edn. Oxford: Oxford University Press.
10. White C, McLean I (2006) Adolescent complainants of sexual assault: injury patterns in virgin and non-virgin groups. *Journal of Clinical Forensic Medicine* **13**: 172–80.
11. Christian CW, Lavelle JM, De Jong AR, *et al.* (2000) Forensic evidence findings in prepubertal victims of sexual assault. *Pediatrics* **106**: 100–4.

FURTHER READING AND RESOURCES

Dalton M (2004) *Forensic Gynaecology.* London: RCOG Press.

Local Safeguarding Children Boards (LSCBs) *Inter-Agency Safeguarding Children Procedures.*

Department for Education and Skills (2006) *Working Together to Safeguard Children: a Guide to Inter-Agency Working to Safeguard and Promote the welfare of Children.* London: HMSO.

Royal College of Paediatrics and Child Health (2006) *Child Protection Companion.* London: RCPCH.

Gray J (2000) *Framework for the Assessment of Children in Need and Their Families.* London Department of Health. ISBN 0113223102.

RCPCH and FFLM (2007) *Guidance on Paediatric Forensic Examinations in Relation to Possible Child Sexual Abuse.* Produced by The Royal College of Paediatrics and Child Health and The Faculty of Forensic and Legal Medicine. A Joint Publication.

Draft Recommendations of Best Practice in the Management of Intimate Images that may become Evidence in Court. (2007) From the Royal College of Paediatrics and Child Health (RCPCH) and the Faculty of Forensic and Legal Medicine.

An expert group convened by the Royal College of Paediatrics and Child Health evaluated growth reference charts in use in the UK, recommending UK90 Centile Charts (see Wright CM, Booth IW, Buckler JM *et al.* (2002) Growth reference charts for use in the United Kingdom. *Archives of Disease in Childhood* **86**: 11–14). They can be viewed at www.patient.co.uk/showdoc/40001849

13

Adult sexual offences

Deborah J. Rogers

Introduction

Home Office figures show that in 2005/06 there were 13 331 recorded offences of rape of a female. This represented an increase of 3% on the previous year. In the same 12-month period there were 23 026 recorded offences of 'sexual assault on a female' and 25 724 recorded offences in the 'other sexual assault' category. The latter includes rape and other sexual offences on males. It is suggested that between 75% and 95% of rape crimes are never reported to the police [1].

Traditionally, the examination of complainants of sexual offences has focused on the collection of forensic evidence. However, it is now recognized that the medical and psychological needs of the complainant have equal importance. Thus the forensic physician has a duty to ensure that all relevant needs are addressed, either at the time of the examination or by appropriate referral. Sexual assault referral centres [2] that provide for forensic, medical and psychological needs of complainants are accessible both to patients who report to the police and those who choose not to.

The forensic, medical and psychological needs of a complainant or suspect of a sexual assault will depend on the nature and timing of the assault. The first, and major, part of this chapter is designed to guide forensic physicians through the potential components of a sexual assault examination and to help them with the interpretation of the findings.

The remainder of the chapter deals with the medico-legal aspects of pregnancy and sexual variations.

Legislation and definitions

The Sexual Offences Act (SOA) 2003 consolidated and improved the existing legislation in England and Wales applicable to sexual offences. The following summarizes the parts of the SOA 2003 that are most pertinent to the forensic physician.

Rape (SOA 2003 section 1)

Rape is the intentional, non-consensual penetration of the vagina, anus or mouth with a penis. The SOA 2003 (section 79) states that 'vagina' includes vulva and that references to a part of the body are also applicable to surgically constructed body parts (for example, following gender reassignment surgery).

Assault by penetration (SOA section 2)

A person commits an offence if he/she intentionally penetrates the vagina or anus with part of his/her body (except the penis) or anything else and the penetration is sexual.

Sexual assault (SOA section 3)

A person commits an offence if he/she intentionally touches another person and the touching is

Clinical Forensic Medicine, third edition ed. W. D. S. McLay. Published by Cambridge University Press. © Cambridge University Press 2009.

sexual and the other person does not consent to the touching.

In Scotland, rape is a crime at common law. The *actus reus* is constituted by the man having sexual intercourse with the woman without her consent and the *mens rea* is present when he knows the woman is not consenting, or at any rate is reckless as to whether she is consenting.

Complainants (complainer in Scotland) and suspects

In this chapter the term complainant will be used to denote persons who report that they have, or may have, been sexually assaulted. Complainants may be male or female. However, as the majority are female, in this chapter the complainant will be referred to by the female pronoun.

A suspect is somebody who is thought to be possibly guilty of doing something illegal. Suspects of sexual assaults may be male or female. However, as the majority are male, in this chapter the suspect will be referred to by the male pronoun.

The role of the forensic physician is to collect all available forensic evidence and provide immediate medical care to all patients whom they encounter in their forensic practice. They must remain impartial when dealing with both complainants and suspects regardless of the nature of the allegation.

Examination facilities

The health and immediate medical needs of the patients should always be considered paramount; any urgent medical treatment must be given priority over any forensic examination. Ill and severely injured complainants requiring hospitalization can only be examined forensically after the responsible hospital doctor has given permission (see [3]).

Most complainant examinations will take place in a specifically designated and equipped examination suite. Conversely, suspects are usually examined in the medical room in the custody suite. Both facilities must have the necessary equipment to provide basic

medical care and to undertake an adequate forensic assessment. The Faculty of Forensic and Legal Medicine and Association of Chief Police Officers (ACPO) Rape Working Group provides guidance on the appropriate furnishings and equipment.

To prevent later allegations of cross-contamination, it is vital to avoid all possible contact between complainant(s) and the alleged assailant(s) from the same incident. Therefore, they should not be examined at the same venue, nor by the same doctor. If this proves impossible, the doctor is advised to shower (including washing his/her hair), completely change his/her clothing and shoes, and arrange for the room to be thoroughly cleaned between each examination. However, even with these precautions, allegations of cross-contamination would be difficult to refute.

Support for the complainant

When a serious sexual assault is reported to the police, in many police areas in the United Kingdom, a specially trained police officer (ideally of the same sex) will be allocated to the case (that is, a sexual offence trained investigator). This police officer will accompany the complainant to the examination facilities, obtain details of the allegation in order to determine the need for forensic samples and further the police investigation, and provide verbal and practical support for the complainant. In sexual assault referral centres a crisis worker will often undertake these duties.

In addition, the police officer/crisis worker can undertake a number of other tasks to improve the comfort of the complainant and facilitate the examination (Box 13.1).

Documentation

The 'Pro forma for post-pubertal female and male forensic sexual assault examination' produced by the Faculty of Forensic and Legal Medicine (FFLM) (www.fflm.ac.uk) (or an equivalent document) should be used to record details of the examination

Box 13.1 Assistance that can be given by the chaperone/crisis worker

Before the examination:
- Arrange a change of clothing
- Obtain urine samples and mouth washings (using the relevant forensic modules)
- Summarize the allegation for the examining doctor

During the examination:
- Collect (as their exhibits) significant clothing and the paper sheet on which the complainant has stood during examination
- Chaperone and assist the examining doctor

After the examination:
- Assist the doctor in the labelling and sealing of forensic exhibits*
- Store/transport all forensic exhibits
- Organize follow-up appointments

Note: (*the doctor retains overall responsibility for ensuring that the samples are correctly labelled and packaged)

Box 13.2 Details of the allegation

The incident
- Date and time of the sexual assault(s)
- Locations: inside/outside (weather wet/dry)
- Number of alleged assailants
- Restraints/weapons and their use
- Injuries sustained by the complainant (when, how and where on body?)
- Injuries sustained by the suspect (e.g. was the assailant scratched by the complainant?)
- Type and number of sexual act(s)/use of condoms/lubricants
- Relative positions during sexual acts
- Site(s) of ejaculation
- Bleeding per vaginam or anum: due to injury or menstruation
- Use and disposal of sanitary pads/tampons
- Other types of contact (e.g. gripping, kissing, licking, biting, spitting or scratching)

Since the incident

Relevant to all recent allegations
- Manner of leaving scene and resulting injuries
- Changed/washed clothing
- Bathed/showered
- Washed/brushed/combed hair
- Alcohol/drugs taken
- Medical treatment received

Relevant to allegations of oral intercourse
- Cleaned teeth/rinsed mouth
- Drank any fluid/ate food

Relevant to allegations of vaginal intercourse
- Consensual vaginal intercourse
- Contraception (particularly condoms) used
- Lubricants used
- Douched
- Vaginal bleeding/pain

Relevant to allegations of anal intercourse
- Consensual anal and/or vaginal intercourse
- Protection (condoms) used
- Lubricants used
- Anal bleeding/pain
- Bowel action

of a complainant. This pro forma is not suitable to be used for suspects (use a fitness for detention/interview proforma instead).

Obtain written consent from the complainant/suspect before recording personal medical information or undertaking any examination. The various pro formas produced by the FFLM include appropriate consent forms. Where an adult complainant lacks capacity to consent, follow the advice in the FFLM document *'Consent from Patients who may have been Seriously Assaulted'* [3]. When obtaining consent for intimate and non-intimate samples from a suspect, follow the advice in the current Codes of Practice of the Police and Criminal Evidence Act 1984 (PACE; but note that PACE does not apply in Scotland) and the FFLM guidelines.

Appraisal of the allegation

The forensic physician needs a summary of the allegation in order to determine which forensic samples (if any) are relevant, to tailor the examination and to address the medical and psychological needs of the complainant.

With regard to complainants, in most cases the accompanying policeman or crisis worker can provide details of the allegation, thus obviating the need for the complainant to reiterate intimate details that have already been relayed. However, if the complainant has not provided information to another person obtain a more detailed account directly from her. Box 13.2 details the key information that may be required from a complainant before the examination can be conducted.

When the information is obtained from a police officer/crisis worker the complainant should be read the summary of the incident and asked to correct verbally any inaccuracies. You should record any corrections in the notes without obliterating the original text. It should be clear who has provided the recorded information.

If the details of the allegation are incomplete, you should ask the complainant specific questions to elucidate the information described above. Wherever possible, both the question and the answer should be recorded verbatim in the medical notes. When asking questions, avoid medical jargon and be sensitive to the fact that some complainants will find certain sexual acts very difficult to talk about.

If injuries are noted during the examination it is appropriate for you to ask the complainant to account for the injury and to record the responses (where possible verbatim). Again, it must be clear in the notes who provided the information.

Suspects should not be asked for any details of the alleged incident (this will be covered in a police interview). Instead, a police officer with knowledge of the case should apprise you of the essential details of the allegation and any significant findings following the examination of the complainant. It is important to note whether (and in what manner) the alleged assailant may have been injured. The police requirements (medical and forensic) should be established, and the samples to be taken discussed. Proceed with the examination in a similar manner to that described for the complainant, after consent has been properly obtained. The Police and Criminal Evidence Act 1984 requires the defendant to give consent to the police for the obtaining of samples. Nonetheless, the doctor should obtain valid consent and

advise the defendant not to incriminate himself (see Chapter 4). However, if either suspect or complainant volunteers information, note it in your contemporaneous medical records.

Current medical problems and medication

Information about current medical problems and medication is required to:

- document any symptoms (e.g. pain) or signs (e.g. injuries) that the complainant/suspect attributes to the incident;
- identify any pre-existing physical· or psychological conditions that could lead the forensic physician to misinterpret the clinical findings;
- determine what aftercare is required and reveal contraindications to any proposed treatment, e.g. emergency contraception;
- reveal vulnerabilities in the complainant (e.g. suicide ideation) that may lead you to arrange more specific aftercare (as opposed to simply referring the complainant to her general practitioner) or support during an interview (for suspects see Chapter 6);
- assist the forensic scientist with the interpretation of the toxicology results.

Past medical history

Although obtaining a detailed medical history is part of standard medical practice, there is a debate regarding how much medical history should be obtained from a complainant of sexual assault [4]. Concerns have been raised about the ability to protect medical confidentiality when the notes are disclosed to third parties and, given that very little of a patient's medical history will be relevant to the deliberations of the jury, there is an argument for restricting the medical history to that considered relevant to the allegation. For example, if the patient complains of anal bleeding following an act of non-consensual anal penetration, it is appropriate to try to determine whether the complainant had experienced similar symptoms prior to the assault. On occasions it may be necessary for the patient to be asked to consent to allowing a medical expert access to her medical records. If consent for disclosure is not forthcoming, a judge can be asked to consider making a court order for their release [5].

A detailed medical history should be obtained from the suspect in order to determine his fitness for detention and, where appropriate, fitness for interview (see Chapter 7).

Sexual and contraceptive history

In cases presenting acutely after a single sexual assault, it is necessary to ask some questions regarding a complainant's recent sexual experiences and contraceptive history to:
- identify any recent sexual activity that could lead the forensic physician or the forensic scientist to misinterpret the clinical or scientific findings;
- determine what aftercare is required and to reveal contraindications to any proposed treatment, for example when considering the need for emergency contraception, information should be obtained about other acts of unprotected sexual intercourse since the last menstrual period.

Suspects should not be asked about recent sexual experiences (if relevant this will be covered in a police interview).

Drugs and alcohol

Following a recent sexual assault the following information will need to be obtained before the blood and/or urine samples are submitted for analysis. These points can be covered either by the forensic physician or by the police officer when the complainant provides a detailed statement:
- was alcohol consumed?
- if yes – the time that drinking began and ended and type and quantity of alcoholic beverages consumed;

- the time of the last urination (prior to the specimen provided in this examination);
- have any drugs (prescribed, over-the-counter or illicit) been used by or administered to the complainant within four days of the examination?
- if yes – detail what was used and when it was used;
- are other substances suspected of having been used/administered, which could be relevant to the offence?
- if yes – detail what provoked the complainant's suspicions and any other available information such as times.

A detailed drug and alcohol history should be obtained from the suspect in order to inform the court and to determine his fitness for detention and interview (see Chapter 7).

Clothing and jewellery

Make a note of clothing and jewellery (if worn at the time of the incident) and appraise the state of the clothing (e.g. torn, stained, wet, worn inside out). However, it is the role of a forensic scientist to interpret any damage to clothing. Consideration should be given to exhibiting or swabbing any jewellery that may be a source of forensic evidence, such as rings through piercings on the vulva, clitoris or penis.

The complainant/suspect should undress on a paper sheet in order to collect foreign matter that may fall from the clothing as it is removed. Each item of relevant clothing and the paper sheet are exhibited separately (see role of chaperone, Box 13.1).

General examination

Your approach must be sympathetic but professional. Time taken to establish a rapport before the examination commences gives the complainant/ suspect the reassurance that you will be understanding and sensitive. The complainant/suspect should be allowed to control the pace at which the examination proceeds and be assured that the procedure can be stopped at any time. At all times, attempt to preserve the dignity of the complainant/suspect and minimize any discomfort. This may be facilitated by the use of screens, disposable gowns and/or single use paper sheets.

The complainant/suspect may be unaware of some injuries resulting from the incident. Therefore, where the incident is purported to have occurred within the preceding 14 days, offer a comprehensive general examination. This recommended timeframe has been chosen to take account of healing and fading of most injuries. However, it should be extended if there is an indication that injuries or scars relating to the assault remain.

The general examination will consist of a methodical inspection of every body surface using a good light source and, where necessary, a magnifying lens. This inspection must include recessed areas such as those behind ears, axillae, breasts, and non-intimate body orifices such as mouth and ears.

The inspection of the body surfaces and relevant body orifices can be done in tandem with the obtaining of forensic samples. However, care should be taken not to destroy any potential evidence or contaminate a body surface. For example, if an injury is covered with blood, whenever possible the wound should be swabbed (with the relevant consent) prior to cleaning and inspection.

Record every significant, or potentially significant, injury or lesion precisely, noting shape, colour, degree of swelling, degree of blanching (assessed by digital compression and release), site (related to a fixed bony point), size and degree of healing (if any) (see Chapter 10). Palpate each injury to identify any induration or more severe underlying injury. Use body charts or diagrams to record the physical findings. In some instances the patient may indicate an area of discomfort that shows no external signs of trauma. To avoid such findings being dismissed as subjective or hearsay, you are advised to distract the examinee and note facial and motor responses (grimaces, withdrawal) when the area is touched. You may choose to return to the area later in the examination to validate the findings.

Note also disabilities, medical conditions, surgical/accident/self-inflicted scars and the patient's demeanour. It is essential that the notes detail all the body surfaces examined, and whether any abnormality was present or not. If the patient declines part or all of the general examination, document this. The dominant hand is relevant when considering the possibilities that injuries are self-inflicted. Examine the fingernails, noting their length, if any are broken and if there is any evidence of debris under the nails. The head hair should be examined, noting stains and evidence of trauma (for example, broken hairs). If substances may have been consumed, make a note of the following:

- speech (rate, content and form);
- behaviour;
- mood;
- alertness;
- orientation;
- pulse rate;
- blood pressure;
- co-ordination.

Whenever possible the height and weight should be measured to assist the forensic scientist with the interpretation of any toxicology results.

Examination of genitalia and anus

The extent of the examination and forensic sampling of these areas should be tailored to the alleged incident. Record the location of all abnormalities with reference to an imaginary clock face represented by 12 o'clock at the mons pubis and 6 o'clock at the coccyx. All areas must be systematically examined, as detailed below, wearing disposable gloves. In acute cases the bed should be covered by the 'couch cover' in the kit, which is then packaged and retained as an item of clothing. *To avoid destruction or contamination of evidence it is imperative that all trace evidence be retrieved before any examination is conducted.*

Position: the partial lithotomy position (with the knees flexed and the heels on the couch) is most commonly used for examination of the female genitalia. Male genitalia are examined with the patient supine. The anal area is usually inspected with the patient in the left lateral position. However, these positions are not prescribed and can be adapted to suit the needs of the patient and/or the examining doctor. The position/s should be recorded.

Inspection of the ano-genital area: inspect the inner thighs and buttocks carefully for evidence of injury or possible stains. Then expose the genital area by gently parting the labia or buttocks. Secretions or stains (blood, seminal fluid, faeces, foreign material) should be noted and swabbed specifically.

Pubic hair: Note the presence, length and colour of the pubic hair. Secretions seen amongst the pubic hairs must be cut or swabbed and exhibited. Combing (with a wide-toothed comb) may reveal foreign bodies or loose hairs which must be exhibited. When control pubic hairs are required, cut them close to the roots. Pubic hair should never be plucked.

Female genitalia

Inspection

When the complainant describes peno-vaginal penetration, inspect the vulva (labia, clitoris, urethral opening, vestibule and posterior fourchette) carefully with a cool light source, and have access to a magnifying lens. A colposcope provides both illumination and magnification, and has the added advantage that if attached to a DVD or still camera (and the patient gives consent) it can be used to provide a permanent, truly contemporaneous, record of any potentially significant genital findings. Toluidine blue dye, used in some countries to highlight small breaches in the stratified squamous

epithelium [6], is not currently advocated in the United Kingdom. After all relevant forensic samples have been obtained, where necessary, a moistened swab or a Foley catheter [6] can be used to tease out any folds in the hymenal tissue and facilitate the inspection of any hymenal injury. Thereafter, undertake internal inspection of vagina and cervix using an appropriately sized, clear, disposable speculum or proctoscope. Record any evidence of discharge (amount and viscosity), bleeding (with the source identified, e.g. the cervical os) and injuries.

Bimanual examination

A bimanual examination is sometimes indicated, after swabs have been taken, for example, to localize pelvic tenderness or prior to prescribing emergency hormonal contraception.

Male genitalia

Inspection

The foreskin (if present) must be retracted and injuries or abnormalities of the foreskin, penile shaft, scrotal sac or testes noted (including evidence of circumcision and vasectomy).

Perianal area

Inspection

When the complainant describes peno-anal penetration inspect the perianal area carefully with a cool light source; you should have access to a magnifying lens. Again, a colposcope may be used. After obtaining all relevant forensic samples, you can use a moistened swab to tease out the perianal folds to facilitate the inspection. Alternatively, gently stretching the skin with gloved fingers may be required. Note abnormalities such as gaping, swelling, reddening, lacerations (tears), fissures, warts, discharge, haemorrhoids, scars, thickening of the skin or flattening of the normally puckered anal verge margin.

After obtaining the forensic samples, undertake an internal inspection of rectum and anal canal, using an appropriately sized, clear, disposable proctoscope. Any evidence of discharge (amount and viscosity), bleeding (with source identified) and injuries should be recorded.

Digital examination

A digital examination should only be undertaken if clinically indicated. Research has shown that digital examination is not a reliable tool to assess accurately the degree of anal tone.

Forensic samples

Forensic samples are usually obtained using specialist kits available from the local constabulary or direct from manufacturers. These kits are modular and include all the necessary swabs and equipment needed for a forensic examination. Standard medical swabs (with or without transport medium) and polypots should only be used in exceptional circumstances where no forensic kit is available.

The following text gives an overview of the persistence of various body fluids and exogenous substances in different sites and describes how those sites should be sampled. Guidance on forensic sampling is always being updated, so forensic physicians should ensure that they are working in accord with current guidance provided by the Forensic Science Committee of the Faculty of Forensic and Legal Medicine (www.fflm.ac.uk).

For ease of reference the text is divided into a number of sexual acts. It is not exhaustive and, consequently, the doctor may have to adapt the stated principles to the particular case. Further information can be found at www.fflm.ac.uk. Labelling and packaging is covered in Chapter 16. Microbiology/virology samples that may have forensic significance should be handled in accordance

with the 'chain of evidence' guidance produced by the Royal College of Pathologists (www.rcpath.org).

Although this section only refers to obtaining samples from the body of the complainant, the practitioner should be mindful that sanitary towels, panty liners, tampons and clothing worn during or immediately after a sexual act, as well as bedding, towels and inanimate objects may be contaminated with forensic material and should be appropriately packaged and retained.

Principles of forensic sampling

Avoidance of contamination

You must wear gloves throughout the sampling process, and change these when sampling different body orifices or surfaces. All used gloves should be retained and exhibited in a single tamper-evident bag except for gloves used to sample the penis, which should be submitted in a separate bag and labelled accordingly.

If you feel that there is a possibility you will cough or sneeze over an unsheathed swab, wear a facemask as the sample is obtained.

Preparation

You and, when relevant, the police officer should discuss and agree which areas of the body are going to be sampled. Thereafter, it is useful to pre-label the swabs with the description of the sample and 'A' or 'B', to indicate the order of sampling. The label should be rechecked as the swab is placed in the sheath.

'Double swabbing'

Although moist stains will be recovered on dry swabs, in practice most visible stains, or potentially contaminated areas of skin or hair, will be dry. Dry skin (and hair) is sampled using the 'double swab' technique originally described by Sweet et al. [7]. When using this technique the first swab should be moistened with three to four drops of sterile water (dripped on the swab head) then rolled with moderate pressure over the relevant area. Then a second dry swab is immediately rolled with moderate pressure over the same area: the theory is that the first, moist swab loosens any cellular material, which is then adsorbed by the second dry swab. The limited research that has been done to date on DNA extraction from skin swabs has found this sampling technique gives the maximal yield of DNA.

Rolling of the swab head

When swabbing an area of skin the whole of the swab head should be used to maximize the surface area available for recovery. This can be achieved by rolling the swab over the relevant area.

Number of swabs

Two swabs are used at all of the sites that are sampled. The swabs are used, one at a time, to sample the same area. However, if a stain remains visible on a body surface following the use of two swabs, the double swab technique (see above) should be repeated until the stain has been removed completely. Swabs from the same site can be placed in the same tamper-evident bag.

Controls for water and swabs

A control for the batch of swabs and any water used is obtained by dripping three drops of water on an unused swab at the end of sampling.

Packaging and labelling

The exhibits should be bagged, labelled, signed, sealed and handed to the police officer or stored in the Sexual Assault Referral Centre (SARC) freezer/fridge. Samples obtained from suspects should be sealed in their presence to reassure them of the security of the samples.

Vaginal intercourse

During the act of vaginal intercourse spermatozoa and/or seminal fluid may be deposited on the vulva or in the vagina. Research [8, 9] has shown that spermatozoa may be identified on vaginal swabs taken from post-pubertal females up to seven days after vaginal intercourse, although the numbers will decrease incrementally during that time. In exceptional circumstances, for example where the woman has been bed bound since the vaginal intercourse, spermatozoa may persist in the vagina for longer periods. Research has shown that when the vaginal intercourse has occurred two or more days before the samples are taken, endocervical swabs are more likely than high vaginal swabs to be positive for spermatozoa [10]. This study found spermatozoa in the endocervix up to ten days after sexual intercourse.

The current UK advice is that when a patient describes vaginal intercourse in the preceding seven days, or anal intercourse in the preceding three days, swabs should be obtained in the order indicated below. Vaginal swabs are requested even when the allegation is of anal intercourse alone as semen can drain from the vagina into the anus, so negative vaginal swabs and positive anal swabs may be used to support an allegation of anal intercourse alone [8].

The samples should be taken even if the patient is menstruating or has douched/washed/showered/bathed.

(a) Cut or swab pubic hair that appears to be stained with secretions (which may represent semen).

(b) Recover any foreign hairs or debris using single-use disposable forceps and place in a tamper-evident bag.

   If the identity of the perpetrator is unknown, comb the pubic hair over a paper sheet – fold and place, with the comb, into a tamper-evident bag and cut 10–20 pubic hairs close to their roots and package as 'control pubic hair';

(c) Swab (A&B) the vulva and perineum; if the vulval skin (or visible stain) appears dry prior to sampling the first swab should be moist. Label as 'vulva'.

(d) If possible, insert a dry swab approximately 3–5 cm into the vagina. Use gentle rotational movements to sample the lower half/third of the vagina. Repeat with second dry swab. If the vaginal mucosa is markedly dry the first swab can be moistened with sterile water (see skin). Label as 'low vagina'.

(e) If possible, pass an appropriately sized, single use, lubricated (with K–Y Lubricating jelly® or Pedicat®) speculum into the lower half/third of the vagina. Rub two dry swabs, one at a time, over the mucosa of the unsampled upper two thirds/half of the vagina, making sure the fornices are sampled. Label as 'high vagina'. *If it is not possible to pass a speculum, attempt to obtain two 'vaginal swabs' instead, inserting them further than the low vaginal swabs. These replace the high vaginal swabs.*

(f) In addition to the high vaginal swabs, if the vaginal intercourse has occurred two or more days before the examination, and it has been possible to pass a speculum, two small swabs should be used, one at a time, to sample the endocervical canal. Label 'endocervical';

(g) If a speculum is used it should either be retained or swabbed (if speculum is dry the first swab should be wet) then discarded, with the swabs labelled as 'speculum'.

Anal intercourse

Research has shown that spermatozoa may be identified on anal/rectal swabs taken up to three days after anal intercourse, even when defaecation has occurred [8]. These samples should be obtained even if an individual has washed/showered/bathed.

The current UK advice is that when a patient describes anal intercourse in the preceding three days the following samples should be undertaken:

(a) Cut or swab any areas of hair around the perianal area that appear to be stained with secretions (which may represent seminal fluid).

(b) Recover any foreign hairs using single-use disposable forceps and place in a tamper-evident bag.

(c) Swab (A-wet & B-dry) the perianal skin in an area of 3 cm radius from the anus. Label as 'perianal'.

(d) Insert two swabs (A-wet & B-dry), one at a time, 2–3 cm through the anal orifice and gently rotate. Label as 'anal canal'.

(e) If possible pass an appropriately sized, single use, lubricated (K–Y Lubricating Jelly or Pedicat®) proctoscope approximately 3 cm into the anus. Remove the obturator and swab (A&B) the lower rectum. Label as 'rectum'.

(f) If it is not possible to pass a proctoscope (for example because of perianal injury or because of the age of the examinee) an attempt should be made to pass two dry swabs, one at a time, into the anus to sample the lower rectum and anal canal simultaneously. Label as 'rectum/anal canal'.

(g) If a proctoscope is used it should either be retained or swabbed (if proctoscope is dry the first swab should be wet) then discarded, with the swabs labelled as 'proctoscope'.

Oral sexual acts

Oral sexual acts may involve oral contact with the vulva/vagina (cunnilingus), anus (anilingus) or penis (fellatio).

During an act of cunnilingus or anilingus saliva may be deposited on the vulval or anal skin. There are no data regarding persistence of saliva on the skin following these sexual acts. However, research looking at persistence of DNA (in deposited saliva) on other areas of skin indicates that the swabs may give a positive result for up to two days [11]. Therefore, if an act of cunnilingus or anilingus has purportedly occurred in the preceding two days, and the patient has not washed in that time, vulval and low vaginal swabs and perianal swabs should be obtained in the manner described under 'Vaginal intercourse' and 'Anal intercourse' above.

Casework has shown that, following fellatio, spermatozoa may persist in the oral cavity for two days [8]. Therefore, when a patient describes having had a penis placed in the mouth in the preceding two days the following samples should be obtained:

(a) Swab (A&B) the whole of the mouth, including all the surfaces of the tongue, the floor of the mouth, all surfaces of the teeth (with particular attention to the interdental spaces), the gum margins and inside the cheeks. Label as 'mouth'.

(b) A control swab of the mouth wash by dripping three to four drops of the 10 ml ampoule of sterile water allocated for the mouth washings on a third unused swab. Label as 'control mouth wash'.

(c) Use the remainder of the sterile water in the ampoule as a mouth wash and put washings into a polypot. The patient must wear gloves if handling the polypot. Label as 'mouth washings'.

During fellatio it is not uncommon for ejaculation to take place over the head, therefore, consideration should be given to sampling the skin on the face and the hair (see Other sexual/physical acts below).

If the patient has been the subject of fellatio (that is, a mouth has been placed around the penis) in the preceding two days the following samples should be obtained:

(a) Swab (A-wet & B-dry) the coronal sulcus. Label as 'coronal sulcus'.

(b) Swab (A-wet & B-dry) the glans of the penis. Label 'penis – glans'.

(c) Swab (A-wet & B-dry) the shaft of the penis. Label 'penis – shaft'.

Other sexual/physical acts

Other sexual acts involve a number of practices whereby body fluids are transferred from one individual to another such as kissing, licking, biting, ejaculation outside a body orifice and manual handling of the female genital region. The limited data available indicate that positive results for DNA may be obtained up to two days after the body fluid has been deposited on the skin [11]; there are even some case reports of skin swabs being positive for spermatozoa after the patient had 'cleansed'.

Cellular material from skin can be deposited on parts of the body that are handled or gripped. However, these areas should only be swabbed if there is a clear indication (for example, reddening or bruising) of the site where the pressure was applied. When relevant, skin or hair should be sampled using the double swab technique described above.

Any areas of head hair that may be contaminated with semen, or other body fluids should be cut or swabbed. When the target 'stain' or potentially stained area is large or in a prominent area on the head swabbing will be the preferred method of sampling to minimize the distress experienced by the examinee. Any foreign hairs or debris in the hair or on the skin should be recovered using single-use disposable forceps and placed in a tamper-evident bag. If there is a possibility that the hair may be contaminated with fibres (for example, when an item of material has been placed over the head) the head hair should be 'taped', using low adhesive tape, which is then stuck to a sheet of acetate (these items may need to be sourced from a crime scene examiner). Control hair samples (relevant only to cases where the assailant is unidentified) may be collected by cutting 10–20 hairs close to their roots.

Ultraviolet light (delivered via a Wood's Lamp – wavelength 360 nm) is not helpful in identifying semen on the skin but, when semen stains are exposed to a high-intensity light source of variable wavelength (e.g. Poliray®, Bluemaxx® and BM500 Polilight®) and viewed through specialist filters incorporated into goggles, the stain may be visible. However, more research is needed before routine use of these light sources can be recommended [12].

If a struggle has occurred or the complainant, or suspect, is believed to have scratched someone during the assault, fingernails should be clipped (the preferred method of sampling) and the fingernail and cuticle should be swabbed. When the fingernails are too short to be cut, or the patient declines to have fingernails clipped, swabs alone will suffice. The hands should be sampled one at a time, over a piece of paper, and labelled accordingly. The 'double swab' technique described above should be used.

Toxicology

Forensic toxicologists advocate obtaining a blood (10 ml) and a urine sample (20 ml) whenever a complainant/suspect presents within three days of an alleged sexual assault. These are used to screen for drugs and alcohol. If the incident occurred between three and four days previously only a urine sample need be obtained. Current advice recommends that when a patient is seen within 24 hours of an assault, two urine samples should be collected, the first obtained as soon as possible and the second from the next urination. Two consecutive samples obtained soon after the assault will allow a toxicologist to estimate the blood alcohol concentration at the time of the assault if the blood sample (which may not be collected until some time after the incident) is negative.

Although this advice relates to incidents in the preceding four days, a urine sample for analysis of drugs may also be pertinent for longer periods – a toxicologist can give advice on this.

Certain drugs are detectable in head hair, but there is only limited information regarding the success of analysis following single-dose ingestion. Therefore, these samples are not collected routinely. If considered pertinent to the investigation, a sample of head hair for toxicology can be harvested four to six weeks after ingestion using specialist kits which give precise instructions on the sampling and packaging requirements.

Products of conception

If the sexual assault results in a pregnancy that is terminated in accordance with legal requirements and after specialized counselling, the complainant should be asked to consent to retention of the products of conception for DNA analysis. The products of conception are placed in a plain container (not previously used for anything else) by a healthcare professional who was present at the time of the medical or surgical termination. A police officer will be required to collect the specimen directly from the healthcare professional to ensure a chain of evidence. The specimen is then either transported immediately to a forensic science laboratory in a cool box or frozen. In such cases control DNA samples are needed from the mother and the purported father for comparison.

Control samples

Control buccal cells are collected in order to determine the DNA pattern of the individual. They should be deferred for 20 minutes after eating, drinking or smoking and for 48 hours following male-to-male fellatio.

The 'Volunteer DNA sampling kit' should be used for complainants and the 'PACE DNA sampling kit' used for the suspects. Both kits contain instructions for use. Complainants should *not* be asked to consent to their sample being loaded in or on the National DNA Database. These samples may be collected by a trained police officer.

Interpretation of general injuries

The absence of injuries does not negate an allegation of sexual assault. There are many reasons why a complainant is uninjured, which include:

- submission of the victim may be achieved by emotional manipulation, fear of violence or death or by verbal threats;
- the force used, or the resistance offered, is insufficient to produce an injury;
- bruises may not become apparent for 48 hours following the assault, and some bruises are never visible externally;
- a delay in reporting the incident will allow minor injuries to fade or heal.

When injuries are sustained, any type or combination of the injuries described in Chapters 10 – *injuries* – and 17 – *bites* – may be identified. Most of the injuries will be minor and will not require first-aid, but even minor injuries may be forensically significant. Any necessary treatment should be provided as appropriate, and patients with serious injuries such as stab wounds, should be referred urgently for secondary care.

Although it is impossible to age an injury accurately, it should be possible for the doctor to form an opinion whether the appearance of the injury is consistent with it having been produced during the incident in the manner alleged.

Genital and anal findings

Less than half of all complainants of sexual assault have injuries to the genital and anal areas. It is important for the examining doctor to be familiar with the reasons why injuries may not occur. These include:

- the alleged sexual act (such as rubbing, touching) was unlikely to result in injuries;
- sexually experienced;
- the natural elasticity of the post-pubertal female genitalia, including the hymen;
- the natural elasticity of the anus;
- the use of lubricants.

Any of the injuries detailed below may be identified following a sexual assault, although their precise forensic significance is limited by the lack of specific research into their relative prevalence following consensual and non-consensual intercourse. Some of the findings may have alternative non-sexual causes with which the doctor must be cognisant. A detailed discussion on genital injuries can be found in the chapter on sexual assault in *Clinical Forensic Medicine. A Physician's Guide* [13].

Reddening

Reddening of the vulva, penis or anal margins, whether diffuse or localized, is a non-specific finding with a wide range of causative factors including consensual sexual intercourse. While it should be noted it cannot usually be assigned any forensic significance.

Abrasions

Abrasions on the female genitalia (vulva, hymen and vagina), penis and anal margin are produced by the dragging of the skin or contact with rough objects such as fingernails.

Bruises

Genital or anal bruising is indicative of trauma to that area if the skin is otherwise healthy. The pattern of the bruising may be very significant, for example when caused by teeth or blunt trauma through clothing. Bruising of the anal skin can be differentiated from prominent anal margin veins as the latter reduce if compressed.

Lacerations

Small lacerations or tears (normally a few millimetres in length) of the vulva, foreskin, frenulum and anal margins may be produced by excessive stretching of the skin, with or without blunt impact trauma, or be related to local irritation or general medical conditions. In the vulval area they are most commonly identified in the regions of the posterior fourchette and fossa navicularis. When located on the anal margin they are called 'fissures'. The lacerations may be single or multiple.

Minor lacerations usually heal completely but if repeatedly traumatized they may leave scarring, for example around the anal margin (although these may be concealed by the anal folds). Anal tags are said to be formed where anal fissures have healed.

Fresh lacerations (tears) of the hymen may be complete or incomplete depending on the original size of the hymenal opening, the size of the penetrating object and the elasticity of the tissues. When fresh, the edges of the transection may bleed but healing in this area is remarkably rapid. The presence of chronic or healed transections may be relevant if the extent of previous sexual activity is questioned.

Lacerations within the vagina are rare findings, most commonly identified at the fornices. They are seen infrequently following consensual intercourse when there may be predisposing factors such as vaginal surgery or atrophic tissues [12]. Some lacerations will bleed extensively, requiring resuscitation and surgical intervention. It is extremely difficult to differentiate a laceration of the vagina from an incised wound as many of the features typically seen in a lacerated wound are difficult to identify in this area. Therefore, the differential diagnosis of a vaginal laceration would have to include causation by a sharp object such as glass.

Deep perianal lacerations that extend through the muscle or into the anal canal/rectum are caused by significant dilatation of the anus and are rarely seen following consensual anal intercourse.

Incisions

Incisions on the genital or anal skin or mucosa are forensically significant as they are indicative of contact with sharp objects such as jewellery. Incisions of the penile skin can be associated with sadomasochistic gratification.

Subsequent to the examination

After completion of the examination procedure, the complainant should be offered the opportunity to bathe and wash her hair. This gives you time to complete notes and finish packaging the exhibits.

When the patient is seen as part of a police investigation it is important that you apprise the police of the relevant findings. A written summary will ensure all parties are clear what has been found. The forensic physician should retain a copy of any written reports given to the police.

Emergency contraception

If the sexual assault has exposed the patient to a risk of pregnancy the forensic physician should discuss emergency contraception with her. Unprotected sexual intercourse includes sexual intercourse with withdrawal prior to apparent ejaculation and when there has been ejaculation upon the external genitalia. Currently in the United Kingdom two methods of emergency contraception are available (see below).

Oral hormonal method (levonorgestrel emergency contraceptive, LNG EC)

Levonelle-1500® (prescription only) and Levonelle One Step® are only licensed for use within 72 hours of an act of unprotected sexual intercourse. However, they may be given between 73 and 120 hours after unprotected sexual intercourse as long as the patient is informed that such use is outside the product licence, that there is limited evidence of efficacy in this period and that an intrauterine device is an alternative [14].

LNG EC is most effective when given within 12 hours of the unprotected sexual intercourse and its efficacy decreases incrementally thereafter. *Therefore, all doctors who examine complainants of sexual assault should have ready access to supplies of Levonelle-1500.*

Most patients only require one Levonelle-1500 tablet. However, patients who are on concurrent liver enzyme-inducing drugs (including St John's wort) should be given two 1.5 mg tablets (total 3 mg) as a single dose (this is unlicensed use) [14].

Patients should be told that if their period does not start within seven days of when it is expected, or is unusual in any way, they should attend a family planning clinic or their primary care physician for a pregnancy test.

Intrauterine devices

A copper-containing intrauterine device can be inserted in the normal way to prevent a pregnancy for up to five days (120 hours) after the most likely expected day of ovulation. That is calculated from the expected date of next menses (based on the previous shortest cycle length) minus 14 and plus 5. The result is given in good faith, based on the patient's menstrual data, and applies irrespective of the number of earlier acts of unprotected intercourse. Intrauterine devices have been estimated to be 99.9% effective in preventing a pregnancy.

Complainants who request or who are considering an intrauterine device should be offered LNG EC (if they present within 120 hours) *and* referred urgently to a family planning clinic where their suitability for an intrauterine device will be discussed.

Sexually transmitted infections (STIs)

The FFLM leaflet 'What Happens Now' (www.fflm. ac.uk) should be used when discussing the following issues with a complainant of sexual assault.

For many complainants of serious sexual offences, the initial physical and psychological trauma is superseded by the fear of acquiring human immunodeficiency virus (HIV). Fortunately, they can be reassured that the risk of contracting HIV during a sexual assault is believed to be extremely low (see Chapter 14). However, there is a risk of acquiring other STIs. The need for STI screening and prophylaxis will depend on the nature and timing of the assault, and any information that is available regarding the assailant. These issues are covered in detail in Chapter 14.

Suspects who have symptoms or signs suggestive of an STI should be advised to attend a genito-urinary clinic. If the suspect is remanded in custody a medical officer at the local detention centre can be asked to organize this. In such circumstances the police seek the consent of the suspect or a court order to obtain the results.

The psychological consequences of sexual assault

The immediate and long-term psychological sequelae experienced following a sexual assault will vary among individuals. However, patterns are now recognized which equate to the reactions following other extraordinarily stressful events such as mass disasters, robbery and war.

Immediate phase

Only some of the complainants of sexual assault are emotionally expressive immediately following the incident (the stereotypical image of a person who has recently been sexually assaulted is a distraught, frightened individual) while others will dissociate themselves from the incident, appearing calm and controlled. Pre-existing or a past history of mental or physical illness or social problems may influence the initial behaviour of the complainant [15].

Heterosexual men are often very distressed that they had an erection and, on occasions, ejaculated during non-consensual anal intercourse. These responses can cause them to doubt their sexual orientation. They can be reassured by the knowledge that this is simply a physiological response and does not necessarily reflect sexual excitement.

Self-reproach is a common theme which can be addressed by the examining physician and advice given.

Long-term response

Most will experience an acute stress reaction in the weeks following sexual assault. The most common are listed in Box 13.3. By definition, post-traumatic stress disorder cannot be diagnosed until symptoms persist for one month. Nevertheless, most women who report rape fulfil the other diagnostic criteria for post-traumatic stress disorder in the first week following the incident. Although many will recover fully, nearly half will continue to suffer from significant psychological problems three months after the assault [16].

The severity of the psychological disturbance appears to be unrelated to the particular sexual act(s) or degree of associated physical assault; complainants of attempted rape and acquaintance rape sometimes experience the most psychological trauma.

A consequence of these psychological sequelae is that the complainants of rape become frequent users of medical services for months, and often years, following the incident. Behavioural responses such as moving home, changing employment and not going out alone may also be found. The combination of behavioural, somatic and psychological reactions following a sexual assault have been termed 'The Rape Trauma Syndrome' [15].

Box 13.3 Recognized responses to sexual assault

PSYCHOLOGICAL REACTIONS	SOMATIC SYMPTOMS
Intrusive thoughts	Sleep disturbances
Avoidance	Anorexia
Heightened arousal	Headaches
Numbing	Nausea
Poor concentration	Abdominal pain
Irritability	Genito-urinary
Fear	discomfort
Sexual dysfunction	
Depression	
Low esteem	
Suicidal ideation	

To minimize the psychological consequences appropriate advice on support and counselling agencies (primary care physician, Victim Support, Survivors, Social Services) should be given in writing together with encouragement to seek emotional and practical support from a trusted friend or family member. The doctor should ask specifically whether or not the complainant wishes her own primary care physician to be informed about the alleged incident.

The medico-legal implications of pregnancy

The medico-legal ramifications of pregnancy and the postnatal period are manifold and extend beyond the immediate brief of this chapter. However, the forensic physician should be familiar with the issues discussed below.

Termination of pregnancy

The Offences Against the Person Act (OAPA) 1861 makes it a criminal offence to attempt, or achieve, a termination of a continuing pregnancy unless the strict requirements of the Human Fertilisation and Embryology Act (HFEA) 1990 are fulfilled; HFEA does not apply in Northern Ireland. Prior to the legislation allowing medical terminations (Abortion Act 1967) illegal abortions accounted for a

significant proportion of maternal deaths (due to vagal inhibition, air embolus, primary haemorrhage, bowel perforations or secondary infections).

Except where there is a genuine medical emergency (when treatment is immediately necessary to save the life of the pregnant woman or to prevent grave permanent injury to her physical or mental health) two registered medical practitioners are required to certify that the decision to terminate is appropriate. All terminations must be notified to the Chief Medical Officer, Department of Health. The products of conception may be required for DNA profiling to determine paternity if the pregnancy resulted from a sexual assault.

Terminations can only take place up to the 24th week of pregnancy where the indication is that '. . . the continuance of the pregnancy would involve greater risk, greater than if the pregnancy were terminated, of injury to the physical or mental health of the pregnant woman (or any existing children in the family of the pregnant woman)'. However, when 'the termination is necessary to prevent grave permanent injury to the physical or mental health of the pregnant woman', or there is a 'risk to the life of the pregnant woman (greater than if the pregnancy were terminated)', or 'there is a substantial risk that if the child were born it would suffer from such physical or mental abnormalities as to be seriously handicapped' there is currently no upper limit for the termination. The Infant Life Preservation Act 1929 states that it is an offence to kill a child which was capable of being born alive, a crime known as 'child destruction'. However the Infant Life (Preservation) Act (never applicable in Scotland) does not apply to terminations after 24 weeks conducted in accordance with HFEA.

Stillbirth

The decreased mortality of very premature infants was also recognized in the Stillbirth (Definition) Act 1992. This Act requires that all children delivered after 24 weeks' gestation, which show no sign of life, be registered as stillbirths.

Concealment of birth

It is a civil offence to fail to notify the birth of a child. It is also a criminal offence under the OAPA for any person to dispose of the body of a dead child secretly, regardless of whether the child died before, during or after birth. In order to trace the mother, investigating officers may require a forensic physician to state whether a suspected female shows signs of recent delivery (Box 13.4). Furthermore, DNA analysis of both the suspected mother and the dead child can be undertaken. Pathological assessment may assist in the determination of fetal age.

Box 13.4 Signs of recent delivery

- Engorged lactating breasts
- Pink striae on the abdomen
- Enlarged uterus
- Fresh tears of the vulva, vagina or cervix
- Bloodstained serous discharge (lochia) from the uterus

In Scotland, by the Concealment of Pregnancy Act 1809, a pregnant woman who conceals her being with child during the whole period of her pregnancy and does not call for, nor make use of, help or assistance at the birth may be charged if the child is found dead or missing.

Infanticide

If it can be shown that a woman has caused the death of her child within one year of its birth, whether by wilful act or omission, she may be charged with murder or, if the balance of her mind can be shown to be disturbed because of the recent delivery or lactation, infanticide (Infanticide Act 1938). Infanticide is analogous to manslaughter in having the advantage of case-dependent, not mandatory, sentencing. Proof that the child had a separate existence from its mother is fundamental to the charge of infanticide. However, there are very few signs that confirm a neonate had a separate existence; the most obvious are food in the stomach or separation of the stump of the umbilical cord.

Sexual variations

Normal sexuality is variously described as behaviour overtly approved of by society, statistically common or biologically desirable in the sense of leading to procreation [17]. Sexual behaviour and gender identity disorders deviating from the norm are considered to be sexual variations or paraphilia (Box 13.5).

Box 13.5 Definitions of sexual variations

Homosexuality	Same gender
Transsexualism	Belief that person is of opposite sex from own bodily sex
Fetishism	Object
Transvestism	Dressing in clothing of the opposite sex
Zoophilia	Animal (bestiality)
Paedophilia	Child
Exhibitionism	Exposure of genitals to opposite sex
Voyeurism	Spying on others undressing or indulging in sexual intercourse
Sexual masochism	Sexual pleasure from receiving pain
Sexual sadism	Sexual pleasure from causing pain
Coprophilia	Faeces
Frotteurism	Rubbing
Telephone scatoglia	Lewdness
Necrophilia	Corpse
Electrophilia	Electrical impulse
Anaesthesiophilia	Using volatile substance, e.g. chloroform, ether, butane

---

Sexual variant behaviour may be illegal if it involves children, animals, sadism, exhibitionism or frotteurism. Unless combined with a recognized mental disorder, sexual 'deviations' (variations) are specifically excluded from the Mental Health Act 1983 (s1.3). Some offences can only be committed by a person of a specific sex.

Some sexual variations involve inherently life-threatening practices. These include autoerotic asphyxia (using strangulation, hanging, gagging, plastic bag asphyxia, inverted suspension), electro-philia and anaesthesiophilia. When accidental deaths do occur in these circumstances associated paraphernalia may be present at the scene, such as evidence of transvestism, bondage, pornographic material or mirrors. Family members or friends who discover the body in these situations may, in an attempt to preserve the reputation of the deceased, remove certain articles. In doing so they may create a scene erroneously considered a suicide or homicide. When the truth is divulged sympathetic explanations are necessary for reassur-ance that these deaths are usually accidental.

REFERENCES

1. HM Crown Prosecution Service Inspectorate (2007) *Without Consent.* Her Majesty's Inspectorate of Constabulary. Available at www.inspectorates.home office.gov.uk/hmic

2. Association of Chief Police Officers Rape Working Group (2003) *Sexual Assault Referral Centres (SARC): 'Getting Started'.* Home Office. Available at www.police. homeoffice.gov.uk/publications/operational-policing/sarcs-getting-started

3. Faculty of Forensic and Legal Medicine (2008) *Consent from Patients who may have been Seriously Assaulted.* Available at www.fflm.ac.uk

4. Walter H, Dalton M (2004) Taking a history. In: Dalton M, ed. *Forensic Gynaecology* London: RCOG Press pp. 66–75.

5. General Medical Council (2004) *Confidentiality: Protecting and Providing Information.* London: GMC.

6. Girardin BW, Faugno DK, Seneski PC, Slaughter L, Whelan M (1997) *Color Atlas of Sexual Assault.* St. Louis: Mosby.

7. Sweet D, Lorente M, Lorente JA, Valenzuela A, Villanueva E (1997) An improved method to recover saliva from human skin: the double swab technique. *Journal of the Forensic Science Society* **42**: 320–2.

8. Keating SM, Allard JE (1994) What's in a name? Medical samples and scientific evidence in sexual assaults. *Medicine Science and the Law* **34**: 187–201.

9. Willott GM, Allard JE (1982) Spermatozoa – their persistence after sexual intercourse. *Forensic Science International* **19**: 135–54.

10. Wilson EM (1982) A comparison of the persistence of seminal constituents in the human vagina and cervix. *Police Surgeon* **22**: 44–5.

11. Sweet D, Lorente JA, Lorente M, Villanueva E (1997) PCR-based DNA typing of saliva stains recovered from human skin. *Journal of the Forensic Science Society* **42**(3): 447–51.

12. Rogers DJ (2004) The general examination. In: Dalton M, ed. *Forensic Gynaecology.* London: RCOG Press, pp. 91–104.

13. Rogers DJ, Newton M (2005) Sexual assault examination. In: Stark MM, ed. *Clinical Forensic Medicine. A Physician's Guide* Totowa, NJ: Humana Press.

14. Faculty of Family Planning and Reproductive Health Care Clinical Effectiveness Unit (FFPRHC) (April 2006) *Emergency Contraception Guidance.* Available at www. ffprhc.org.uk

15. Burgess AW, Holstrom LL (1974) Rape trauma syndrome. *American Journal of Psychiatry* **131**: 981–6.

16. Rothbraum BO, Foa EB, Riggs DS, Murdoch T, Walsh WA (1992) Prospective examination of post traumatic stress disorder in rape victims. *Journal of Traumatic Stress* **5**: 455–75.

17. Faulk M (1988) *Basic Forensic Psychiatry.* Oxford: Blackwell Scientific Publications.

14

Management of at-risk exposures and infection control in custody

Felicity Nicholson

Introduction

This chapter provides information on the preva-lence of hepatitis B, hepatitis C and human immunodeficiency virus (HIV) – collectively referred to as blood-borne viruses (BBVs) – in risk groups, identifies the risks of specific body fluids and the routes of transmission. It further acts as a guide to the immediate management of at-risk exposures from BBVs both for the recipient and the contact, and any follow-up management this may entail. It will also cover some basic infection control guidance that will be helpful in the safe and practical day-to-day running of a custody suite. Although not exhaustive, it aims to cover the more commonly raised concerns and how best they should be managed.

Prevalence of BBVs: at-risk groups, body fluids and routes of transmission

Hepatitis B

Around 350 million people worldwide are chronic-ally infected with hepatitis B and are therefore at risk of developing chronic liver disease. There are around 180000 people in this category in the UK. In general the world can be divided into three broad areas by prevalence of chronic infection

(Table 14.1). About 75% of the world's population live in areas of high prevalence.

The virus can be transmitted through contact with body fluids (blood, saliva, semen, vaginal fluids, sweat, breast milk and any other if blood-stained) via percutaneous or mucosal exposure. In areas of high prevalence, infection most commonly occurs perinatally or in early childhood. In areas of intermediate prevalence, needle sharing, acupunc-ture, tattooing and body piercing are also important modes of transmission. In the UK the number of acute cases of hepatitis B peaked in 1982 with 2000. Since then the number has declined, reaching a low of 512 in 1992. Since 1993 the number of cases per annum ranges from 600 to 800 with 97% of acute infections occurring in people over 15. The highest incidence is in the 15–29 age-group. Most people become infected through injecting drug use or sexual intercourse, with homosexual transmission being higher than heterosexual transmission. Around 12% of cases are travel-related to areas of high or intermediate prevalence mainly through sexual contact or medical treatment. In England and Wales the most reliable data are from 2003 due to a decline in the quality of reporting in 2004 and 2005. This showed that injecting drug use was the main risk factor for hepatitis B infection, accounting for 38% of those with a known risk factor in England, 27% in Wales and 6% in Scotland (2003–5). Overall it is estimated that more than one

Clinical Forensic Medicine, third edition ed. W.D.S. McLay. Published by Cambridge University Press. © Cambridge University Press 2009.

Table 14.1. Prevalence of chronic infection
of hepatitis B by world areas

Prevalence	Areas
Low <2%	Most of Western Europe (including UK), North America, Australia (excluding Aborigines), New Zealand
Intermediate 2–8%	Mediterranean, the Amazon Basin, most of the Middle East, Japan, the Indian subcontinent and southern parts of Eastern and Central Europe
High >8%	Sub-Saharan Africa, most of Asia and the Pacific Islands

Table 14.2. Exposure categories of HIV infections
diagnosed in the UK in 2003 (% of total)

MSM	Heterosexual	IDU	Mother → infant	Other/ undetermined
26%	58%	2%	2%	12%

in five injecting drug users have been infected with hepatitis B and new cases are still occurring with the prevalence of hepatitis B core antibody (anti-HBc) increasing from 3.4% in 1997 to 7.1% in 2005 in those who started injecting in the previous three years. Unlinked anonymous surveys conducted in England, Wales and Northern Ireland in 2005 showed that there was a higher prevalence amongst those injecting crack cocaine than in those who did not [1]. Most newly reported cases of chronic hepatitis B infections in England and Wales occur among immigrants (6571 versus 269 in non-immigrants in a survey conducted from 1995 to 2000).

Hepatitis B vaccine coverage continues to increase, with the majority of intravenous drug users (IDUs) in contact with drug treatment agencies and prison services having taken up the offer of vaccination. In England, 126 of 143 prisons reported offering vaccination at the end of 2006. The Scottish Prison Service introduced a hepatitis B vaccination programme to all inmates in 1999, and since then there have been no outbreaks of acute hepatitis B infection among IDUs in Scotland.

Blood and the aforementioned body fluids containing hepatitis B surface antigen (HBsAg) are considered infectious. This may be as a result of acute or chronic infection. The degree of infectivity depends on the presence or absence of other markers. The highest infectivity occurs when the

person is HBsAg and hepatitis B e antigen (HBeAg) positive; intermediate infectivity occurs if HBsAg is the only marker, and low infectivity when HBsAg is accompanied by hepatitis B e antibody (HBeAb). The risk of acquiring hepatitis B from a single needlestick exposure varies from <10% to 40% depending on the status of the source.

Human immunodeficiency virus (HIV)

By the end of 2003, the number of people aged 15 or over living with HIV in the UK was estimated at 53 000. Some 14 300 (27%) of these were unaware that they were infected. In terms of risk groups, 46% of the cumulative total since 1993 were men who have sex with men (MSM) and 26% of these were unaware. Heterosexual men and women living in the UK formed the highest risk group (48.9% of the cumulative total since 1993) with nearly 30% being unaware of their status. Black African men and women had the highest prevalence and formed 62% of this group with 45% unaware. Heterosexual intercourse accounted for 58% of all new diagnoses reported in 2003 (Table 14.2) compared with 31% in 1994. Although there has been a steady increase in the prevalence of previously undiagnosed HIV acquired through heterosexual intercourse occurring in those born in the UK, three quarters of all new diagnoses were probably acquired in Africa. Conversely 84% of new cases occurring in MSM were probably acquired in the UK [1, 2].

The main focus of the HIV epidemic continues to be in London, where 52% of the diagnoses made in 2003 were among London residents. Surveys conducted show that the incidence of HIV is still increasing despite efforts to educate and reduce risks. In MSM the incidence in 2003 was estimated at 3.7% seroconversions (appearance of antibodies) per year. On a more positive note the uptake of voluntary confidential testing within this group has increased from 47% in 1998 to 64% in 2003 in those attending 16 genito-urinary medicine clinics in England and Wales.

The prevalence of HIV among IDUs in England and Wales has increased in recent years with an estimate of 1 in 50 being infected by mid 2006. The rate in London is higher at 1 in 25 (4%), but the highest change has occurred elsewhere in England and Wales with current estimates at 1 in 65 compared with 1 in 400 in 2003. In Scotland, about 1 in 110 IDUs are probably infected with HIV. There is still evidence of on going transmission of HIV in the UK among IDUs, but the proportion acquired abroad has declined. Surveys conducted anonymously found that more than half of the IDUs who were HIV positive were unaware of their status. This is twice the level seen in 2003 [1].

Since 1984 five cases of occupationally acquired HIV infection have been reported in healthcare workers (HCWs) in the UK with one case seroconverting despite post-exposure prophylaxis (PEP) with triple therapy. A further 14 HCWs have been found to be HIV positive with no risk factors other than their occupation to account for their infection. However, baseline blood samples were unavailable to corroborate the findings. Eleven out of the 14 had worked in sub-Saharan Africa and all had worked in countries with a higher HIV prevalence than the UK.

The risk of acquiring HIV following a single needlestick exposure with fresh blood is estimated at 0.3%. The risk is increased with hollow bore needles, where the contact has a high viral load at the time of seroconversion or in later stages of HIV disease and where the needle is visibly bloodstained or has been in an artery or vein. The risk of acquiring HIV through mucous membrane exposure (mouth/eye) is estimated at 0.09%. High-risk body fluids include blood, or other blood-stained body fluids. Urine, vomit, saliva or faeces are generally considered low or no risk unless they

Table 14.3. Risks of HIV transmission

Type of exposure	Estimated risk of HIV transmission per exposure (%)
Blood transfusion (one unit)	90–100
Sharing injection equipment	0.67
Needle stick injury	0.3
Mucous membrane exposure	0.09
Receptive anal intercourse	0.1–0.3
Receptive vaginal intercourse	0.1–0.2
Insertive anal intercourse	0.06
Insertive vaginal intercourse	0.03–0.09
Receptive oral sex (fellatio)	0–0.04

are bloodstained. A summary of the risks of HIV transmission following an exposure from a known HIV-positive individual is shown in Table 14.3 [3].

Hepatitis C (HCV)

The HCV was first discovered in 1989. It is estimated that around 200000 people in England have chronic hepatitis C. In the UK, the major route of HCV transmission is through sharing equipment for injecting drug use, most commonly through blood-contaminated needles and syringes. The current estimate is that one in two IDUs are infected in the UK and, whilst this is still low compared with other countries, evidence suggests that it is continuing to increase. The highest areas of prevalence are in London, Glasgow and North West England (more than half infected) with Wales and the north east of England having the lowest prevalence of one in four or less. Spoons, filters and water may also transmit infection if contaminated with blood. Current guidelines from the Department of Health recommend that drug users should not share any part of their equipment.

Other routes of infection are as follows:

- Receiving a blood transfusion or blood products prior to September 1991 when screening was introduced in the UK. This has been shown to account for the majority of cases of post-transfusion non-A, non-B hepatitis.

- Transmission from mother to baby is estimated at around 6%, but this can increase to around 15% with concomitant HIV.
- Sexual transmission occurs but is not common, with estimates of around 5% or less in sexual partners of those with HCV. There is an increased risk for those with multiple sexual partners.
- The risk through occupational exposure following a single needlestick injury with an HCV RNA positive source is estimated at 1.8%.
- Tattooing, acupuncture, ear or body piercing with unsterilized equipment.
- There are no data of the risk of hepatitis C through a bite. With saliva alone the risk is considered to be very low. However, if there is blood in the mouth the risk increases and could be taken to be about the same as that following a single needlestick injury.

The average time from exposure to onset of symptoms is about six weeks, with seroconversion at around eight to nine weeks. This can be delayed as long as nine months and may be absent in immunocompromised patients, those with renal failure or hepatitis C virus cryoglobulinaemia. This is important when testing contacts, as it may be necessary to test for viral RNA using molecular amplification techniques (see investigations below).

Around 75–85% of people develop chronic infection indicated by persistently raised or fluctuating liver function tests (LFTs). Chronic infection often goes undetected for years unless accidentally identified during routine screening. Cirrhosis develops in about 10–20% of patients after 20–30 years and between 1% and 5% will develop hepatocellular carcinoma.

Factors associated with a more rapid progression to severe liver disease include being over 40 at the time of initial infection, the level of alcohol consumption, being male, co-infection with HIV or hepatitis B and immunosuppressive therapy.

Around one third of HIV-positive people have concomitant infection with HCV. Improved treatment regimens for HIV have led to an increase in survival rates and this has led to a rise in the number of cases in end-stage liver failure secondary to HCV infection with rapidly progressive fibrosis and cirrhosis.

Immediate management following an exposure to BBVs

The immediate management following a potential exposure depends not on the virus but on the route of infection. The routes can be divided into three broad categories:

1. parenteral exposure, e.g. needlestick, bites or other sharps injury;
2. mucous membrane exposure, e.g. mouth and eyes;
3. contamination of non-intact skin (< 24 hours old).

Where there has been a penetration of the skin or contamination of an open wound, encourage gentle bleeding from the site. Then wash the wound with soap and warm running water, but do not scrub or apply antiseptics. Mucous membranes should be irrigated copiously with sterile water. If the recipient is wearing contact lenses then they should be removed and the eyes irrigated again.

It is important to gather as much information as possible from the recipient about the exposure. This is summarized in Table 14.4.

This follows the WHEN, HOW and WHAT principles. WHEN did it occur (date and time); HOW was the exposure caused (bite, spit, needlestick, contamination of broken skin); and WHAT body fluids were involved (blood, bloodstained fluid, saliva)?

Other information should also be sought as to the health of the recipient, specifically asking if they are immunosuppressed, if they are on any medication or have previously received medication for any of the BBVs. This would include antiretroviral treatment for hepatitis B and HIV, and ribavirin and interferon therapy for hepatitis C. Check whether they have been vaccinated for hepatitis B and if so how many doses they received and when, and whether their antibody levels were checked at

Table 14.4. Summary of information required following a potential exposure

Date and time of incident				
Nature of incident	Bite	Spit	Splash*	Needlestick injury (NSI)
Material	Blood	Bloodstained fluid		Saliva
Site of injury	Skin	Mucosa	Eye	Mouth
Injury type	Puncture	Laceration		
If NSI	Fresh	Discarded	Visible blood	
	Hollow	Solid		
Injury through	Gloves	Clothes	No protection	

Note:
*Contamination of broken skin.

any time. All these factors will play a part in the decision-making process for further management (see Follow-up management, below).

The final piece of information required is WHO – referring to the contact. If the contact is known, again gather as much information as possible. Ideally the healthcare professional should talk with and examine the contact, with valid consent. Ask about specific risk behaviours such as injecting drug use whether current or historic; a detailed sexual history; country of origin; history of blood transfusions and/or surgical procedures including when and where they were carried out. Ask the contact the same questions as the recipient about health, medication and vaccination. Elicit details of any time spent in prison or contact with drug treatment agencies. If this is done in a sympathetic and non-judgemental way, explaining why this information is needed, one can often be successful in gaining trust and receiving honest answers. It is also worth asking the arresting or investigating officer for any useful background information.

A sample of clotted blood (ideally 10 ml but not less than 0.5 ml) should be taken from the contact and placed in a yellow top tube. The sample can only be taken with specific consent for testing for HIV, hepatitis B and hepatitis C. A consent form should be completed and sent with the blood to the designated hospital. An example of a consent form is shown in Fig. 14.1. Further details about the use of the consent form are given later in the section on specific management of HIV.

Follow-up management

Specialist management of any potential exposure is required to ensure that the optimum treatment is given where relevant. This would be handled at the same time for all the viruses, but it is easier to discuss them as separate entities. It is important that all police personnel be aware of the importance of reporting at-risk incidents immediately. A system of 24-hour cover should be in place. This could be primarily occupational health during working hours, and accident and emergency (A&E) departments after hours. The A&E staff should have access to on-call expert advice. Such experts could be consultants in virology, microbiology, infectious diseases, HIV medicine, genitourinary medicine or occupational health. They could also include public health physicians, namely consultants in communicable disease control (consultants in public health in Scotland). The occupational health departments for the different constabularies should also be involved acting either as a point of referral or to collate information about police personnel following any exposure.

Specific management for hepatitis B

Hepatitis B, unlike HIV or hepatitis C, can be prevented before exposure by administering hepatitis B vaccine. Pre-exposure vaccination is used for those who are at increased risk of hepatitis B because of their lifestyle, occupation or other factors. The

---

Part 1

I, ... having discussed with
.... who is a Forensic Medical Examiner/Healthcare
Practitioner to the ....(insert Constabulary), hereby consent to give a sample of my
blood for testing for hepatitis B virus, hepatitis C virus and human immunodeficiency virus
(HIV). I also authorize the testing laboratory to inform the Senior Physician in Occupational
Health, ...(insert Constabulary), of the results of the tests and agree that the
results may also be released to ....(insert name and shoulder
number of police officer (recipient)). If I so wish, the results may also be communicated to
the Healthcare Practitioner/Primary Care Physician named in Part 2 of this form.

I do/do not* wish to be informed of the results.

Signed.....................................   Address....................................

                                            ....

                                            ....
                                            Contact No. ....

Signature
witnessed by.............................   ....

Countersigned
by FME...................................   ....

*Delete as applicable
Part 2
I would also like the result of the test to be communicated to the Healthcare Practitioner/
Primary Care Physician named below.
....

THIS FORM SHOULD ACCOMPANY THE BLOOD SAMPLE

Fig. 14.1 Consent form.

following groups of people ideally should be offered
vaccination:
- IDUs (including their sexual partners and children, and non-injecting users living with current injectors)
- MSM and male and female commercial sex workers
- Close family contacts of a case or an individual with chronic hepatitis B infection
- Families adopting children from countries with a high or intermediate prevalence of hepatitis B
- Some foster carers
- Recipients of regular blood or blood products and their carers

- Patients with chronic renal failure or chronic liver disease
- Inmates of custodial institutions
- Those with learning difficulties in residential accommodation
- Travellers to areas of high or intermediate prevalence
- Individuals at occupational risk

Hepatitis B vaccine was originally licensed to be given at 0, 1 and 6 months and can still be used where rapid protection is not required. However, for pre-exposure prophylaxis in high-risk groups or where compliance may be difficult to achieve with the longer schedule, and for post-exposure prophylaxis (PEP), an accelerated schedule with doses at 0, 1 and 2 months should be used. A fourth dose given a year later is recommended for those at continued risk, and is considered to produce similar response rates as with the original course. More recently, Engerix B has been licensed for a very rapid schedule of three doses at 0, 7 and 21 days with a further dose at one year. This is recommended for adults over 18 who are at immediate risk and could include IDUs and prisoners. This schedule, although unlicensed, may also be used for those aged 16–18 where there is a need for rapid protection and better compliance.

Hepatitis B surface antibody (anti-HBS) levels are used as an indicator of vaccine response. This blood test should be carried out 1–4 months after the primary course. Levels over 100 mIU/ml are considered to show an effective response, although most people consider a level of 10 mIU/ml or more to be adequate to protect against infection. The reason for the discrepancy is that some assays are not particularly specific at lower levels and therefore levels of 100 mIU/ml give greater confidence.

Ten to fifteen per cent of adults fail to respond or are poor responders to vaccination. Factors that are associated with a poor or no response include: >40 years, obesity, smoking, alcoholics with advanced liver disease, immunosuppressed or those on renal dialysis. Table 14.5 gives a summary of the guidelines following a primary course of hepatitis B vaccination in immunocompetent individuals [4].

Table 14.5. Summary of the guidelines following a primary course of hepatitis B vaccination in immnuocompetent individuals

Titres (1–4 months post primary course)	Management
≥ 100 mIU/ml	Boost at 5 years
10–100 mIU/ml	Boost at time of result and boost at 5 years
< 10 mIU/ml	Non-response to vaccine. Test for current or past markers of infection. Repeat course of vaccine. Retest after 1–4 months Still < 10 mIU/ml and no markers require HBIG post exposure

Note:
HBIG, hepatitis B immunoglobulin.

Regardless of previous antibody titres those who have been exposed to a known hepatitis B-positive contact or have had a high-risk exposure should be given a dose of vaccine.

Post-exposure prophylaxis (PEP) for hepatitis B

National guidance in the UK gives detailed advice on the use of hepatitis B vaccine and specific hepatitis B immunoglobulin (HBIG) for PEP [4]. Vaccination is not needed for those known to be HBsAg positive or who have had past infection, but vaccination should not be delayed if test results are not rapidly available. Hepatitis B immunoglobulin provides passive immunity and is given together with hepatitis B vaccine unless the recipient is known to be a non-responder to hepatitis B vaccine. It is used only in high-risk exposures when the recipient has not been or has been incompletely vaccinated, or in non-responders. Ideally it should be given within 48 hours but may be considered for up to a week after exposure. The HBIG used in the UK is derived from plasma sources outside the UK due to the theoretical risk of variant Creutzfeldt–Jakob disease.

Table 14.6. Hepatitis B prophylaxis following exposure incidents

HBV status recipient		Significant exposure			Non-significant exposure	
	HBsAg +ve source	Unknown source	HBsAg −ve source	Continued risk	No further risk
≤1 dose HBV pre-exposure	Accelerated course of HB vaccine HBIG X 1	Accelerated course of HB vaccine	Initiate course of HB vaccine	Initiate course of HB vaccine	No HBV prophylaxis
≥2 doses HBV pre-exposure (anti-HBs not known)	One dose of HB vaccine + 2nd dose 1 month later	One dose of HB vaccine	Finish course of HB vaccine	Finish course of HB vaccine	No HB prophylaxis Reassure
Known responder to HBV (anti-HBs ≥10mIU/ml)	Consider booster dose of HB vaccine	Consider booster dose of HB vaccine	Consider booster dose of HB vaccine	Consider booster dose of HB vaccine	No HB prophylaxis Reassure
Known non-responder to HBV (anti-HBs <10 mIU/ml 2–4 months post-immunization)	HBIG X 1 Consider booster dose of HB vaccine	HBIG X 1 Consider booster dose of HB vaccine	No HBIG Consider booster dose of HB vaccine	No HBIG Consider booster dose of HB vaccine	No prophylaxis Reassure

Notes:
- A baseline clotted blood sample (yellow tube) should be taken at initial assessment for storage. Anti-HBs should be requested if there is any history of HB vaccination.
- An accelerated course of vaccine comprises three doses at 0, 1 and 2 months. A booster dose should be given at 12 months to those at continued risk of exposure to HBV. A standard course comprises three doses at 0, 1 and 6 months.
- Test for anti-HBs (clotted blood) 6–8 weeks after the last dose of the accelerated or standard course. If recipient already immune or a previous known vaccine responder and only needs a booster dose, no further tests required.

HBIG, hepatitis B immunoglobulin.
Anti-HBs, hepatitis B surface antibodies.
Source: Source [5].

This means supplies are scarce and so should only be used as indicated. When used in conjunction with hepatitis B vaccine HBIG should be given in a different site (usually the upper outer quadrant of the gluteus muscle) with the vaccine usually being given in the deltoid muscle. The use of hepatitis B vaccine and/or HBIG for PEP is summarized in Table 14.6.

Specific management for HIV

Robust systems of reporting and effective protocols for referral are paramount in the management of potential exposures to HIV to increase the likelihood of PEP being given appropriately and maximize the chance that it will work. The decision to give PEP and the need for follow up depends on the nature of the exposure. This is summarized in Table 14.7 [5]. The decision on which drugs to use for PEP will be made by the expert, but most commonly will include the following:

Combivir – One tablet bd. (zidovudine 300 mg and lamivudine 150 mg)

Plus

Kaletra – two tablets bd. (lopinavir 400 mg and ritonavir 100 mg).

Table 14.7. Guidelines for administration of PEP follow up after potential HIV exposure

Exposure incident (Contact – Recipient)	Risk of HIV infection in source individual (contact)		
	HIV negative, no known risk factors or unknown risks	HIV risk factors but status unknown	Known or strongly suspected HIV infection*
Saliva – intact skin	No PEP, no follow up	No PEP, no follow up	No PEP, no follow up
Blood – intact skin	No PEP, no follow up	No PEP, no follow up	No PEP, no follow up
Saliva – mucous membrane	No PEP, no follow up	No PEP, no follow up	**Offer and follow up
Bite – no contact blood	No PEP, no follow up	No PEP, no follow up	**Offer and follow up
NSI – discarded	No PEP, no follow up	No PEP but follow up	**Offer and follow up
Bite – contact blood	No PEP, no follow up	**Offer and follow up	Yes and follow up
Blood – fresh cut	No PEP, no follow up	**Offer and follow up	Yes and follow up
Blood – mucous membrane	No PEP, no follow up	**Offer and follow up	Yes and follow up
NSI – fresh	No PEP, no follow up	**Offer and follow up	Yes and follow up

Notes:

*Where possible test contact for HIV antigen/antibody or RNA viral load if suspected seroconversion.

**Recommend initial dose(s) if source blood sample available for testing with consent.

However, the final choice of antiretroviral drugs will depend on whether the source has previously taken any of the drugs and there may be resistance. The regimen also has to account for whether the recipient is allergic to one of the drugs, if she is pregnant, or if there is any interaction with other medications being taken. The standard course should be taken for four weeks unless there are valid reasons for stopping.

Ideally PEP should be given within one hour but may be considered up to two weeks. Post-exposure prophylaxis guidance has been created, based on the risks following occupational exposure in the healthcare setting [6]. There are no clear-cut rules for advice outside of the healthcare setting, and so guidance will be made on an individual basis, which in part depends upon information about the source. The healthcare practitioner plays a key role in collating this information and obtaining a sample of blood from the source. In the healthcare setting it is appropriate and required to give pre-test counselling, but this is rarely possible or practicable in custody [7]. In this instance, to obtain valid informed consent from the source is

considered enough providing that adequate measures are in place for post-test counselling if the detainee wishes to know the results and they are positive. This can be achieved by ensuring all relevant contact details are provided on the consent form, which should accompany the blood sample. The detainee, the healthcare practitioner and an independent police officer (most usually the custody sergeant) must sign the consent form in order for the testing laboratory to conduct the tests. The blood sample and the consent form should be taken to the testing site by an independent police officer to ensure integrity of the sample. True continuity of evidence is not needed in this instance, but would be relevant in cases where blood samples are required as part of a criminal investigation.

The recipient should go immediately to the agreed referral department where an initial baseline clotted blood sample is taken. When follow-up is advised, EDTA blood for HIV RNA viral load and clotted blood for HIV antigen and antibody is taken at six weeks and again at three and six months for HIV antigen and antibody if the first test is negative.

If PEP is given, a final blood sample will be taken six months after treatment has ceased. Anyone receiving PEP will have their full blood count, liver function and urea and electrolytes checked every week. They will also be advised of possible side effects. Whether or not PEP is given, all recipients should be advised to report any acute illnesses – rash, fever, myalgia, fatigue, malaise and lymphadenopathy – occurring during the follow-up period. They should also be advised about protected sex and not donating blood or semen until they are cleared.

Specific management for hepatitis C

As stated previously, the risk of acquiring HCV following a single needlestick exposure with an HCV RNA positive source is estimated at 1.8%. No post-exposure vaccine is currently available and no immunoglobulin or antiviral agent has been shown to work. For HCWs or other personnel who have an exposure to a source known to be HCV positive or deemed high risk, a sample of clotted blood for serum should be taken after the initial contact and stored. Further samples are taken at 6 weeks for HCV RNA, at 12 weeks for HCV RNA and hepatitis C antibodies (anti-HCV), and again at 24 weeks for anti-HCV only. Testing for HCV RNA at an early stage will give some reassurance if the result is negative.

Follow-up blood samples for anti-HCV may also be considered at 12 and 24 weeks following an unknown or low-risk contact and exposure if the recipient is concerned. Blood from the source with suspected HCV infection should be tested for anti-HCV using the most up-to-date assay. The third generation ELISA (enzyme linked immunosorbent assay) is over 97% sensitive, but cannot distinguish between acute, chronic or resolved infection. However, like any screening test it has a poor positive predictive value in populations with a prevalence of <10%.

Those who are positive for anti-HCV or those at risk of infection with negative or equivocal results require a test for viral RNA using amplification techniques (polymerase chain reaction (PCR)).

A positive result indicates that they have a current viraemia and are therefore infectious. A positive anti-HCV but negative PCR sample needs further investigation to confirm or refute the result.

Liver biopsies are becoming increasingly important in the management of HCV infection. They indicate the degree of inflammation, progression of fibrosis and the presence or absence of cirrhosis unlike LFTs – poor predictors of both necro-inflammatory and fibrosis scores. Liver biopsies have been used to assess suitability for treatment, although more recently the need for a biopsy as a treatment guide has been questioned. Biopsy is recommended for those found to be PCR positive regardless of the LFTs. An experienced pathologist should examine the biopsies and apply a standard histological scoring system to ensure uniformity of histology reports.

Quantitative measurement of HCV RNA and genotyping is required to determine the duration of treatment and gives prognostic information on the potential response to such treatment.

Those diagnosed with hepatitis C should be referred for the appropriate diagnostic and therapeutic options to a specialist. They should also received counselling from an experienced HCW on the implications of being HCV positive, risk reduction and the risk of transmitting infection. They should not donate blood, tissues, organs or semen. Barrier contraception is not advised in stable monogamous relationships, but is encouraged for those with multiple sexual partners. They should also be encouraged to abstain from drinking alcohol, or at least to reduce intake to below current UK guidelines for a healthy adult. Screening for suitability for treatment with peginterferon alfa and ribavirin is mandatory in accordance with the current National Institute for Health and Clinical Excellence (NICE) guidelines. Treatment is usually recommended for those 18 and over with moderate to severe chronic HCV [8] and may also be recommended for those aged 18 or over with mild chronic hepatitis C [9]. The duration of treatment is dependent on the genotype of HCV. Types 2 or 3 should be treated for 24 weeks.

Types 1, 4, 5 or 6 are treated initially for 12 weeks. If at this time they show a reduction in viral load to <1% of the starting load, treatment will be continued to 48 weeks. Otherwise treatment is discontinued.

If ribavirin is contraindicated or not tolerated, peginterferon alfa monotherapy is advised. Regardless of the genotype, viral loads should be measured at 12 weeks and treatment would only be continued if the load is <1% of the starting load. The duration of treatment is 48 weeks.

For those patients in whom a liver biopsy is contraindicated, treatment can be given on clinical grounds alone.

Treatment is not recommended for those under 18, or who have chronic HCV recurrence after liver transplantation, or who have previously been treated with combination therapy using peginterferon alfa.

Trials with interferon alfa in IDUs have not shown such good results, however, this may be due to the drop-out rate. There is evidence that where compliance is achieved the success rates are similar to other patients.

Infection control

There is a need to protect detainees from acquiring infection from other detainees, and staff from acquiring infection from detainees. However, since it is not always possible to identify people who may spread infections to others, universal precautions should be followed at all times. This practice applies to both healthcare practitioners and custody personnel involved in the care of detainees. It also reduces the need to disclose sensitive information about the health of detainees except in particular circumstances and with their consent. Infections may be transmitted through a variety of routes, summarized below; with examples of infections.

- Blood-borne – hepatitis B, hepatitis C, HIV
- Respiratory – tuberculosis (TB), meningococcal meningitis

- Contact – methicillin-resistant *Staphylococcus aureus* (MRSA), lice, scabies, fleas, bed bugs, chickenpox etc
- Faeco-oral – hepatitis A, whole host of diarrhoea-causing viruses (e.g. rotavirus, Norwalk virus etc – the sort that cause rapid outbreaks within hospitals and on board cruise ships)

There is a constant throughput of detainees in custody who may carry any number of diseases. Hand decontamination is recognized as the single most effective method of controlling infection. It should be carried out before and after physical contact with each detainee and after handling contaminated items such as wound dressings, clothing and blankets. Good practice would also include removal of jewellery before hand washing and ensuring that fresh cuts and abrasions are covered with a waterproof dressing. Visibly soiled hands should be thoroughly washed with liquid soap and water before using an antiseptic to disinfect. Antiseptics include chlorhexidine, povidone-iodine or alcohol hand rub. Particular attention should be given to the tips of the fingers, thumbs and finger webs. After disinfection, hands should be rinsed thoroughly and dried using disposable paper towels, unless using an alcohol hand rub when it is not necessary. Single use non-powdered gloves conforming to European Community standards should be used. Hands should be washed before and after use as described above. Gloves should be disposed of as clinical waste.

Sharps handling and disposal

All needles and other sharp objects should be disposed of in sharps containers. These containers must comply with (UN 3921/BS7320) standards. They should be labelled with the work area (e.g. Medical examination room Bromley police station) and dated and signed when assembled and when closed. They should never be filled beyond the safety line and should always be placed on a firm surface – never on the floor or above shoulder height. Sealed units should be removed to a

Table 14.8. Summary of cell management and handling of laundry

	Cell	Laundry
Blood/bloodstained body fluids, vomit, urine, faeces, saliva	Specialized cleaning	Handle with gloves and launder at $>60\,^{\circ}\text{C}$ (or incinerate)
Scabies, body or head lice	No special cleaning required	Handle with gloves and launder at $>60\,^{\circ}\text{C}$ (or incinerate)
Fleas	Specialized cleaning	Handle with gloves and launder at $>60\,^{\circ}\text{C}$ (or incinerate)
Bed bugs	Specialized cleaning	Handle with gloves and launder at $>60\,^{\circ}\text{C}$ (or incinerate)
Active TB	Specialized cleaning and ventilation	Handle with gloves and launder at $>60\,^{\circ}\text{C}$ (or incinerate)
MRSA	Specialized cleaning	Handle with gloves and launder at $>60\,^{\circ}\text{C}$ (or incinerate)

designated place and removed by a professional company.

Spillage management

In the event of small spills of blood or other body fluids it is acceptable to use commercially available spillage kits. These should be kept in a designated place and checked that they are in date. For larger spills and cell cleaning commercial cleaning companies should be used.

Cleaning protocols

Routine cleaning

It is neither practical nor cost effective for the cell to be cleaned after every detainee. However, some basic principles apply. Cells should be cleaned on a daily basis with hot water, detergent and, ideally, an antimicrobial agent. Cleaning extends to door handles, cell wickets, floors and toilets. Blankets should be changed between detainees, and pillows and mattresses should be wiped with an antimicrobial agent or exchanged. The rest of the custody area, including the medical examination room, should also be cleaned daily. The golden rule for minimizing the risk of cross-contamination is to work from the cleanest area (medical examination room) to the dirtiest area (cells – leaving the toilets until last). Good practice would entail colour coding of the cleaning materials (mops, buckets, cloths, gloves) in accordance with the Safer Practice Notice published by the National Patient Safety Agency.

Specialized cleaning

Cells need to be isolated and cleaned professionally in certain situations (see Table 14.8).

Surfaces including door handles, cell wickets, floors and walls should be cleaned with hot water and detergent followed by 0.1% chlorine-releasing compound such as 1000 ppm sodium dichloroisocyanurate (Precept, Haztabs) or 1000 ppm sodium hypochlorite (1 part bleach to 10 parts water). Alternatively Atichlor Plus, combining a detergent and chlorine agent can be used.

Clinical waste handling and disposal

Waste legislation in England has been updated in line with that in Europe. More detailed guidance [10] can be found in the relevant Department of Health Technical Memorandum. Waste should be correctly bagged in appropriate colour-coded bags which must be UN-approved with BS EB 7765:2004 and BS EN ISO 6383:2004. Double bagging is only needed where the exterior of the bag is contaminated or the original bag is split. Bags should be securely sealed and labelled with coded tags once they are three quarters full or less. They should be placed in the designated clinical waste collection point. Arrangements for regular collection should be made to ensure that hazardous waste is not accumulating unnecessarily and acting as a potential source of infection. Legislation is in place to prevent accidents at work; if these laws are breached the constabulary responsible could be held accountable.

Screening questions

When seeing detainees, ask about symptoms indicating that they are an infectious risk to others (see Box 14.1).

Box 14.1 Symptoms suggestive of infectious risk

- Recent or long-term cough – productive or dry – bloodstained?
- Recent weight loss
- Fever
- Malaise
- Vomiting and diarrhoea
- Skin rash

Remember to ask about foreign travel, particularly within the previous six months but even up to one year, to exclude malaria.

Immunization of staff

Consideration should be given to vaccinating police personnel and other staff who come into contact with detainees against hepatitis B, meningitis ACWY, tetanus and diphtheria (Revaxis comprises tetanus, diphtheria and polio as an all-in-one vaccine lasting ten years). It would be difficult to defend a claim against a constabulary if an employee acquired an infection through work unless they had been offered and refused to have

the vaccines or, in the case of hepatitis B, had failed to respond to the vaccine.

Methicillin-resistant *Staphylococcus aureus* (MRSA)

The epidemiology of infections by MRSA is rapidly changing. What was primarily a hospital-acquired (HA) infection has, over the past ten years, emerged in the community. Less than 2% of *S. aureus* carry the Panton-Valentine leukocidin (PVL) toxin that destroys white blood cells and occurs both in methicillin-sensitive (MSSA) and -resistant (MRSA) strains. Although most PVL-related infections in the UK have been caused by MSSA, strains of MRSA containing the PVL gene have appeared in the community. Like all forms of *S. aureus* infection they are more frequently associated with soft tissue and skin infections, but they can cause more severe invasive infections, including septic arthritis, bacteraemia, endocarditis or community-acquired (CA) necrotizing pneumonia. Hospital-acquired infections occur most commonly in the elderly or very ill patients, whereas CA strains tend to affect previously healthy children and young adults. As yet there is no evidence to suggest that PVL-producing MRSA is more dangerous or more transmissible than some other types of MRSA. The principal risk factor for CA infections is through personal contact, especially where the skin is broken. Overcrowding (as in prisons), playing close contact sports and sharing contaminated items such as towels and razors may result in such infections [11].

Staphylococcus aureus infections are common among IDUs and are usually methicillin sensitive. However, between April 2003 and March 2006 a total of 50 cases of injecting drug use related sepsis due to MRSA were identified from geographically distinct areas in England and Wales. The clone has been identified as ST1-MRSA-I – one of the commonest CA strains in England and Wales. However, whilst more than 50% (28/50) of the cases had localized wound infections or abscesses, 13 presented with bacteraemia, 4 with endocarditis and

1 with pneumonia even though the clone does not encode the PVL toxin [1]. These more serious presentations could be a reflection of their immune status. At present it is not felt to be due to a drug contamination problem, but continued surveillance is required to further the understanding of the pathogenicity and epidemiology.

This has implications for the management of IDUs with infected injection sites or abscesses in custody. However, it must also be remembered that anyone may be colonized with MRSA, so providing reservoirs of infection.

The main mode of transmission is via hands and standard precautions must be applied to minimize the risk of cross-contamination. Such precautions include hand washing with an antimicrobial agent after contact with blood, body fluids, secretions, excretions and contaminated items such as soiled dressings. Wear single use gloves whenever possible and practicable and remove immediately after use. Gloves and soiled dressing should be discarded into designated clinical waste bags and hands washed again. Gowns may not be considered necessary in custody, but masks should be available in the event of any procedure likely to generate splashes or sprays of body fluids. Blankets and clothing should only be handled with gloves and should be incinerated or laundered at 60°C. Wherever possible, detainees with MRSA should be discouraged from moving around between cells or in the custody area. Once they have left the cell it should be isolated until it has been professionally cleaned.

Methicillin-resistant *S. aureus* has been shown to survive for up to 90 days on plastic and other surfaces. This could include handcuffs, desktops, cell furniture and the medical examination room. Clear protocols should be in place to deal with potentially contaminated handcuffs and management of cells after a detainee leaves. Alcohol-based hand rubs are easy to use and very effective in killing all forms of *S. aureus*. Acceptable for use by healthcare practitioners, it may not be considered appropriate for use by other police personnel in police stations where evidential breath machines are used. Washing hands with soap and water or using a non-alcohol-based antimicrobial agent should be encouraged.

Managing detainees with suspected pulmonary tuberculosis

Tuberculosis is a leading cause of morbidity and mortally worldwide. An estimated two million deaths from TB occur every year, with 98% occurring in the developing world, mostly sub-Saharan Africa and South Asia. In the UK, TB has moved from being a disease that occurred in all parts of the population to one that is mainly in specific population subgroups. Rates are higher in communities with connections to higher prevalence areas of the world and those with endemic factors, such as homelessness and alcohol and other substance misuse. Around 8000 cases of TB are recorded annually in the UK (surveillance data from England, Wales and Northern Ireland) [12]. However, there has been an 11% rise in the number of cases recorded in 2005 compared with 2004. The London region accounted for 43% of cases in 2005. Between 2000 and 2005 the rate of TB among the UK-born population was relatively stable. However, there has been an annual increase in the non-UK-born population, with 78% of these cases in 2005 occurring in people who had arrived in the UK two or more years prior to diagnosis. In 2005, the BCG vaccination policy changed from a universal schools-based programme to one targeted to particular risk groups. The Joint Committee on Vaccination and Immunisation (JCVI) reviewed this advice in early 2007 and it was agreed not to reintroduce the school vaccination programme [13]. The BCG is not usually recommended for people aged over 16 unless the risk of exposure is great. This could include healthcare or laboratory workers at occupational risk or where vaccination is indicated for travel. This may have implications for staff working in the custody environment, as with time, fewer will have had BCG through schools. Nevertheless the risk of acquiring TB in custody is still considered low. Only cases of pulmonary TB are infectious and among those who have pulmonary TB about 90% remain well or have only a minor or transient illness and it is only the 10% of cases with active disease who are a potential risk.

Healthcare practitioners should ask detainees about specific symptoms including cough, weight loss, dyspnoea and chest pain. These may occur over weeks or months. Consideration should also be given to the assessment for multi-drug resistant TB (MRTB) – see Box 14.2.

Box 14.2 Factors suggestive of multi-drug resistant TB

- Previous history of drug treatment for TB
- Contact with a known case of drug resistant TB
- Born in countries outside the UK with high incidence of TB
- London resident
- HIV positive
- Male
- Aged between 35 and 44 years

Detainees with TB can be managed in custody, unless clinically ill, and are usually only a risk to others if they have a productive cough and have not received at least two weeks of treatment. This may not be sufficient time in cases of MRTB. Simple measures include asking detainees to cover their mouths when coughing and preferably coughing into a tissue. Used tissues should be disposed of as clinical waste. Blankets should be laundered in a hot wash. Staff who have not had BCG vaccine should avoid contact with suspected cases if they have a productive cough or, if this is not possible, they should wear a mask.

Diagnosis and treatment of scabies

Scabies is widespread in Europe and North America and is endemic in the developing world where treatment is expensive. It is highly contagious, being spread via close personal skin-to-skin contact. In adults transmission is often through sexual contact. It may also be spread from clothing or bedding though this is rare, and only if freshly contaminated. Infestation occurs when the pregnant female mite burrows into the skin and lays eggs. Two to three days later the larvae emerge and dig new burrows. The larvae mature, mate and repeat the cycle every two weeks. Scabies can continue for months if left untreated. It may recur even after treatment either due to incorrect or incomplete application by the individual or by reinfestation from an untreated contact. Symptoms of a primary infestation usually occur within two to six weeks and within 48 hours of a reinfestation.

The most common symptom is pruritus, often worse at night, but the absence of itching does not rule out scabies. The classical burrows most easily found on the hands and feet may be missed if the skin has been scratched, has become secondarily infected or is masked by eczema. Eczema may be either a pre-existing condition or develop as a result of scabies infestation. Secondary bacterial infections with *Staphylococcus* and/or *Streptococcus* may occur. Itching may continue for up to six weeks after treatment.

Sites of infestation include web spaces, fingers and flexor surfaces of the wrists, axillae, the abdomen especially around the umbilicus and the lower buttocks and genital areas. Itchy papules on the scrotum or penis are almost pathognomonic and in women itching of the nipples associated with a generalized itchy papular rash is characteristic. In adults the face and neck are very rarely involved, which is the converse of that found in children and babies.

Definitive diagnosis requires the microscopic identification of mites or eggs, but treatment should not be delayed.

Patients with HIV or other forms of immunosuppression or neurological disease are more likely to develop crusted scabies (Norwegian scabies), which is even more infectious. The treatment of choice in the UK is permethrin 5% dermal cream, being well tolerated and having a low toxicity. Malathion is second choice and should be used in an aqueous form in children. Permethrin should be applied twice to the whole body except the head and neck, a week apart. In children two years or less, the elderly or the immunocompromised, the scalp, face, ears and neck should be included. The treatment should be washed off after 12 hours. For optimum success, the affected household and sexual contacts should be treated at the same time.

Management in custody

It is often not practicable or possible to treat suspected cases in custody. Personnel wearing gloves should remove blankets after use; they should be bagged and sent for laundering or incineration. It is not necessary to clean the cell after use. Scabies is highly infectious, but prolonged skin contact is needed before it is deemed a risk. Police personnel can usually be reassured that they are not at risk of catching scabies – even though some seem to start itching at the first mention of it.

REFERENCES

1. PHLS Hepatitis Subcommittee (2005) *Shooting Up. Infections Among Injecting Drug Users in the United Kingdom 2005.*
2. Health Protection Agency (2004) *Focus on Prevention. HIV and other sexually transmitted infections in the United Kingdom in 2003. An update November 2004.* Available at www.hpa.org.uk/webw/ HPAweb&HPAwebStandard/HPAweb_c/ 1203496898041?p=1158945066450
3. Fisher M, Benn P, Evans B, *et al.* (2006) UK guideline for the use of post-exposure prophylaxis for HIV following sexual exposure. *International Journal of STD & AIDS* **17**: 81–92.
4. Department of Health (2006) Hepatitis B. In: *Immunization Against Infectious Diseases* pp. 161–84. Available at www.dh.gov.uk/en/Publicheath/ Healthprotection/Immunisation/Greenbook/ DH_4097254
5. Department of Health (2000) *HIV Post-exposure Prophylaxis. Guidance from the UK Chief Medical Officers' Expert Advisory Group on AIDS.*
6. Department of Health (2004) *HIV Post-exposure Prophylaxis. Guidance from the UK Chief Medical Officers' Expert Advisory Group on AIDS*, 2nd edn. Available at www.advisorybodies.doh.gov.uk/eaga/ publications.htm
7. Department of Health (1996) *Guidelines for Pre-test Discussion on HIV Testing.* [PL/CMO/(96)1]. Available at www.advisorybodies.doh.gov.uk/eaga/ guidelineshivtestdiscuss.pdf
8. NICE (2004) *Technology Appraisals; Hepatitis C – pegylated interferons, ribavirin and alfa interferon (TA75).* Available at www.nice.org.uk/Guidance/TA75
9. NICE (2006) *Technology Appraisals, Hepatitis C – pegylated interferon alfa and ribavirin for treatment of mild chronic hepatitis C (TA106).* Available at www. nice.org.uk/nicemedia/pdf/TA106 publicinfo.pdf
10. Department of Health (2006) *Environment and Sustainability – Health Technical Memorandum 07–01: Safe Management of Healthcare Waste.* 2006. Available at www.dh.gov.uk/en/Publications and statistics/ Publications/Publications Policy And Guidance/ DH_063274
11. Health Protection Agency (2007) *Interim Guidance on Diagnosis and Management of PVL-Associated Staphylococcal Infections in the UK* (last modified 13 March 2007). Available at www.dh.gov.uk/en/ Aboutus/Ministers and DepartmentLeaders/ ChiefMedicalOfficer/Feature
12. Health Protection Agency (2006) *An Update – October 2006.* Available at www.hpa.org.uk/infection/ topics_a-z/injectingdrugusers
13. http://www.advisorybodies.doh.gov.uk/jcvi/

15

Scenes of crime

Ian Hogg

The solution of many crimes (and certainly all major ones) depends to a large extent on scientific support for the investigation team. This can cover a wide spectrum of specialisms both inside and outside the police service, and includes the police surgeon. Initial crime scene examination is mainly carried out by police or civilian scene examiners supplemented by other experts where their specific knowledge and expertise is required. The formation of scientific support departments within police forces has varied greatly from force to force but most incorporate personnel responsible for photography, fingerprint, marks/impressions and forensic examination either as individual or multi functional disciplines. In Scotland, these along with ballistic and suspect document examination fall within the remit of the Scottish Police Services Authority Forensic Services.

Detailed analysis of trace elements left at a scene by the perpetrator, and subsequent comparison with samples taken from a suspect, will frequently solve a case; therefore it must be ensured that a complete and comprehensive examination of the scene is carried out and that all material seized is properly packaged and preserved for future analysis. The potential value of the information gained from such a careful examination is so important that those who have access to the scene for whatever purpose must appreciate the severe consequences of displaying a careless or haphazard attitude. In order that all the disciplines present at a scene accomplish their full potential a recognized order of examination is followed or, where conflict occurs, proper discussion is held with the crime scene manager (CSM) and senior investigating officer (SIO).

Preservation of the scene

Scientific support in some form has always been an integral part of crime scene investigation, but with advances in latent fingerprint development techniques, photography and forensic science, particularly DNA, the importance of evidence gleaned from a scene by scene examiners and forensic scientists has become in some cases the lead investigative tool rather than taking a 'support' role. In order that all available evidence can be taken from a scene the integrity of the location concerned is of paramount importance.

The initial steps taken by the first officer attending can thus greatly assist an enquiry. Careful thought has to be given to the circumstances which present themselves to the officer. External locations present the greatest challenge. Control and preservation of evidence can require fast and decisive action because of the weather. Where death has occurred, the immediate area surrounding a deceased may have to be protected from the elements, with particular attention being paid to preserving any access route. Internal locations generally present the officer with a more controlled

Clinical Forensic Medicine, third edition ed. W. D. S. McLay. Published by Cambridge University Press. © Cambridge University Press 2009.

environment, but that still puts vital importance on the immediate area surrounding the deceased and the entrance and egress routes of the perpetrator. These include paths, common entrances, back courts/gardens, pavements and even roadways. The officer has to be aware of the damage he/she can do or allow others to do while the locus is under his/her control and, to this end, he/she has to form a protected/controlled area as quickly as possible and identify a common route or path to be used by all personnel approaching and leaving the scene. Thereafter, access to this area must be restricted to essential personnel until the arrival of the photographer, scene examiner and, where relevant, the forensic scientist. Those who have no specific task to perform, no matter what their rank or position, must be excluded from the scene. At times, overriding considerations, such as the need to save life or prevent further injury, to ascertain that life is extinct and to search the premises for further victims or perpetrators, justify contravening this principle, but this should be strictly controlled.

Experience over the years has identified a number of areas where actions at a scene have destroyed potential evidence or introduced cross-contamination. Examples are shown in Box 15.1.

Where any action has been taken which disturbs the scene, even inadvertently, it should be brought to the attention of the CSM or SIO. Close control must be maintained of all persons entering a scene. At major incident scenes large numbers of personnel from a variety of departments can require access. These can include police, fire service, ambulance, utility services, regional/district employees, service personnel. Detailed logs are kept, noting arrival and departure times of all persons and are generally situated at the access to the controlled area. The activities of all these people must be co-ordinated in order that the actions of one does not prejudice the actions of another, and it is for the CSM, having considered the requirements of the case, to programme operations in such a way as to maximize the benefits he/she can gain from the disciplines present.

Box 15.1 Scene contamination

Use of telephone	Addition/obliteration of fingerprints
Use of washing facilities	Obliteration of blood stained fingerprints on and around basins; flushing of possible evidential material from sink trap.
Use of toilet facilities	Flushing of possible evidential material from toilet; addition/obliteration of fingerprints.
Use of towels	Cross-contamination
Smoking at scene	Addition of cigarette stubs and ash
Unnecessary handling of weapons	Addition/obliteration of fingerprints/DNA; possible injury
Use of bare hands to open doors	Addition/obliteration of fingerprints/DNA
Careless use of gloved hands	Obliteration of fingerprints/DNA
Standing on footwear/tyre impressions	Obliteration
Standing on wet blood	Additional footwear impressions
Moving the body or clothing of deceased	Photographs should be taken first
Covering body with blanket	Introduction of extraneous fibres
Entering crime scene without protective clothing/footwear	Cross-contamination

---

Techniques used at the scene

Photography

Photographs taken at a crime scene, used as evidence in subsequent court proceedings, give a visual impression of the location concerned, and detail particular aspects of the scene, yielding specific information required by the investigation officer. It is important, therefore, not to disturb the scene before the arrival of a photographer, enabling him/her to capture a true record of the scene as left by the perpetrator. The photographs also assist witnesses (including the police surgeon) to recall the scene and their actions.

On arrival at a scene, the photographer consults the CSM and/or SIO to determine which views must be taken. The SIO is ultimately responsible for deciding which photographs to take, but the photographer, using his/her professional knowledge and experience, will offer advice and ensure that sufficient images are taken.

Normal practice is to record progressively as the photographer enters, in order to capture the scene undisturbed and to maintain continuity. Crime scene photographs fall into three main categories:

1. Long views: showing general location and conditions.
2. Intermediate views: showing more detail of general areas and highlighting specific sections to relate close-up photographs to the general scene.
3. Close-up views: detailed perspective of potential evidential material.

Long and intermediate views should always be taken using a standard 50 mm lens guaranteeing that no distortion is present in the photographs and, where possible, taken from eye level so ensuring that witnesses can relate to any views they would have seen there. Close-up views can be taken with a variety of lenses or close-up attachments.

Long views illustrate the general situation, and several shots may be required to cover a large area. In difficult locations aerial photography is frequently used to complement the ground shots. Where the crime takes place within premises it is common practice to photograph the exterior of the building and the surrounding area.

Medium views cover the general area surrounding the deceased, showing conditions in general and relating the overall scene to specific items and places. If located indoors, all the rooms are photographed with views taken from each of the four corners. Views of the deceased from a variety of angles are taken using a standard 50 mm lens and must be recorded before any disturbance has been caused. Where possible a photograph of the deceased's face is taken to assist identification.

Close-up views are used to record particular items of evidence at the locus, or visible wounds, bruises, discoloration and abrasions on the deceased; if, during an examination, the doctor notices any of these features he/she should draw them to the attention of the photographer. More detailed photographs of all injuries are taken at the post-mortem on the directions of the pathologist.

Injury photographs are taken at right angles to the subject using a scale, so ensuring that prints can be reproduced to actual size. In certain circumstances, ultraviolet photography can be used to image injuries months after the visible signs have disappeared.

Most police forces video major crime scenes; although these are occasionally produced in court their main function is to provide a comprehensive record of the scene for briefing and debriefing purposes.

A number of forces also use 360-degree panoramic photography to capture complex scenes fully. This technology can be linked to other scene images to produce a comprehensive multimedia package for briefing and court presentation. Where the offence is one of assault, cruelty or rape, the doctor may consider requesting photographs to be taken, although he/she should remember that – to the police – the purpose of photography is to compile an image presentation for production in court; because of this the views requested, particularly in cases of a sexual nature, should be suited to the court, rather than a medical lecture.

Fingerprinting

The examination of a crime scene for visible and latent finger and palm print impressions by scene examiners can lead to an expeditious identification of the person responsible. Many major crimes are solved exclusively by the identification of fingerprint marks from the locus attributable to one specific person, so placing them at or near the scene of the crime.

Techniques available to the scene examiner are always developing, but aluminium and other powders are still widely used at the locus in examining dry, smooth surfaces. These powders are brushed over the surface, and any resultant impression photographed or lifted by means of a low impact adhesive tape then placed on a clear acetate mount and retained for comparison and subsequent court proceedings.

Many other surfaces can also be examined for latent impressions using a variety of individual or sequential chemical treatments to give results which, a few years ago, would have been impossible (see Box 15.2).

Box 15.2 Developing latent impressions from different surfaces

Surface	Related treatments
Paper/cardboard	Ninhydrin
Wet paper	Physical developer
Hard plastics	Superglue
Polythene bags	Metal deposition
Adhesive tape	Powder suspension
Vinyl/rubber/leather	Superglue
Raw wood	Ninhydrin
Bloody surfaces	Amido Black
Fabric	Radioactive sulphur dioxide

In addition to these treatments, surfaces can be examined by the use of laser or conventional fluorescence. This involves examination of an article using a high-intensity light source to produce a fluorescent effect from either naturally occurring chemicals in a fingerprint or ones which have been introduced during treatment.

It can be seen, therefore, that contamination of any surface within a crime scene, even with gloved hands, must be avoided to ensure that the scene examiners do their work in the best possible conditions.

Articles most likely to come to the attention of the doctor include weapons and medicine bottles which should not be handled without consulting a qualified scene examiner. If a doctor has handled any item either by necessity or accident he/she should notify the scene examiner or, in his/her absence, a police officer at the locus.

Firearms

Examination of the scene of a shooting incident will reveal a great deal about the type of weapon used, the distance over which it was fired, the position of the firer and, often, whether what happened was accidental, suicidal or homicidal.

When a shot is fired from close range the clothing and the skin of the victim can disclose various features which, by subsequent ballistic testing using the weapon concerned, help to estimate the range and direction of shot. Accordingly, it is important that any such marks or injuries be photographed (with a scale, as in Fig. 15.1a and b) for future analysis, and that extra care be taken with the victim's clothing to preserve any residue, particles of propellant or projectiles.

Projectiles come in an enormous variety of shapes and sizes. What is found seldom conforms to the normal idea of a bullet shape. Bullets and other projectiles deform very readily on impact, often shattering into many pieces of such diverse shape that they are recognizable as projectiles only to the informed eye. For example, the copper/nickel jacket of a pistol or rifle bullet can separate from the lead core; unless care is taken to recover all parts, the possibility of matching the bullet to a specific weapon could be lost. Photographs of bullets, projectiles and cartridge components appear as Fig. 15.2.

Documents

Document examination and handwriting does not normally come within the scope of a scene of crime examination, but police surgeons should be aware

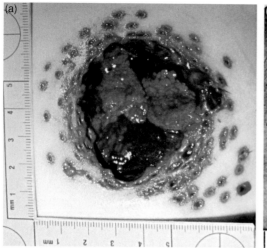 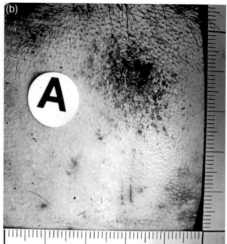

Fig. 15.1 (a) Shotgun injury. (b) Bullet injury with powder tattooing. (Photograph reproduced with permission of Scottish Police Services Authority (SPSA) Forensic Services.)

that injudicious handling of paper material could cause difficulties.

One of the examinations carried out on paper uses the ESDA (electrostatic detection apparatus) which will visualize very fresh fingerprint impressions, footprints and indented writing on the paper. This evidence is easily destroyed. Paper is also subjected to chemical treatments to raise latent fingerprints. Careless handling with bare hands may impart further impressions, wholly or partially obliterating the writing on the document, so preventing handwriting comparison. Even to fold or smooth paper may interfere with analysis.

The doctor at the scene

The primary reason for your attendance as a police surgeon is to pronounce life extinct and this should be done as soon as you arrive. Where death is obviously due to foul play this may be the only function, but where the circumstances surrounding the death are not clear a preliminary examination may be required at the scene.

Before gaining access to the immediate area surrounding the deceased confirm with the senior officer present any requirement to wear protective clothing such as a forensic suit, boots, gloves and mask, if a designated route into the scene has been established and whether the scene has been photographed. Care must be taken in approaching the deceased, even along a predetermined route, in order not to destroy footprints, fingerprints and other forensic trace evidence. If you find signs of life, subsequent actions to revive the patient should take priority but you should bear in mind the preservation of evidence where possible.

If the deceased has not been photographed, delay movement of the body, clothing or surrounding items, but where circumstances dictate and you have disturbed the scene, inform the photographer and officer in charge of the enquiry: it will be recorded that the photographs do not represent the scene as found. Do not attempt to return the scene to its original state for photography. If, during an examination, you declare a death suspicious, stop what you are doing and have the scene photographed.

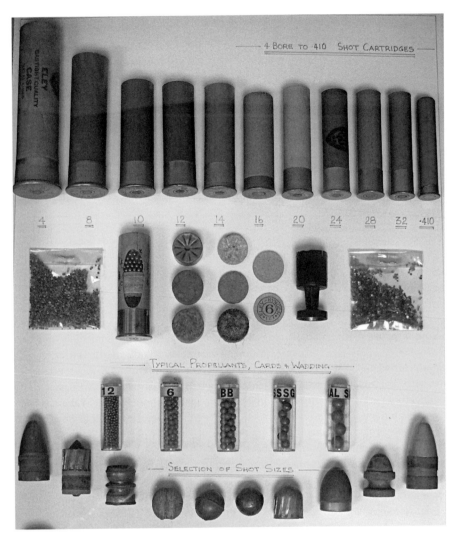

Fig. 15.2 Shotgun cartridges, calibres and missiles. (Photograph reproduced with permission of SPSA Forensic Services.)

Even where initial evidence points to a sudden death, subsequent post-mortem examination may reveal foul play, initiating a murder enquiry. You should, therefore, ensure that in all circumstances you have carried out a satisfactory examination and paid attention to evidence preservation. Professional litter such as discarded gloves and instrument wrappings must be removed from the locus for disposal.

16

Forensic science

Ian C. Shaw and Julie Mennell

The role of the forensic scientist is to carry out appropriate scientific examinations in support of the investigation of crime. Through advances in science and technology and with less reliance being placed on other types of evidence such as admissions or witness evidence, forensic science has become one of the principal means of investigating crime.

Traditionally, forensic science has been associated with providing objective corroborative evidence that supports or refutes other forms of evidence so often seen as being more subjective. However, forensic science is being used increasingly to support the early stages of an investigation by providing forensic intelligence. It is this use of forensic science, principally through DNA analysis and the use of DNA databases, which has seen a significant increase in the use of forensic science by police forces in the UK.

While most of the work of the forensic scientist is carried out at the laboratory, the forensic scientist may also undertake examinations at the scene of crime (see previous chapter). Examinations at the scene may be vital in helping to establish exactly what went on. The interpretation of bloodstains can help to identify the location and nature of an attack. The identification of several seats of burning may establish the cause of a fire as arson. Attending the scene also allows the forensic scientist to select the most appropriate material for detailed examination at the laboratory. Most laboratory examinations are, however, carried out on material selected and recovered by others such as crime scene examiners (CSE), police officers, the pathologist or the forensic physician. In many instances the forensic scientist may have little knowledge of the circumstances of the case beyond those provided on the case submission form and associated documents such as medical examination forms.

The importance of a relevant and complete picture of the alleged circumstances, together with a clear requirement in terms of what the investigator is seeking to establish, cannot be overemphasized. Using this information, the forensic scientist will assess how best to approach the examination, which scientific methods to employ and how to interpret the findings and reach conclusions that address all the relevant points of the case. The importance of proper case assessment and interpretation and the need to consider alternative hypotheses has seen many forensic scientists adopting a 'Bayesian' approach to the consideration of forensic evidence. The Bayesian approach considers the likelihood of the evidence obtained, given not only the hypothesis that the alleged suspect is the source of the evidence, but also the alternative hypothesis that the evidence may have come from someone other than the suspect.

When interpreting findings, the forensic scientist also considers what is known as the 'hierarchy of

Clinical Forensic Medicine, third edition ed. W. D. S. McLay. Published by Cambridge University Press. © Cambridge University Press 2009.

propositions'. The hierarchy of propositions recognizes that forensic science can address propositions at three levels:

- level 1 – source
- level 2 – activity
- level 3 – crime

At the most basic level, forensic science can be used to provide evidence that identifies a 'source' such as a person through a DNA profile, or a garment through matching fibres. In the past, forensic scientists have often concentrated on this most basic level. It is now recognized that while evidence of 'source' is very important, the use of forensic science to provide evidence of 'activity' adds considerably to its contribution to an investigation. The presence of blood on the shoes of a suspect that matches the blood of the victim (level 1 – source) may have an innocent explanation. If, in addition, the pattern of bloodstaining suggests that the blood has arisen as the result of an assault (level 2 – activity) the potential value of this evidence is very much greater. The third level relates to forensic science evidence that addresses the proposition that the suspect committed the crime. While forensic science can undoubtedly be of great value in addressing the proposition of guilt or innocence, it is the role of the court to establish guilt or innocence, not the forensic scientist. The hierarchy of propositions from *source* to *activity* through to *crime* should be recognized by forensic scientists both when assessing a case before starting work and when interpreting the findings arising from the subsequent examinations. While it is not the role of the forensic scientist to address level 3 propositions, it is the duty of the scientist to maximize the evidence to the benefit of the investigation. This means that, wherever possible, forensic scientists should seek to address propositions at the 'activity' level and not restrict their considerations to the level of 'source'. Further information on interpreting evidence, the Bayesian approach to evidence and the hierarchy of propositions can be found in the work of Roberston and Vignaux [1] and Cook *et al.* [2]

The type of scientific evidence employed in the investigation of crime covers a wide range of scientific expertise from molecular biology to metallurgy. In the past, laboratories have tended to be organized by scientific discipline.

Instead of being organized into divisions such as 'Biology' or 'Chemistry', the modern forensic science laboratory is more likely to consist of units based around crime types such as volume crime (mainly burglary, theft, criminal damage), serious crime (such as homicide, robbery, sexual offences) and drug offences. Each unit will consist of scientists who, together, embrace all the knowledge and skills necessary to investigate the types of case allocated to their unit. Supporting these crime-based units will be service units providing specialist analytical support such as chemical analysis or DNA profiling.

The types of scientific examination undertaken in the laboratory may be broadly categorized into biological, physical, drugs and toxicological.

Biological examinations

In the past, biological examinations have been associated primarily with providing corroborative evidence in cases of violent crime. Changes in the way that crimes are now investigated, coupled with new scientific developments, have resulted in the evidence from biological examinations being applied to a much wider range of crimes and to all stages of the investigative process. However, of greatest importance to the forensic physician will be the types of evidence associated with violent crime.

By its very nature, violent crime may often result in close, prolonged, physical contact between the suspect and the victim, the scene of crime and weapons or implements that may be associated with the crime. The interrelationship between all these elements is shown in Fig. 16.1.

Depending on the type of the crime, the degree of contact and the nature of the scene, there are opportunities for the transfer of a wide variety of

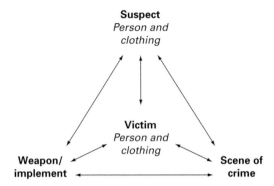

Fig. 16.1 Inter relationship between the suspect, the victim, the scene of the crime and weapons/implements implicated.

evidence types. In addition, other aspects of evidence, such as bloodstain distribution or damage to clothing, may be present. The type of trace evidence of greatest significance to the forensic physician is perhaps that derived from body fluids.

Body fluids

The forensic scientist is able to identify and analyse a number of body fluids. Some fluids, such as blood and semen, can be identified with certainty, whereas the forensic scientist may be able to provide only an opinion on the likely origin of certain other materials, such as saliva or vaginal secretions. While most body fluids encountered in casework are human, the forensic scientist is also able to provide an opinion on the species of origin of animal material.

The identification of blood and semen involve the initial use of presumptive tests locating likely stains. Semen is confirmed by identifying spermatozoa on slides that have been stained, usually with haematoxylin and eosin. In the absence of spermatozoa, perhaps as a result of vasectomy, the presence of other components such as choline and the seminal plasma protein P30 can be used to confirm semen.

The identification of spermatozoa on internal vaginal swabs is of particular importance as it can confirm recent sexual intercourse. However, care must be taken in using the findings from vaginal swabs to indicate time since intercourse. Spermatozoa may persist in the vagina for up to 72 hours, and on rare occasions even up to a week. The presence of bleeding does not prevent the taking of swabs or the identification and subsequent analysis of semen; it can, however, affect the survival of spermatozoa in the vagina. It is important for the forensic physician to obtain a recent sexual history from the subject, as such information may be vital in helping to interpret the scientific findings.

In cases of oral sex, semen may be recovered from face and mouth swabs and mouth rinses. Similarly, semen can be recovered from skin swabs or clippings of matted pubic hair. In cases of buggery, semen may be recovered from anal swabs. It has been reported that an ultraviolet (UV) light source may be useful in locating possible semen stains at the scene, on clothing and even on the person. Experience shows that this method cannot be relied upon to visualize semen and its use is not recommended. Strong UV sources can also have a deleterious effect on DNA, although with the sensitivity of current DNA techniques this is not likely to be a significant issue.

The examination of vaginal or anal swabs for lubricants may be important where the attacker has used a condom or has used a lubricant to aid penetration. Penile swabs can also be examined for traces of lubricants as well as vaginal material, faeces, saliva and blood. As well as being the source of lubricants, a discarded condom can link the attacker to the crime through the analysis of the semen contents and vaginal material and/or blood from the outer surface. Swabbings from bite marks may yield traces of saliva.

A number of methods are available to the forensic scientist for establishing the likely donor of body fluids. Tests for blood groups, polymorphic red-cell enzymes and serum proteins have been used in the past, but these methods have now been completely superseded by DNA profiling.

DNA profiling

Deoxyribonucleic acid profiling has revolutionized forensic science since its introduction in 1986. Based on the discovery of Professor Sir Alec Jeffries at Leicester University in 1984, the original multi-locus probe technique (MLP) offered a significant advance on the conventional blood grouping techniques that were then the order of the day.

Although DNA profiling has been used to investigate crime for only a little over 20 years, several changes in technology over these years have led to the techniques available today becoming, to a large extent, standardized across the world.

In 1994 the Forensic Science Service (FSS) launched a new method of DNA profiling in the UK, which analysed areas of DNA known as short tandem repeats (STRs). The STR method uses, as part of the analytical process, a technique known as polymerase chain reaction (PCR). The technique of PCR utilizes the ability of DNA to replicate itself. By making millions of copies of the target DNA the crime material can be 'amplified' to enable the smallest amounts of DNA material to yield DNA profiles. The current implementation of STR (known as SGM-Plus®) analyses for ten separate independent STR loci together with a locus that determines sex: together these have a combined frequency of occurrence of one in greater than one billion (1 in 10^9). In other words, with a profile from a crime stain, the chance of obtaining that evidence, given that it matches the suspect, is not less than one billion times more likely if the DNA comes from the suspect than if it comes from some random unrelated individual. It must be recognized that, if there is a chance that the DNA material originates from someone related to the suspect, the chance of a relative having the same STR profile as the suspect is much greater than one in one billion, with the likelihood of a chance match increasing as the degree of relatedness increases. In the case of identical twins, both individuals would, of course, share the same STR profile.

The greater chance of a match between related individuals has led to what is know as 'the brothers defence' where it is sometime argued in court that the DNA originated not from the suspect but from a close relative. To counter such a defence it is important for the investigator to close off this option by eliminating relatives of the suspect as possible sources of the crime DNA. Where the 'brothers defence' is invoked it is usually a simple matter of refuting the claim by analysing the DNA of the 'brother'.

Short tandem repeat results may be obtained from any material that can yield chromosomal DNA. Small bloodstains, traces of semen, saliva from cigarette ends and envelope flaps, a single hair root, can all give results. A measure of the sensitivity of the technique can be gauged by the fact that results have even been obtained from spermatozoa recovered from microscope slides prepared many years earlier from material in rape cases. Even though the material on the slides had been fixed, stained in haematoxylin and eosin and mounted in a xylene-based mountant, STR profiles were still obtained. Profiles have also been obtained from histological preparations, including cervical smears.

The use of semi-automated equipment coupled with computer-aided analysis and interpretation of results means that it is now possible in urgent cases to obtain DNA profiles in under eight hours compared to the 14 days for the original MLP method. Automation, which also helped to reduce the cost of analysis, combined with computerization enabled the FSS to introduce the world's first national DNA database (NDNAD) for criminal investigation purposes.

The National DNA Database

A DNA database has been the goal of forensic scientists and the police since the introduction of DNA profiling in 1986. The improvements in technology, combined with the recommendations of the 1993 Royal Commission on Criminal Justice, led to the establishment of the NDNAD in April 1995. The introduction of the database was supported by changes to the Police and Criminal Evidence Act 1984 (PACE) codes which included the reclassification of mouth swabs as non-intimate samples and confirmation that plucked hairs (excluding pubic) are also non-intimate samples. Such samples could now be taken by a police officer, without consent, where the subject had been charged or reported for, or convicted of, a recordable offence.

Since 1995, several further changes to the law in England and Wales now permit the compulsory sampling of individuals on arrest (that is, without the need for them to be charged or reported). In addition, the retention of samples on the NDNAD where the case is discontinued or the suspect is found not guilty is also permitted. Even where a suspect has been arrested but is not subsequently charged, the profile remains on the NDNAD unless it can be shown that the arrest was unlawful. Individuals can now volunteer to have their samples placed on the NDNAD. However, in the case of intelligence-led screens (see below) volunteers can require that their profiles be used only in the case for which they have provided a sample and not subsequently entered on the NDNAD. Where a volunteer agrees that his/her sample can be included on the NDNAD that individual waives the right to have the sample removed from the database at some later date. Samples from suspects, known as criminal justice or 'CJ samples', are retained on the NDNAD for 100 years. The changes in the law in relation to DNA samples have also been extended to the taking and retaining of fingerprints.

Custodianship of the NDNAD rests with the Home Office and is discharged through the National Policing Improvement Agency established in April 2007. A number of forensic science laboratories, both public and private sector, are authorized by the custodian to analyse samples, both from suspects and from crime stains, and to upload the results to the NDNAD.

Comparison of profiles from suspects and crime stains is a continuous process. As the result from each new suspect is added, that person is searched against all the outstanding crimes on the database.

Similarly, as the result from each new crime stain is added that sample is searched against all suspects. As well as linking a suspect to a crime the database also links crimes. It does this by matching the results from different crimes committed by the same person, even if that individual is not on the database.

Having established a link between a suspect and a crime the police are informed. Should the police wish to pursue the case using DNA evidence they are usually required to take a further 'evidential' sample from the suspect. It is the results from this evidential sample that will be put before the court as evidence to connect the suspect with the crime. However, if the defendant accepts the evidence of the link established through the NDNAD a further evidential sample may not be required. In England and Wales, the Crown Prosecution Service (CPS) has now authorized the police to charge a suspect on the basis of a match against the NDNAD without the requirement to wait for the outcome of the evidential sample.

Deoxyribonucleic acid profiling has also proved to be an effective and economic way of eliminating people from an enquiry. Where the police have a DNA profile in a major crime such as a homicide or rape, but there is no individual matching that profile on the NDNAD, the police will consider setting up an 'intelligence-led screen'. Such screens are best applied where the police have additional information that constrains the potential pool of suspects, such as a likely geographic area or age group. In such cases the police will call upon members of the public within the target group to volunteer to provide samples of DNA so they can be eliminated from an enquiry quickly, cheaply and with certainty. As mentioned above, people volunteering samples through an intelligence-led screen can insist that their profiles are not retained on the NDNAD.

Before embarking on an intelligence-led screen, the police will now usually request that 'familial' searching is carried out against the NDNAD. Familial searching utilizes the fact that closely related individuals are much more likely to have similar

DNA profiles than unrelated individuals. The NDNAD can therefore be searched, not just for exact matches but for what are in effect 'near misses'. Searching algorithms have been developed based on the likelihood of siblings, or parents and their children, having very similar DNA profiles. Familial searching will produce a list of 'near misses' that can be further refined by applying geographic filters to provide investigators with a list of people who may be related to the perpetrator. The use of familial searching has led to the resolution of a number of high profile crimes including several undetected over many years.

In recognition of the importance of DNA profiling, between 2000 and 2005 the Government made available over £250 million of additional funding to police forces through the DNA Expansion Programme. The outcome of this funding, together with the changes to the law bringing more individuals within the scope of the NDNAD, means that the UK now has the largest DNA database for criminal investigation purposes in the world. The NDNAD is not just the largest in respect of the number of individuals held on the database but also in terms of the proportion of the population on the database. As of July 2007, over four million individuals are on the NDNAD, representing a very large proportion of the active criminal population.

'Low copy number' or 'touch' DNA

The use of PCR to 'amplify' DNA in theory permits the preparation of a DNA profile from a single copy of DNA. In practice, this potential to obtain profiles from the very smallest amounts of DNA is not usually exploited with the number of copying cycles in the PCR process being limited to 28. However, when required, the number of PCR cycles can be increased, usually to 34, resulting in many more copies of DNA being produced. An increased number of PCR cycles is often combined with enhanced DNA extraction resulting in a technique with much greater sensitivity than 'standard' DNA profiling. The low copy number (LCN) technique

can produce STR profiles from items that do not appear to have any visible biological material on them. Using the LCN technique, DNA profiles can be obtained from items that have merely been handled without any apparent material such as blood, semen or saliva having been deposited. Where profiles have been obtained from items that have just been handled it is likely that the DNA is present in the form of epithelial cells shed from skin.

The ability of the LCN technique to yield profiles from the smallest amounts of starting material has proved to be of considerable benefit across a wide range of cases. When first introduced, LCN was restricted to high profile cases, given the considerable costs then associated with the technique. However, the technique has now found much wider use across a range of crimes, including vehicle crime, where it has been used to obtain DNA profiles from, for example, car ignition systems. The sensitivity of the LCN technique is not, however, without some attendant problems. That it may no longer be possible to say what the DNA profile came from (for example, blood or semen) can be a limitation. Because the technique is so sensitive, it often yields results that are a mixture of profiles from more than one individual; this can cause possible interpretation problems.

Problems of contamination, always a potential issue in forensic science, are only exacerbated by increasing the sensitivity of a technique. It has been demonstrated that DNA profiles can be obtained from an item where an individual has picked up the DNA from another person, through either direct or indirect contact with that individual, and has then deposited that other person's DNA on that item. This potential problem, known as secondary transfer, together with an increased likelihood of obtaining mixed profiles, means that the use of LCN DNA is best limited to situations where both the risk of secondary transfer and the likelihood of mixtures are reduced. When choosing items for possible LCN DNA analysis, items that are likely to have been touched or handled by a limited number of individuals are the best items to select. For example, in cases of distraction burglary where the perpetrator is masquerading as a 'water board official', swabs taken from items such as doorknobs that may well have been handled by the perpetrator, but also likely to have been handled by many other people, should be avoided. However if, as may be the case, the perpetrator has handled the mains water stopcock, a swab from this item, which is likely to have been handled by many fewer people, may yield a usable result.

The sensitivity of DNA techniques, both 'standard' and LCN, mean that all individuals who are involved in the process of the location and recovery of evidence need to be mindful of the risks of contamination and secondary transfer. Crime scene examiners now wear not just disposable scene suits and gloves, but also head coverings, disposable masks and boots; forensic physicians visiting a scene need to be similarly attired. Disposable gowns, masks, gloves and head coverings are also worn by laboratory personnel during the initial examination of items for the location and recovery of evidence. In addition, the very layout of laboratories has been redesigned with former open-plan laboratory areas giving way to a greater number of smaller examination rooms with ventilation systems designed to minimize the risk of contamination. Hygiene and cleansing routines have also been revised in response to the risks of contamination and the design and operation of modern medical examination suites also recognizes the greater potential for contamination.

Despite all precautions, the sensitivity of DNA techniques means that the possibility of accidental contamination remains a real risk. In acknowledgement of this risk, DNA samples from police and scientific staff are held on the NDNAD Police Elimination Database (PED). The PED is used solely for the purpose of eliminating police and forensic personnel as the possible source of DNA in an investigation. Searches of the PED are not made on a routine basis in an enquiry but only as and when it is considered necessary by the senior investigating officer (SIO). Since April 2003, providing a sample for inclusion on the PED has been a

requirement for all newly recruited police officers and for those support personnel where it is a condition of their employment. For staff in post before April 2003 inclusion on the PED is voluntary. Searches of the PED are only made on the basis of a comparison of a specific crime profile against a named individual's profile. While at this time samples from forensic physicians are not included on the PED, many police forces now require, as part of the contract with their doctors, that they be prepared to provide a DNA sample for comparison purposes if required.

While the use of SGM-Plus is not universal across the world, countries using DNA profiling all use some form of STR profiling. For example, in the USA, the Federal Bureau of Investigation (FBI) uses a combination of 13 separate STR components, or loci. However, countries using STR analysis for DNA profiling purposes all use certain loci in common. There is now an international standard, agreed through Interpol known as the Interpol Standard Set of Loci (ISSOL), whereby member states have agreed to include within the set of STR loci used by their country, seven STR loci in common. This means, for example, that a DNA profile obtained in Britain can be compared against profiles obtained in the USA by searching using the ISSOL markers. In addition to searches made through Interpol, arrangements now exist that enable certain states within Europe to access each others' criminal investigation databases, including DNA and fingerprint databases through the recently negotiated Prüm treaty.

While STR profiling using SGM-Plus remains the method of choice for criminal investigations, samples are sometimes encountered where other types of DNA profiling may be used. Despite the sensitivity of LCN DNA, there remain certain samples such as hair shafts (as opposed to hair roots) where it may not be possible to obtain a STR profile. From such samples it can be possible to obtain a profile from mitochondrial DNA (mtDNA). It should be recognized that mtDNA profiles cannot be compared using the NDNAD and that the discriminating power of mtDNA is many orders of magnitude less than that of SGM-Plus. As mitochondria from spermatozoa are not transferred to the ovum during fertilization, mtDNA profiles are inherited through the maternal line and remain largely unchanged within family groups. Mitochondrial DNA cannot be used, therefore, to identify a suspect but only to confirm that a suspect is related to whoever deposited the DNA at the crime scene.

A number of STRs located on the Y chromosome have been exploited for forensic science purposes. As with mtDNA profiles, Y chromosome STR profiles cannot be compared against profiles held on the NDNAD, so the application of Y chromosome STR profiling is limited to cases where there is a need to compare a crime profile against a given individual. Y chromosome STR profiling may be of occasional value where it is necessary to obtain a DNA profile that relates specifically to a male. Such cases may include samples that may be a complex mixture of male and female material where the female component predominates and there is no possibility of eliminating the female DNA using preferential extraction techniques.

The wider application of DNA profiling

The use of DNA profiling is not restricted to demonstrating the link between an individual and material arising from the commission of a crime. A DNA profile is, of course, a combination of components of the profiles of one's parents, so DNA profiling can be used to investigate paternity. While most paternity investigations will be in support of civil cases involving disputed paternity, issues of probate or immigration, they may also be used in criminal cases to establish incest or to support the identification of the remains of a victim where more conventional means have failed.

The area of casualty identification in mass disasters is one in which DNA profiling is being used increasingly. The benefits of STRs, which can often yield results from poor quality DNA, come into their own when applied to badly burned or decomposed human remains. If no soft tissue remains, results may be obtained from bone or teeth.

Deoxyribonucleic acid technology and the methods of DNA profiling have changed considerably since its introduction into forensic science over 20 years ago. Techniques such as the analysis of single nucleotide polymorphisms (SNPs) have been advanced as a possible future method of DNA profiling. Analysis of a number of different SNPs in combination would be able to match the current discriminating power of SGM-Plus and also have the potential to provide information about various physical characteristics such as hair colour. However, the success of current profiling methods and the investment that has been made in facilities and technology such as the NDNAD make it very unlikely that the current method of DNA profiling using STRs will be replaced in the foreseeable future.

Physical examinations

Physical examinations cover evidence types ranging from particulate evidence, such as paint, glass and soil, to marks such as footwear and tool marks. The type of physical evidence associated with a crime will depend on the nature and circumstances of that crime. For example, while evidence such as glass may often be associated with cases such as burglaries where entry has been gained by breaking a window, and cases of assault where broken glass has been used as a weapon, glass may be associated with any type of crime. However, irrespective of the crime, the one type of physical evidence that is available at every crime scene is footwear evidence. Depending on the quality of recovered marks and the presence of sufficient unique wear and damage characteristics it is possible to link a footwear mark back to a specific shoe. In cases where the forensic scientist is unable to match a mark to a shoe conclusively it will often be possible to give some indication of the likelihood of a match. Given its ubiquitous nature, the value of footwear marks as a source of forensic intelligence that can link crimes as well as connecting marks to suspects' shoes has become recognized increasingly. The potential for forensic intelligence from footwear marks means that forces are now putting much greater effort into the location and recovery of this type of evidence and the forensic physician should be mindful of the need not to leave footwear marks at the scene. When entering a scene the forensic physician should stick to any designated pathway and use stepping plates where provided.

As the value of forensic evidence depends on a number of factors, simply listing types of physical evidence in the order of their potential evidential value may not be helpful. However, types of physical evidence that can yield conclusive results include footwear marks, tool marks where a mark may be able to be associated with a specific tool, and complex multi-layer paint fragments.

Even where an evidence type may not normally be considered to provide conclusive evidence, conclusive evidence can possibly be provided through what is known as a physical fit (also sometimes known as a mechanical or jigsaw fit). For example, in the case of a road traffic accident it is sometimes possible to fit fragments of paint from the scene back to an area of damaged paintwork on the recovered suspect vehicle. In a case of assault, glass recovered from the wound of a victim may fit back to the broken bottle used as a weapon in such a manner that the scientist can state that the glass recovered from the victim came from that bottle.

In the absence of physical fits, the value of evidence associated with material such as glass or paint depends not only on the nature of the material, such as how common or rare it might be, but also on factors such as where it is found and how much of it is present. The finding on the sole of the suspect's shoe of glass that matches the broken window at the scene of the crime may be of little or no value if it is shown that the suspect could have picked up the glass innocently by walking past the scene. However, the finding of matching glass fragments in hair combings taken from the suspect would be much less likely to have an innocent explanation. How much evidence is found may also be of significance. Again, using glass as an example, the finding of a single fragment of glass on the upper clothing of a suspect that matches the glass from the crime scene will have much less significance than the finding of several fragments of matching glass. Studies have shown that particulate evidence such as glass is often lost quickly from clothing, so the finding of a significant number of glass fragments on a suspect may point to that person having been in recent contact with broken or breaking glass.

The value of fibre evidence also depends on the rarity of the material and how much of it is present. The finding of blue denim-type cotton fibres on the clothing of a suspect that could have come from the victim's jeans may be of little value, given the ubiquitous nature of blue denim. However, the finding of a number of different coloured man-made fibres on the clothing of a suspect, all of which match the clothing of the victim in terms of chemical composition, structure and colour would be much more significant. In the case of fibre evidence, particularly in cases where there has been prolonged physical contact such as rape, it is often possible to find fibres on the clothing of both the victim and the suspect that could have come from the other person. This two-way transfer can greatly increase the value of such evidence.

As with any forensic science examination, the process of physical examinations begins with the location and recovery of evidence. In the case of particulate evidence and fibres, the nature of the material is such that it is usually not possible to locate the material visually. Methods of examination have been developed that recover trace evidence even where it is not visible. In the case of particulate evidence this may involve the careful shaking and brushing of items over large sheets of brown paper from which any material can be recovered easily and further examined. In the case of fibres, the normal practice of recovery involves the use of adhesive tape that is carefully pressed against all parts of the item to recover extraneous surface fibres. The adhesive tapes can then be examined using low power microscopy to recover any fibres of interest for subsequent detailed comparison.

It should always be remembered that one type of evidential material can carry other types of evidence. A piece of glass submitted for comparison against other pieces of glass may also bear other types of evidence such as blood, fibres and marks such as fingerprints or even fragments of footwear marks.

It is not possible to list all the possible types of physical evidence that might be encountered by the forensic physician. When conducting any examination of a victim or suspect the forensic physician, just like the forensic scientist, needs to be fully aware of the alleged circumstances of the offence and to conduct the examination with due regard for the potential for all types of forensic evidence.

Drugs and toxicological examinations

Most drug examinations are in connection with the Misuse of Drugs Act 1971 and Misuse of Drugs Regulations 2001. The Act covers more than 100 controlled substances including cannabis, diamorphine (heroin) and morphine, cocaine and 'crack' cocaine, LSD (d-lysergic acid diethylamide), amphetamine and MDMA (ecstasy; 3,4, methylene-dioxymethamphetamine).

In addition to basic identification, detailed examinations may be carried out to establish the concentration of the drug and the presence of adulterants or impurities. Such detailed examinations may be important in helping to substantiate charges of supply or possession with intent to supply. A range of other forensic examinations may also be carried out to establish links between seizures, including the comparison of material, such as cling film or polythene bags, used to package the individual 'wraps'. Forensic scientists are often called to the scene of illicit laboratories. Their

involvement in such cases is crucial, not only to confirm what is being manufactured but also to establish the method and scale of production. A scientific presence at such scenes is also vital in ensuring that the manufacturing process is shut down safely.

While the downgrading of cannabis from a Class B drug to Class C in 2004 has resulted in many fewer forensic examinations for the possession of cannabis there has been a significant increase in the illegal cultivation of cannabis. Using modern hydroponic growing methods, combined with specially selected varieties of the plant, it is possible to produce cannabis in the UK which more than rivals that smuggled in from abroad in terms of both yield and strength. These 'home-grown' varieties are often referred to as 'skunk' owing to their pungent smell.

Toxicology investigations generally involve the analysis of body fluids for alcohol, drugs and poisons and may be associated with sudden deaths, poisonings or the effect on behaviour arising from the use of these substances. Sudden death may be suicidally, accidentally or deliberately induced. In the case of the living, toxicology examinations may be associated with offences against the Road Traffic Act and involve driving under the influence of alcohol and/or drugs. Examination for alcohol and drugs is frequently requested for the suspects and victims in other serious offences such as assault, rape and homicide. The use of drugs to stupefy victims of rape has been commonly claimed, but there is little scientific evidence to support the suggestion of their widespread use in facilitating such crimes.

Tests to screen saliva and urine for the presence of a number of controlled drugs are now used routinely by several police forces to support drugs intervention programmes whereby, from April 2006, the police can test offenders for heroin, cocaine and crack cocaine on arrest for certain acquisitive offences such as street robbery and burglary. Those who test positive are required to attend a drug assessment carried out by a specialist drug worker.

The medical examination: the forensic science requirements

Contamination

We have already seen how important it is that the forensic physician take all possible care to avoid contaminating evidence at the scene of crime. The same care needs to be taken when examining patients and taking samples. Ideally, any doctor who visits the scene of the crime or who examines the victim should not examine any suspects in the same investigation. If different doctors are not available the examiner must be able to show that different outer clothing was worn for the examinations of the various parties. Similarly, it is important to use different examination rooms. Protocols need to be in place and adhered to regarding the protection and cleansing of surfaces in the medical examination room to minimize the risk of cross-contamination. Any instruments used to collect samples or assist in the taking of samples (for instance, proctoscopes) must be new, disposable ones. All these necessary precautions are mirrored in the laboratory where different scientists in different rooms within the laboratory will conduct the initial examinations of the items from the victim and the suspects.

Information

The importance of information to the forensic scientist has been referred to earlier. In sexual offences the vehicle for this information is the series of MEDX1A–C forms. These forms will accompany the laboratory submission and should provide the scientist with the necessary background information. Of particular importance are relevant dates and times such as the date and time that samples were taken and the date and time of the last act of intercourse within the previous ten days. In cases where a MEDX1 form is not required, you should ensure that the investigating officer is aware of any information that may be relevant to the forensic scientist.

Samples

The samples to be taken will depend on the type and nature of the crime. Table 16.1, based on a table from the *Scenes of Crime Handbook* [3], and reproduced by kind permission of the Forensic Science Service Ltd, provides a check list of the more usual samples associated with certain types of crime. You should discuss beforehand with the investigating officer, or with the officer present at the medical examination, exactly what is known about the case and what samples are required. If there is any uncertainty about the need for a particular sample it may be better to take it, as there is unlikely to be a second opportunity. If a sample considered necessary cannot be taken for medical reasons, that reason should be recorded.

Swabs

Use only plain, sterile untreated swabs. Never use charcoal- or albumen-coated swabs. Swabs should never be placed in transport medium. Make sure that the swab stick is returned to the same tube that it was taken from. All swabs should be frozen as soon as possible following the examination.

Vaginal, anal and mouth swabs

To maximize the recovery of material take at least two swabs from each chosen area (e.g. two external vaginal swabs, two internal anal swabs).

Penile swabs and swabs from bite marks

Unless the site is already moist, the swab should be pre-moistened with sterile distilled water: do not use saline.

Reference samples for DNA profiling

Reference samples are needed to establish the DNA profiles of the various parties in an enquiry. These are normally taken using buccal scrape kits or the scrapes provided in sex offences kits.

Table 16.1. Samples required for examination

Examination Type	Samples Required		GBH Affrays	Murder suspects	Drug/drink driving	Armed robbery	Burglary	Suspect poisoning/drugging	RAPE Female victim	RAPE Male suspect	BUGGERY Female victim	BUGGERY Male victim	BUGGERY Male suspect	PACE Notes
Clothing/paper	Clothing & sheet of paper		✓	✓		◆	◆		✓	✓	✓	✓	✓	Authority of the Custody Officer needed to remove clothing.
Intimate	Urine (Preserved)		◆	◆	◆	◆	◆	◆	◆	◆	◆	◆	◆	Written Consent.
	Blood (Preserved) For alcohol/drug/solvent abuse		◆	◆	✓	◆		✓	◆	◆	◆	◆	◆	Written consent of victim needed.
	Penile swab			◆						✓		✓	✓	To be taken by a Doctor ONLY.
	Anal swab	External		◆							✓	✓	✓	
		Internal		◆							✓	✓	✓	
	Vaginal swab	External		◆					✓		✓			
		Low internal		◆					✓		✓			DETAINED/CHARGED PERSON
		or High internal		◆					✓		✓			Authority of Superintendent or
	Cervical	if 2+ days after offence		◆					◆		◆			higher rank needed for ALL intimate
	Pubic hair	Combings (Comb to be submitted with combings)		◆					✓	✓	✓	✓	✓	samples.
		Cut		◆					◆	◆	◆	◆	◆	
Non-Intimate	Fragments	Paint, glass, etc. from wounds	◆	◆		✓								
	Nose swabs	for firearms residues		◆		◆								
	Mouth rinse			◆									◆	WRITTEN CONSENT NEEDED FOR:
	Buccal scrape	For DNA for reference - not for NDNAD*	✓	✓		◆	◆		✓	✓	✓	✓	✓	Samples to be taken from:
		Not for DNA		◆					✓		✓	✓	◆	VICTIMS - Doctor only
	Mouth swab			◆		◆								
	Skin/hair samples	For firearms residues		◆										NO WRITTEN CONSENT NEEDED
	Head hair combings	(Comb to be submitted with combings)		◆					◆		◆	◆	◆	FOR:
		For alien hair	◆	◆		◆	◆		◆		◆	◆	◆	CHARGED/REPORTED/CONVICTED/
		For paint, glass etc.		◆		◆	◆		◆		◆	◆	◆	DETAINED PERSON
		For fibres	◆	◆		◆	◆		◆	◆	◆	◆	◆	
	Head hair - reference	Cut	◆	◆		◆	◆							Police Officer ONLY to take samples.
	Fingernail samples			◆					◆	◆	◆	◆	◆	Authority of Superintendent or higher
	Body fluid traces on skin		◆	◆				◆	◆	◆	◆	◆	◆	rank needed where suspect has
	Cosmetic traces on skin			◆										not been charged, reported or
	Medical Examination Form			◆					✓	✓	✓	✓	✓	convicted of recordable offence.

Notes:

✓ Essential samples – always take.

◆ These samples may be required – consider taking.

* (NB samples for the NDNAD will automatically be taken from arrestees).

Source: This table is based on a table taken from *The Scenes of Crime Handbook* [3] and is reproduced by kind permission of the Forensic Science Service Ltd.

Alcohol and drugs

Blood for alcohol

Blood for alcohol should be stored in vials containing fluoride/oxalate *at the concentration specified for blood alcohol analysis.* Vials supplied for specimens of blood taken under the Road Traffic Act (RTA) are suitable for this purpose. 'Hospital' fluoride/oxalate containers may not contain preservative at the preferred concentration of not less than 1.5% sodium fluoride.

Blood for drugs

A sample preferably not less than 10 ml should be taken. If there is no requirement for alcohol, a 10-ml sample taken into a vial containing an anticoagulant, should be sufficient for most purposes. Where there may also be a requirement for alcohol as well as drugs a RTA vial should also be used. No more than 4 ml of blood should be added to the standard RTA vial. The remaining blood can be placed in a larger vial containing a suitable anticoagulant.

Urine for alcohol and drugs

Urine, preferably not less than 20 ml, should be placed in vials containing preservatives at the concentration specified for urine alcohol analysis. Containers as supplied for specimens of urine taken under the RTA are suitable for this purpose.

Miscellaneous

Mouth rinse

The mouth of a victim of oral sex should be rinsed with sterile water and the washings retained in a suitable sterile plastic container. The sample should be frozen as soon as possible following the examination. Where oral sex is suspected, mouth swabs should be taken before taking a mouth rinse sample.

Head hair

The primary purpose of a hair sample is to provide a reference for microscopical comparison against hairs recovered during the course of laboratory examination. As the characteristics of a person's hair may vary along the length, complete hairs are required. The sample should consist of a minimum of 10–20 hairs which should be cut next to the scalp. The hairs should be representative of the subject and may need to be taken from more than one point on the head. Prior to the taking of reference samples, the advisability of taking hair combings and/or hair tapings for foreign material such as glass and fibres should be considered. Recent history of drug taking can also be determined from the analysis of hair and if this is likely to be a requirement an additional hair sample should be taken for this purpose.

Pubic hair

A minimum of 10–20 hairs is required, cut close to the skin. Any matted pubic hair should be cut off and packaged as a separate sample. Prior to taking reference samples the advisability of taking hair combings and tapings for alien hairs and fibres should be considered.

Fingernail samples

When the intended laboratory examination is to examine for traces of blood, nail clippings should be taken in preference to nail scrapings. This is because the patient's own DNA from material sloughed off by scraping may swamp any DNA from a foreign source. Clippings/scrapings from each hand should be packaged separately.

Clothing

Dry clothing should be packaged in paper bags or sacks. Paper sacks with polythene inserts may be available and these offer the dual benefit of a container from which any residual moisture can escape, combined with a means of viewing the article without opening the bag. If clothing is wet it should be packaged in polythene bags. Items which are to be examined for solvents or accelerants should be sealed in nylon bags.

Other items

Sharp items such as knives, pieces of glass or syringes should be packaged in rigid containers to prevent injury to anyone handling the package. Special tamper-evident bags may be available for packaging controlled drugs.

Labelling

All samples taken by the doctor must be labelled and sealed in a particular and precise way, otherwise difficulties arise at court about the origins of samples produced. With items such as containers, tubes and swabs, it is good practice to use an adhesive label in addition to the police CJA (Criminal Justice Act 1967) exhibit label as this label may become detached from the container. Do not use fountain pens or other types of pen where the ink may run should the label become damp.

Each label should bear the following:

Name of patient

Date, time and place taken

Type of sample

Person taking sample

Other details required on the CJA label

The CJA exhibit labels should also bear a reference number which is usually formed from the initials of the person taking the sample, followed by a serial number. For example, the first samples taken by Dr ABC would be ABC/1 the second ABC/2, and so on. Where multiple samples, such as swabs, are taken from the same location, the order in which the samples were taken should be indicated, e.g. ABC/1**A**, ABC/1**B** etc. If more than one person is examined in a particular enquiry, then item numbers should continue in series. No two samples in an enquiry should bear the same number, even if taken from different people on different days.

Exhibits are described as productions in Scotland. The police officer who corroborates the evidence of the doctor who takes the samples is responsible for completing labels and assigning numbers to them. You must sign the label in the appropriate space. Initial containers with their own labels, adding the date and time.

Sealing

Sealing packages and containers safeguards the integrity of evidence by preventing any material from escaping or entering. The presence of a seal also serves to indicate if there has been any attempt to open the container.

When sealing bags, turn over the top 3 cm or so, then turn the flap created over again, securing it with adhesive tape long enough to fasten the ends on the reverse of the bag and seal any gaps at the edges. Any seams in paper bags should also be taped to preclude the possibility of material entering or leaving the bag through a faulty seam. All seals should be 'signed across' so that any subsequent tampering will be evident.

Swabs and blood samples should be placed in polythene bags sealed in the fashion described above. Where samples are to be stored frozen or refrigerated, the use of special freezer tape is advised. If special 'tamper-evident' bags are available these should be used. Specimens of blood and urine taken under the RTA have special arrangements covering the security of the samples that must be complied with fully.

Forensic science in the UK

England and Wales

The provision of forensic science in England and Wales underwent considerable change in the 1990s. Prior to 1991 the Forensic Science Service (FSS) was funded centrally as part of the Home Office. In 1991 the FSS was established as an executive agency of the Home Office and required to recover its full economic costs through direct charging.

The introduction of direct charging led to the creation of a market place for forensic science where the police as customers were free to choose how to make the most cost-effective use of forensic science. At the same time the FSS gained the freedom to offer its services to a wider customer base. An expanded FSS was formed in April 1996 following the merger of the Metropolitan Police Laboratory with the original FSS laboratories creating a national service covering the whole of England and Wales. At the end of 2005 the FSS became a Government Company, thereby establishing it as a commercial enterprise.

The creation of a forensic market place has seen the entry of other general providers, such as LGC Forensics, Key Forensic Services and Scientifics. In addition there are also specialist providers, such as Orchid Cellmark specializing in DNA analysis, Document Evidence Ltd specializing in questioned documents and handwriting analysis, and a number of companies that specialize in computer forensics and the recovery of evidence from mobile telephony. There are also several companies that concentrate on providing expertise to the defence.

In July 2007, the Government announced arrangements for the establishment of the Office of the Forensic Science Regulator under the Home Office. The role of the Regulator will be to advise the Government and the Criminal Justice System (CJS) on quality standards in the provision of forensic science. This will involve identifying the requirement for new or improved quality standards; leading on the development of new standards where necessary; providing advice and guidance so that providers will be able to demonstrate compliance with common standards, for example, in procurement and in courts; ensuring that satisfactory arrangements exist to provide assurance and monitoring of the standards and reporting on quality standards generally. The Regulator will be supported by a Forensic Science Advisory Council whose members will be drawn from key stakeholders, expert bodies and others with a particular interest in the provision of forensic science to the CJS.

Northern Ireland and Scotland

In Northern Ireland, 'Forensic Science Northern Ireland' operates as an executive agency of the Northern Ireland Office and is funded through direct charging, its principal customer being the Police Service of Northern Ireland.

In Scotland, forensic science, crime scene examination and fingerprints now come under the direction of the Scottish Police Services Authority (SPSA), a non-departmental public body established in April 2007, providing an integrated crime scene examination and forensic science service that is unique in the UK. There are forensic science laboratories in Glasgow, Edinburgh, Dundee and Aberdeen. All four laboratories are able to provide general forensic science provision with certain specialist services being provided by one laboratory on behalf of the service as a whole. For example, the processing of 'CJ samples' for entry onto the NDNAD is carried out by the Dundee laboratory and the Glasgow laboratory provides a firearms examination service for all Scotland. The Scottish forensic science services are funded through the transfer of funds from the eight Scottish police forces to the SPSA on the basis of an agreed level of usage.

REFERENCES

1. Roberston B, Vignaux G (1995) *Interpreting Evidence – Evaluating Forensic Science in the Courtroom.* Chichester: John Wiley & Sons.
2. Cook R, Evett I, Jackson G, Jones P, Lambert J (1998) A model for case assessment and interpretation. *Science & Justice* **38**(3): 151–6
3. *The Scenes of Crime Handbook* (2003) Version 4. Chorley: Forensic Science Service.

17

Forensic dentistry

Judith A. Hinchliffe

Introduction

Forensic dentistry (forensic odontology) can be regarded as a marriage between the dental and legal professions – the correct management, interpretation, evaluation and presentation of dental evidence for criminal or civil legal proceedings.

Disasters, whether man-made or natural continue to claim lives, acts of terrorism are an ever-increasing threat, and human aggression and abuse persist worldwide.

The last decade has seen much progress in the world of forensic dentistry. The discipline has striven to become more scientific, evidence based, standardized and accountable so that from call out to court the evidence is as reliable as possible. All those involved in the subject should be appropriately qualified, build up personal experience of the field, adhere to a professional code of conduct and be responsible for their continuing professional development. As in all the different forensic disciplines, the goal is to produce carefully considered conclusions free from personal bias – miscarriage of justice and incarceration of an innocent person (or release of the guilty) may be the result of getting it wrong. The responsibility of the forensic expert is great indeed.

Major uses of forensic dentistry

Most frequently the forensic dentist is involved with:
- Identification of the deceased, both individual and in mass disaster.
- Age estimation of both the living and deceased.
- Bite mark analysis, to include cases of homicide, sexual assault, fights and abuse issues.
- Fragment comparisons.
- Archaeological discoveries.
- Cold cases.

The forensic dentist and forensic physician are most likely to work together when biting injuries are present or abuse is suspected, but a general understanding of the role of the forensic dentist can only assist in creating better understanding and teamwork between the forensic disciplines.

Bite marks

Bite marks are complex and challenging injuries that require the skills of an experienced forensic dentist. Biting injuries may establish a link between the bitten person and the potential biter – teeth can be used as weapons of offence and defence and provide both physical and biological evidence.

Two of the most concise definitions for biting injuries are:

- A bite mark is a patterned injury caused by teeth and may include injury from other mouth parts.
- A representative pattern left in an object or tissue by the dental structures of an animal or human.

Based on studies of the dentition in large populations, it is believed that the size, shape and pattern of the biting surfaces of the upper and lower front teeth within the dental arches are specific to the individual. It is, therefore, possible to produce an identifiable pattern that may be reproduced in/on a bitten surface/object. How well this detail is recorded in the bite pattern on the skin (or other medium) varies between cases: the more detail present, the likelier it is that comparisons can be made between the bite mark and the dentition of the biter, and the evidentiary value of the bite mark increases. Where there is sufficient detail it may be possible to identify the biter, or, of equal importance, exclude suspects who have not caused the bite mark. However, there is incomplete understanding of the behaviour of skin during the dynamic biting process – more research is needed.

Human bite marks can be found on the skin of the deceased or living, adult or child, victim or suspect. Inanimate objects can also yield bite marks, for example foodstuffs, styrofoam cups, cannabis resin. Human bites are often associated with violent crime: homicide, sexual assaults, abuse, domestic and other fights. We must also beware the self-inflicted bite and the so called amorous or 'love' bite (Fig. 17.1).

The forensic dentist may also be called upon to distinguish an animal bite from those caused by the human dentition.

Medical personnel will most likely become involved with biting injuries to human skin and often be the first to examine the injury or injuries. It is, therefore, of the utmost importance that the responder has some knowledge about the examination, documentation, collection and preservation of bite mark evidence. Delays in recording the evidence may cause valuable information to be

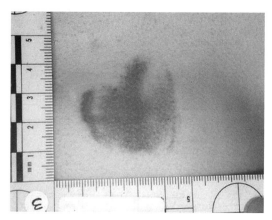

Fig. 17.1 Biting injury or 'love bite'? American Board of Forensic Odontology (ABFO) No. 2 scales in place. A colour version of this figure can be found on the book website at www.cambridge.org/9780521705684.

diminished or lost, especially in the living victim (but also in the deceased). If in doubt ASK and DISCUSS with a forensic dentist.

Considerations

- Is it a bite mark?
- Is it human?
- Are there features in the bite mark that can be compared to the dentition (teeth) of a potential biter?

Early involvement of the forensic dentist will assist in answering the above questions and estimate the potential forensic significance of a confirmed bite mark. Discussion with investigating officers will determine the course of action and how much time, effort and financial commitment will be made available for the case.

Sites bitten

Human bite marks have been recorded on almost all anatomical parts of the body, making a thorough examination absolutely essential. It has been noted that the location varies depending on the type of crime, sex and age of the bitten person.

Studies show that females are bitten more often than males: frequent sites are the breast, arms and legs during sexual attacks. Males are commonly bitten on the arms, shoulders and back [1]. When the victim is attempting defence actions, the hands and arms are commonly the sites of bites.

In an informal survey conducted by the author in the UK, there was agreement with the above results but also a high number of biting injuries were recorded on the face and general head and neck area of both children and adults. Thorough examination is necessary to reveal any/all potential biting injuries.

Recognition of bite marks

Bite marks may present as diffuse or specific bruising, abrasions or lacerations through to complete avulsion of tissue – often a combination of the above. They usually comprise two opposing (facing) U-shaped arches that may be separated by open spaces, or as a ring of marks. The overall diameter of the injury typically ranges from 25 to 40 mm [2]. The arches may comprise individual bruises, abrasions or lacerations that reflect the size, shape and arrangement of the various characteristics of the contacting surfaces of the human dentition. Central bruising is often present and is caused by compression (positive pressure) of the soft tissues between the teeth, or by suction and tongue thrusting (negative pressure). Additional detail may be caused by the palatal/lingual surfaces of teeth imprinting the soft tissues.

Marks from several of the upper front teeth and lower front teeth are sometimes found in the bite mark, but variations can and do occur – sometimes premolars and molars are involved. There may be a partial bite mark caused by one arch, one or a few teeth, or teeth from one side of the jaw only. The dynamic nature of the biting process means that marks made by the teeth scraping across the skin may also be present. There may be multiple bites at separate locations or they may overlap, making interpretation difficult (Fig. 17.2).

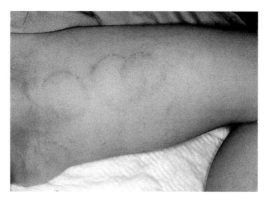

Fig. 17.2 Multiple, overlapping bite marks on the thigh. (Permission from Greater Manchester Police.) A colour version of this figure can be found on the book website at www.cambridge.org/9780521705684.

Differential diagnosis

To further complicate the investigation, other objects can leave circular or elliptical injuries that have sometimes been mistaken for bite marks and should be excluded after careful consideration. Examples are: ECG electrodes, heel marks and door knobs. Also, some conditions of the skin may mimic bite marks, for instance pityriasis rosea. Beware the medical condition that may predispose to bruising.

Collection of evidence

As soon as possible!

Early recognition and action is essential to maximize the dental evidence – healing may occur and the marks may quickly fade or change (in both the living and the dead). Even if the bite mark has little evidential value it is best to record all evidence under the assumption that there may not be another opportunity to record the injury.

From the victim

Evidence collected from the victim does not usually involve informed consent – but it is prudent to explain your intentions and record consent, just in case.

Investigating officers and attending physicians will record a thorough history. The physical appearance of the injury should also be carefully documented, for example: colour, size, shape, location/orientation, type of injury (bruising, abrasion, etc.). Is it on a curved surface of the skin? Can two distinct arches be seen? Body diagrams are useful, but photographic images are necessary to facilitate measured comparisons with the teeth of a potential biter and full analysis. Photographs are also invaluable when evidence is of a perishable and transient nature.

In biting incidents it is important to consider whether clothing was worn when bitten as this may be a useful salivary DNA source, or there may be tears and holes that support the biting theory.

Photography

Photographs should be taken by someone with experience and skills in this field. The forensic physician should be sufficiently aware of the techniques used that, in the absence of the forensic dentist, he can discuss what is required with a photographer, so ensuring that photographic evidence is recorded and not lost. If in doubt, contact the forensic dentist for advice and instruction – do not risk losing the best evidence. The injury may change dramatically over a period of hours/days – it may give more clarity on day one or a few days later or fade and disappear. Repeat photography may be necessary to capture the image with most detail – every 24 hours for three to five days has been shown to be effective.

Photography should be undertaken *before* any other procedures so that evidence is not changed or affected by them. The only reason to vary this (and take swabs first) is when there might be considerable delay in getting photographs taken. If the area is soiled, photographs should still be taken before the site is cleaned and then re-photographed. Labels should be included to

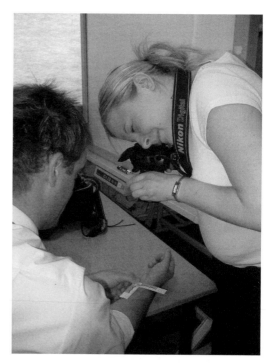

Fig. 17.3 Bite Mark Photography Workshop – getting the correct camera position. (Permission from Greater Manchester Police.) A colour version of this figure can be found on the book website at www.cambridge.org/9780521705684.

indicate the date and time, case number, photographer's initials and number of the bite if there is more than one.

Take photographs to help locate anatomically and orientate the bite(s). A living victim may be able to pose so that the bite is in its original position, minimizing distortion as it is photographed. Close-up views without a reference scale ensure that nothing is hidden beneath the scale. Close-up views with reference scales in the same plane as the bite and clearly visible in the photograph are then taken. The scales must be close to, but not obscuring any part of the bitten area. Position the camera over the bite and scales so that the long axis of the camera lens is perpendicular to the bite to reduce perspective distortion (Fig. 17.3). The ABFO No. 2 scale is recommended – it is small, L-shaped and has a circle so that distortion from incorrect camera angulation can be checked and minimized.

If the bite is on a curved surface (for example around the wrist, over a breast) it may be necessary to photograph the marks made by the dental arches separately.

When bites are on hairy areas, it may be necessary to trim the hairs with scissors – but photographs should be taken before trimming and again after trimming.

Most police forces and medical illustration departments use digital photography, but conventional film photography is still in use (in this case colour and black and white photographs should be taken).

Saliva swabs

Saliva can be deposited on the skin (and inanimate objects) through biting and sucking in sufficient quantity and quality to enable polymerase chain reaction (PCR)-based typing of DNA. This DNA

---

can then be compared with the DNA sample from any potential biter. Swab the area using the double swab technique [3].

Ensure that the area around the arch is swabbed where the lips may have contacted the skin. A DNA sample should be taken from the victim at the same time to provide a comparison sample – this could be a buccal swab or whole blood sample. Swabs should be submitted to the laboratory as soon as possible – if there is delay, paper evidence bags or boxes are recommended to allow air to circulate, and the swabs should be frozen. Correct labelling and storage of the swabs is essential. (See also Chapter 16.)

Dental impressions of the bitten site

An impression of the bitten area will record surface detail produced by the teeth: cuts, indentations and so on. This can be taken by an appropriately trained crime scene examiner or the forensic dentist. A low-viscosity impression material is used first, followed by a stiffer layer to act as a support, giving dimensional stability and reducing the risk of distortion. The impression should be marked to assist with orientation when removed from the skin, for example the letter H can be used to designate the edge facing the head and M to indicate the midline of the body. The impression is then labelled, cast and orientation markers transferred to the model.

Note: when the injury could have been self-inflicted, impressions of the dentition of the bitten person are taken to confirm or refute this.

Tissue excision

Removal of the bitten tissue for further investigation is undertaken only in certain circumstances and only on the deceased! *It is mentioned here for completeness.* Permission of the appropriate legal authority, the coroner or procurator fiscal in the UK, should always be obtained for this procedure. Skin with underlying dermis is removed and preserved

---

> **Box 17.1** Check list for the forensic physician
>
> - History.
> - Examine and describe injury – document.
> - Photograph as soon as possible – using an experienced photographer. If unsure get advice/assistance from the forensic dentist.
> - Note: if injured area dirty, photograph first, then swab, clean and re-photograph.
> - Bitten person in same position as when bitten if possible.
> - General location photographs without scales.
> - Close-up photographs without scales.
> - Close-up photographs with scales.
> - May need to photograph each arch separately.
> - Repeat photographs daily until injury disappears if necessary.
> - Remember – scale in same plane as injury, and camera lens perpendicular to injury.
> - Swab for saliva using double swab technique.
> - Ensure correct labelling, documentation, continuity of evidence.

in formalin. Transillumination of the excised tissue may allow examination of the pattern and bruising impossible to see with the tissue *in situ*. The correct anatomical shape must be maintained to prevent distortions.

Collection of evidence from the potential biter

All evidence must be collected in accordance with the legal obligations of the jurisdiction and with appropriate authority. Continuity of evidence is vital. The forensic physician may examine and take saliva swabs from a potential biter in custody. The general medical and dental history of the biter will be noted, remembering to find out whether he/she has had dental treatment since the incident. Following this, a dental examination will be undertaken by the forensic dentist.

Photographs of the full face and intra-oral photographs are taken to include the upper and lower arch biting surfaces, lateral and anterior views of the teeth. Reference scales are included to facilitate measurements of individual teeth.

Dental impressions, with a bite registration, are taken of any potential biter – once out of the mouth the impressions are rinsed in water to remove obvious saliva and debris and should be disinfected (minimizes potential pathway for cross-infection) before casting into hard dental models.

The models are labelled and stored until needed. In England, Wales and Northern Ireland a dental impression of a suspect in custody is deemed an intimate sample: in accordance with the Police and Criminal Evidence Act 1984 (PACE) it cannot be taken by force and requires authority and consent.

Foodstuffs

Objects such as apples, cheese or chocolate should be sealed in an airtight container and refrigerated (not frozen) until the forensic dentist can examine them. The bitten area will be photographed, swabbed and an impression taken. The impression

is taken last as the procedure might damage the material.

Comparisons

The pattern and characteristics of the biting edges of the teeth (individually and collectively) are compared with life-size photographs (or computer images) of the bite mark pattern using transparent overlays that have been computer generated – this has proved to be the most reliable and accurate method [4]. Despite efforts to standardize the comparison procedure and conclusions, much is still dependent on the expertise and experience of the forensic dentist.

Those at risk from human biting

Certain occupations may be at an increased risk from biting injuries, such as medical personnel and those working in the police, prison services and other institutional settings (along with victims and perpetrators of crime). It has been reported that human bites have a higher incidence of infection than bites from dogs or cats. It should also be noted that there is potential for the transmission of blood-borne diseases such as human immunodeficiency virus/acquired immune deficiency syndrome (HIV/AIDS) and hepatitis. Personnel should be aware of this risk, and protocols for prevention, treatment and management need to be in place (see Chapter 14).

Non-accidental injury (abuse)

Bites and injuries to oral structures are also related to abuse of vulnerable adults and children. Over 60% of physical injuries to children involve the head, face and mouth. Dental practitioners and their teams need to be vigilant for signs of abuse and be familiar with management and reporting procedures.

The forensic physician should be aware of potential injuries in and around the mouth (see Box 17.2).

Box 17.2 Look for:

- Injuries to the palate, floor of mouth, inner aspect of the lips and cheeks, or other soft tissues that may be caused by force feeding or insertion of other objects.
- Burns may suggest force feeding with hot or caustic substances.
- Fraenal tearing in the non-ambulatory child (in toddlers this may simply be the result of an accident whilst learning to walk).
- Signs of dental trauma, including tooth fractures, avulsed teeth, soft tissue bruising and laceration, bone fractures.
- Bite marks.
- Signs of neglect (or simply ignorance) may need addressing, for example, the need for urgent dental care (rampant decay, multiple abscesses).

Dental identification

Background

Today individuals travel widely, there are many man-made and natural disasters and a constant threat of terrorist attack, making identification complicated, international and with the potential to involve large numbers of fatalities. The forensic dentist has a major role in individual and multiple fatality identification.

For relatives, friends and colleagues of the deceased, proof of identity is necessary for many reasons: social, legal, financial and body disposal. The end of hope may be devastating, but it is believed that a positive identification allows for the grieving process and closure – getting the identification wrong causes confusion and distress. Investigations into and following the death may be instigated once a positive identification has been confirmed. These investigations rely upon thorough examinations and team work.

The teeth can survive most conditions of nature that can damage or change other body tissues: even in fires the posterior teeth (Fig. 17.4) and sometimes acrylic dentures may survive, protected by the facial and oral structures. Identification through

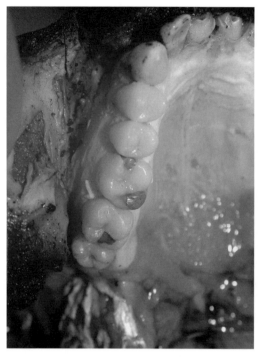

Fig. 17.4 Posterior teeth and fillings preserved in a fire victim. (Permission of South Manchester Coroner.)
A colour version of this figure can be found on the book website at www.cambridge.org/9780521705684.

visual appearance has proved to be unreliable, or unacceptable, particularly when there is severe decomposition, skeletalization, burning, drowning, mutilation and fragmentation. Personal effects may assist with identification, but dentistry, fingerprinting, medical information and DNA are the most reliable methods.

Dental identification involves the collection and interpretation of antemortem and post-mortem dental information and comparing the findings. For example, the following will be recorded:
- Dental arch shape and alignment.
- Number and position of teeth present and missing.
- Size, shape, position and material of any restorations, or presence of decayed surfaces.
- Denture and other appliance design and material.

- Individual tooth characteristics, for example: tooth wear, fractures, anomalies of size, shape and colour.
- Soft tissue (if present) status, abnormalities or pathologies.
- Any other findings of interest, or clues to age, race, diet, occupation, etc.

Antemortem and post-mortem information must match, or any discrepancies should be explainable, perhaps by the passage of time, or attendance at another dental practice or hospital. For example: if a particular tooth is absent in the post-mortem record but present in the antemortem record, it may have been extracted; however, if the tooth is absent in the antemortem record but present at the post-mortem record then an exclusion can be made.

It must be remembered that no tissue can be removed from the body for further examination/specialist tests without the permission of the relevant authority (coroner in England and Wales or procurator fiscal in Scotland).

The dental record

The antemortem dental record may include written notes, charts, radiographs, clinical photos, study models, referral letters, laboratory prescription, results of special tests and any other communications or useful bits of information. Records may be computer generated and radiographs may be film or digital. Good quality dental records are an essential part of patient care and a medico-legal requirement. However, the quality of the antemortem record varies between dentists, areas and countries. Different charting systems with different terminology used by various countries still cause delays and confusion. When dealing with large numbers of fatalities it is practical and sensible to use a standardized, international form to record antemortem and post-mortem data – the Interpol Disaster Victim Identification (DVI) form is currently widely used, and being updated at the time of writing this chapter, so that all dentists from around the world use the same 'language'. Further complications may occur because the record is:

- Inaccurate
- Incomplete
- Not transferable (in contrast to the medical record)
- Lost or damaged

Not everyone regularly attends for dental treatment and there are many persons without records. In the last decade, the dental team has focused on oral health and prevention, so there are individuals with little or no dental treatment; this may not preclude identification by dental methods, but may complicate the situation. Clearly, it is easier to confirm identity when there has been much dental intervention with multiple fillings, crown and bridgework, prostheses or implants. For example, victims of the Asian Tsunami (Boxing Day December 2004) with numerous and complex dental treatments were quickly identified and returned to their families.

Comparisons

When comparing dental antemortem and post-mortem detail there is no minimum number of concordant points, and it may be that a positive identification can be achieved from a few teeth or even a single tooth if there are sufficient unique features. The training and experience of the odontologist will enable conclusions to be made that can be justified in court. Conclusions comprise:

- Positive identification
- Probable identification
- Possible identification
- Insufficient evidence
- Exclusion

Dental profiling (reconstructive identification)

In many situations the coroner or investigating officer wants confirmation of a putative identification following the post-mortem dental examination. If there is no clue to identity or no antemortem record available at the time of examination, the forensic dentist will record all the post-mortem dental findings in case an antemortem record becomes available in the future. However, when antemortem dental records don't become available or are non-existent, the forensic dentist may help narrow the population search by contributing information on the age, sex and ancestry of the deceased. This is sometimes referred to as post-mortem dental profiling [5] and is often performed in close partnership with the forensic anthropologist. It may be possible to provide further information on behavioural habits (e.g. tooth grinding), systemic disease, occupation, smoking status and dietary habits (e.g. dental erosion may be caused by diet, eating disorders, alcohol, substance abuse or gastric disorders).

Denture marking

In some countries (not the UK at present) the marking of full dentures with an identifying number or name is mandatory. Not only is this useful for nursing homes, hospitals and other institutions, but it is yet another method that would assist in establishing identity should the wearer be involved in an accident, crime or mass disaster. The marker should ideally withstand most conditions (water, fire, etc.), be acceptable to the patient, not weaken the denture and be easy and cheap to produce. The most resilient markers are those incorporated into the denture when it is made.

Additional dental information

Where records are not available or are of poor quality, good quality, smiling photographs showing the positions and angles of the anterior teeth may play a part in dental identification. It may be necessary to use facial superimposition or to reconstruct the facial appearance and release this to the public and hope that information will be forthcoming.

Dental fragments, for example pieces of tooth or restorations found at crime scenes may link the victim or perpetrator to the scene. Other scientific resources may be necessary to recognize and differentiate tooth structure from other material, for example microscopy or scanning electron microscopy and energy dispersive X-ray spectroscopy (SEM/EDS).

Teeth and DNA

Teeth are an excellent source of DNA [6]. The PCR technique with amplification of DNA material revolutionized sample size. Mitochondrial DNA (maternally inherited) might be useful if genomic DNA cannot be analysed because it is too degraded. The forensic dentist is best qualified to assess the dental evidence and leave the rest to the forensic scientist! Despite the advances with DNA technology, there are situations when it cannot be used and dental methods still contribute hugely to the identification process, currently being faster and cheaper.

Disaster situations

Dental identification methods are fundamentally the same whether there is one fatality or many, but the problems are magnified with larger numbers, when there may be burning, fragmentation (Fig. 17.5), mutilation and commingling of remains as seen, for example, following the London and Sharm el Sheikh bombings, both incidents in July 2005.

Disasters may be closed (known information or list of those involved), open (little or no idea at first who may be involved) and mixed (combination of open and closed).

Preparation and organization of an appropriately skilled and trained DVI team (before a disaster strikes) is essential, with readiness to deploy, wherever and whenever necessary, following an assessment of the situation. All involved must be prepared to learn from the problems and any mistakes made. It must be remembered that different countries have different jurisdictions, beliefs and cultures and each situation must be handled with sensitivity. Each situation is different and has its own problems and pitfalls (see Chapter 19).

Dental teams will usually be involved with antemortem and post-mortem dental information collection, interpretation and comparisons. Ideally the

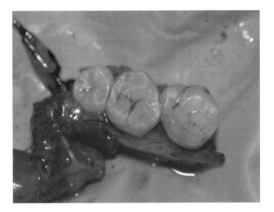

Fig. 17.5 Fragment showing maxillary teeth, following bomb attack. (Permission from Centre for International Forensic Assistance (CIFA)). A colour version of this figure can be found on the book website at www.cambridge.org/9780521705684.

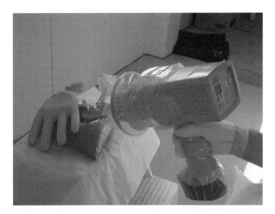

Fig. 17.6 Portable, hand-held X-ray unit in use. (Permission from CIFA.) A colour version of this figure can be found on the book website at www.cambridge.org/9780521705684.

remains will be photographed, dentally examined, radiographed and teeth may be removed for DNA analysis at a later date. Resection of the jaws (with appropriate permission) for improved access, or for further investigation, is performed *when necessary* – sensitivity is needed for different cultural and ethical issues. Body parts must be labelled, photographed and returned to the body. If the deceased is suitable for viewing, care should be taken that any dissection does not damage the features.

Computer programmes to assist with identification of large numbers of fatalities are constantly being developed and updated but it must be remembered that the final decision lies with a person! PlassData was used in the Asian Tsunami and glitches ironed out by skilled computer personnel as the identification process continued. Win ID is currently used in the USA.

The new portable, hand-held, lightweight (less than 3 kg), mains or battery-powered X-ray machines have proved to be extremely useful in the disaster situation (Fig. 17.6). These machines can be linked to digital sensors (as well as used with conventional X-ray film) and are very tolerant of hand-shake when numerous views are taken during the session! As with all radiographic procedures,

guidelines for the safety of the operator and colleagues must be followed.

Age estimation from teeth: a brief overview

Generally, neonates, children and young adults can be aged to within narrower ranges than adults by dental methods.

Age estimation may be very useful because emphasis on prevention and the use of fluorides has led to some children in the western world having little or no caries (decay) and consequently no restorations, making dental identification difficult, especially where large numbers of fatalities occur. Very few young children have had radiographs taken, unless perhaps for orthodontic assessment and treatment, in which case the records will be available. Also, the dentition of the child is continually changing with the 20 deciduous (baby) teeth being lost, and the permanent teeth erupting (Fig. 17.7) until around 12–13 years of age when all teeth except the wisdom teeth are potentially present.

The order of eruption of the teeth into the mouth may give an approximate age, but there is

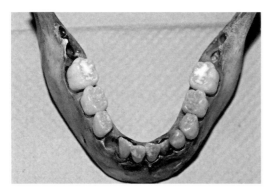

Fig. 17.7 Mixture of deciduous and permanent teeth, with eruption visible. (Permission from South Manchester Coroner.) A colour version of this figure can be found on the book website at www.cambridge.org/9780521705684.

considerable variation and it is not the most accurate method. It is, however, the least invasive technique requiring only a visual inspection and may have some use in the living child.

A more reliable method is to compare the developmental stages of the teeth with published developmental charts, requiring radiographs (and/or histology in the deceased). With these methods the conclusions are usually accurate to approximately ±1.5 years of age, and stages of development are illustrated for easy consideration in, for example charts by (1) Schour and Massler, (2) Gustafson and (3) Moorrees, Fanning and Hunt [7].

Third molar (wisdom tooth) development has been used for age estimation in middle to late teens and those in their early twenties. Most dental practitioners will be aware of the variability of development of these teeth and that not everyone has all four wisdom teeth. However, despite the limitations, it may be one of the few methods available for this age group. The question from investigating officers is usually 'has this person reached 18 years of age?' a milestone age for the courts (when dealing with crimes and illegal immigrants).

It is more difficult to age an adult accurately once third molar development is complete. Progressive changes in the teeth, such as the amount of attrition, periodontal status, root resorption, pulp size,

secondary dentine and dentine translucency, may all be used in various combinations, but require the removal and sectioning of teeth – once more not acceptable in the living subject! Laboratory facilities will be needed to detect and analyse biochemical changes in teeth reflecting the ageing process, such as amino acid racemization.

Radiographic techniques are most suited to the living person, provided that there is consent and it remains acceptable to the dental governing bodies. However, research must continue for different populations and ethnic groups because there are many variables. Because of the variables, it is good practice to use more than one method before reaching a conclusion and offering an age range.

Summary

There is a wealth of information to be gained from the teeth and dental structures for the purpose of identification and bite mark analysis. Careful examination of a scene for dental fragments and bitten objects must not be forgotten. For best results, teamwork is hugely important. Together we owe a duty of care and dignity to the injured or deceased, and to assist investigations and the justice systems with thorough and competent examination, evidence collection, interpretation and conclusions.

REFERENCES

1. Pretty IA, Sweet D (2000) Anatomical locations of bite marks and associated findings in 101 cases in the United States. *Journal of Forensic Science* **45**: 812–14.
2. Sweet D, Pretty IA (2001) A look at forensic dentistry – Part 2: teeth as weapons of violence – identification of bite mark perpetrators. *British Dental Journal* **190**(8): 415–18.
3. Sweet D, Lorente JA, Lorente M, Valenzuela A, Villaneuva E (1997) An improved method to recover saliva from human skin: the double swab technique. *Journal of Forensic Science* **42**: 320–2.
4. Sweet D, Parhar M, Wood RE (1998) Computer-based production of bitemark overlays. *Journal of Forensic Science* **43**: 1046–51.

5. Pretty IA, Sweet D (2001) A look at forensic dentistry – Part 1: The role of teeth in the determination of human identity. *British Dental Journal* **190**(7): 359–66.

6. Sweet D, Hildebrand D, Phillips D (1999) Identification of a skeleton using DNA from teeth and a PAP smear. *Journal of Forensic Science* **44**: 630–3.

7. Moorrees CFA, Fanning EA, Hunt EE (1963) Age variation of formation stages for ten permanent teeth. *Journal of Dental Research* **42**: 1490–502.

FURTHER READING

Dorion RBJ (2004) *Bitemark Evidence*. New York: Marcel Dekker.

Herschaft EE, Alder ME, Ord DK, Rawson RD, Smith ES (eds.) (2006) *Manual of Forensic Odontology*, 4th edn. New York: ASFO (American Society of Forensic Odontology) publication.

Whittaker DK, MacDonald DG (1989) *A Colour Atlas of Forensic Dentistry*. London: Wolfe Publishing.

18

Investigation of death

Peter Dean

Since the last edition of this book several significant events, notably the conviction of Dr Harold Shipman for the murder of a number of his patients and separate concerns about organ retention following inquiries into events at Alder Hey Hospital and elsewhere, have focused the attention of the general public and the legal and medical professions on the systems in place for the investigation of sudden death. Much notice was directed to the fact that Dr Shipman himself was able to certify the deaths as natural, thereby avoiding referral to and scrutiny by the coroner service. At the present time, coroners can legally respond only to referrals, and lack the legal powers to screen all deaths proactively.

Since the conviction of Dr Shipman, three separate inquiries into different aspects of the investigation and certification of sudden death have been held. Some of the resulting proposals will be looked at later but, despite the publication of a draft Coroners Bill in 2006, at the time of writing the law remains unchanged, as stated below. The coronership continues to respond to and investigate those deaths which have been referred to it for a wide variety of reasons (approaching nearly one half of all deaths in England and Wales, an increase from the previous level of just over one third), rather than screening all deaths that occur, whether in the community or in hospital, and then determining which ones should be subjected to further scrutiny.

It is clearly to the benefit of the community as a whole to investigate thoroughly any sudden, unnatural or unexplained death. A range of medical and legal factors and their implications must be considered. The first step is to determine that a death has actually occurred; this may often be very obvious indeed, but merits further discussion.

Confirmation of death

The United Kingdom, unlike some countries, does not have a legal definition of death, and the diagnosis of death is therefore entirely a matter of clinical medical judgement. Colloquially, reference is often wrongly made to 'certifying death' in these circumstances, whereas the doctor is actually confirming that death has occurred. The separate process of issuing a Medical Certificate of Cause of Death will be described later.

The point at which death can be said to have occurred may not always be immediately apparent. Numerous medical consequences flow from this, such as the implications for organ donation and transplantation, but there may also be significant legal consequences, both civil and criminal. In a multiple fatality such as an aeroplane or car crash, the sequence in which deaths have been

Clinical Forensic Medicine, third edition ed. W.D.S. McLay. Published by Cambridge University Press. © Cambridge University Press 2009.

determined to occur in a family group may have profound effects on inheritance. There has recently been debate and proposed legal reform concerning the unavailability in England and Wales of a murder charge for an assailant whose victim survives on a ventilator for more than a year and a day.

Knight [1] notes that there is wide variation in the rate at which different tissues and organs die, resulting from their range of vulnerability to oxygen deficiency. He observes that skin, bone and muscle may survive hypoxia for a long time, whereas nervous tissue is very vulnerable to it, and that the motility of white blood cells for at least six hours after cardiac arrest makes the concept of 'vital reaction' (that is, evidence of cellular activity equates with persistent life) less certain.

Clinically, the fact of death is usually confirmed after determining the absence of carotid pulse and heart and breath sounds, with additional possible signs such as segmentation changes in the retinal vessels. Care must be taken to listen to the chest for an adequate period of time, minutes rather than seconds, and to be aware of and to avoid the pitfalls presented by hypothermia, overdoses of drugs such as barbiturates, apparent drowning, cachexia and coma, and electrocution. Attempts at resuscitation should, of course, commence if there is any doubt, and in some circumstances ECG or EEG confirmation may be necessary.

Where organ donation is an option, cardiopulmonary function is maintained artificially, and the concept of brain death becomes important. Brain death should be diagnosed by a consultant (preferably the one in charge of the patient's clinical care) and confirmed by another doctor of senior level who is clinically independent of the first. This is discussed further in the relevant Code of Practice [2]. In these circumstances, the time of death is recorded as the time at which death was conclusively established, and not earlier at the time of the original injury or insult, or later at the time at which artificial support is withdrawn or the heartbeat finally ceases.

Examination of the body and estimation of time of death

Where the doctor is called to the scene of a death occurring some time previously, these questions arise:
- was the death natural or unnatural?
- if unnatural, accidental or intentional?
- if intentional, suicidal or homicidal?

The estimation of time of death is the source of a great deal of debate both in and out of court and, in common with much in the medico-legal field, is an area where extreme care must be taken not to over interpret what one sees, and not to make dogmatic, unsupportable and potentially inaccurate statements, for these may inadvertently mislead a murder investigation, or lead to a miscarriage of justice. Time of death will be considered with the examination of the body, but further and more detailed reference material on changes in the early post-mortem period is recommended in the reading list at the end of this chapter.

In keeping with basic medical principles, first take all available history, before considering any useful evidence derived from initial examination of the scene. Detailed scene examination has already been dealt with (Chapter 15) but be mindful of any local physical or environmental factors, such as the presence of fires and domestic heating, open windows or recent ambient temperatures, affecting the rate of change in the early post-mortem period. To avoid losing or disturbing evidence, any detailed examination of the body at the scene of a suspicious death, including the route by which the body is approached, should only be undertaken after discussion with the officer in charge of the investigation, and after appropriate photographic recording of the scene.

The initial flaccidity of the body after death is replaced after a very variable period by rigor mortis. This may commence in the first 2–4 hours, more noticeably in the smaller muscles such as those around the jaws and fingers, become established by 9–12 hours, and start to wear off after 24–36 hours as the muscle protein starts to break down.

Its onset is due to the failure to resynthesize adenosine triphosphate (ATP) from adenosine diphosphate as the muscle's store of glycogen reduces after death, leading to the overlapping actin and myosin fusing, with resultant muscle stiffness and loss of elasticity.

The onset is delayed while residual glycogen stores allow for the resynthesis of ATP, so it follows that this latent period will be influenced by the amount of glycogen present initially. The onset of rigor will be influenced, therefore, by the nutritional state and the amount of activity in the period preceding death, and it may develop sooner, for example, in a death following a struggle or convulsions. Its duration and subsequent reduction as muscle decomposition proceeds is dependent on temperature and will, therefore, also be very variable. The marked variability of onset and duration of rigor mortis reduce its usefulness in estimating time of death. Cadaveric spasm, an extreme variant where rigor appears instantaneously after death, is much less common and less well understood. Consideration should also be given to other effects of temperature on the tissues, such as extreme cold freezing the joints and muscles, and extreme heat causing contractures as in the pugilistic attitude sometimes seen in fire victims.

Post-mortem hypostasis or lividity results from the gravitational pooling of blood, particularly of erythrocytes, in vessels. Its onset is also very variable, and it may start to appear in the first hour after death, become more fully established over the following six to nine hours, and remain until putrefaction supervenes. It is seen in dependent areas, although there may be paler areas of sparing if pressure of the body on a firm underlying surface empties the vessels in those compressed areas. If seen in non-dependent (so inappropriate) parts of the body, it indicates that the body was moved after death. This effect, however, may not be long lasting and the old concept of hypostasis fixing in one position is no longer felt to be correct. The onset of hypostasis is too variable to be of any great use in estimating time of death, and it may be difficult to see if the person has a lot of fat or has lost a lot of blood. Take note of its colour, which may be cherry red due to carboxyhaemoglobin in carbon monoxide poisoning, pink due to undissociated oxyhaemoglobin in hypothermia, a deep red due to blood remaining fully oxygenated in cyanide poisoning and grey-brown in methaemoglobinaemia.

Temperature loss from the body after death has long formed the basis for much discussion, opinion and research when considering the time elapsed since death. The traditional concept of an estimate of time based on the body temperature declining at 0.9°C (1.5°F) per hour after death is modified because bodies cool at different rates if clothed or naked, thin or obese, indoor or outdoors (dependent on factors such as the presence or absence of wind, rain, ambient temperature or immersion). Moreover, body cooling progresses in a sigmoid rather than a linear manner. The picture is further complicated by lack of knowledge of what the body temperature was at the time of death, for example raised through illness or physical activity or reduced through hypothermia, and the presence of a plateau of a few minutes to a few hours before body cooling starts which, because of its variability, is of unknown duration in any individual case.

Should the temperature be taken at the scene or in the mortuary, by whom and from what orifice or location? The temperature of exposed skin will clearly be more susceptible to environmental factors than the rectal temperature, but if a rectal temperature is taken, photographs and relevant swabs and samples should be taken beforehand to avoid interference with potentially vital evidence. This may, therefore, be more appropriately conducted in the mortuary, but even with considerable care in controlled circumstances recording errors may still arise, for example from the thermometer or probe being inadvertently sited in a bolus of faecal material. Much experimental work has been conducted using sequential measurements in different sites, and results have been the subject of complex analyses in order to try to improve the level of accuracy.

Other research methods have looked at biochemical changes in blood, cerebrospinal fluid and ocular fluid, in particular at an approximately linear post-mortem increase in potassium in the vitreous humour, and other tissue changes, such as post-mortem muscle excitability, have been examined.

Other physical findings that have traditionally been looked for include the early colour changes in the right iliac fossa due to putrefaction, which may be present after the second day depending on temperature, and eye changes such as corneal opacity due to desiccation after approximately 12 hours, and dark marks on the sclera known as *taches noires sclérotiques*. The various forms of insect life to be found on the body after death may, if the opinion of an expert in forensic entomology is sought, give much useful information about time and season of death and whether the body has been inside or outside; in cases of suspected poisoning, toxicological examination of maggots found on a decomposing body has proved revealing.

Injury has been dealt with in Chapter 10 but clearly, subject to the constraints imposed by access to the body at the scene and consultation with the senior officer as to the extent to which the body may be touched or disturbed, examination should include assessment and recording of any injuries present, noting any features of particular forensic significance such as the presence of tentative cuts on the neck or wrists, or the presence of defence injuries. The position of clothing may be of significance, and the relationship of the body to any relevant objects in the vicinity, such as weapons, furniture if inside, and any particular items such as medication containers that may be of relevance should also be documented.

After a consideration of the body at the scene, one must consider the legal framework in which sudden, unexplained, violent or unnatural deaths are investigated, the responsibilities that these impose on the medical practitioner, the procedures for disposal of bodies and how these systems developed. In England, Wales and Northern Ireland, the coroner has the statutory duty to enquire into these deaths, and in Scotland, as will be discussed later, they are investigated by the procurator fiscal.

Historical aspects

The history and development of medical jurisprudence in general and death investigation in particular are closely linked, and the office of coroner has evolved over the eight centuries since the office was formally established in 1194, from being a medieval official concerned with protecting royal revenues to an independent judicial officer charged with the investigation of sudden, violent or unnatural death for the benefit of the community as a whole.

The early coroners performed a variety of functions and investigated any aspect of medieval life that had the potential benefit of revenue for the Crown. Suicides were investigated as the possessions of those found guilty of the crime of *felo de se* or 'self-murder' would be seized by the Crown. Suicide continued to be classed as a crime until the Suicide Act of 1961 (in common parlance people still refer to 'committing' suicide) and aiding and abetting remains one. The standard of proof required by a coroner to record a verdict of suicide remains the criminal standard of 'beyond reasonable doubt' rather than the civil standard of 'a balance of probabilities' required for most other verdicts.

The early coroners also investigated a wide variety of other features of medieval life, ranging from shipwrecks and fires to the discovery of buried treasure in the community which, as 'treasure trove', remains a statutory duty of the coroner under s30 of the Coroners Act 1988, although in modern times it is for the purpose of preserving antiquities rather than for any financial benefit to the Crown. This fact was recognized in the enactment of the Treasure Act in 1996, which has served to increase the role of the coroner here, but has also undoubtedly helped to preserve antiquities which might otherwise have been lost to the nation in an age of increased use of metal detectors and online auctions!

From the earliest days of their office, coroners were involved with the investigation of sudden death, although for very different reasons from those of today. In the years after the Norman Conquest, to deter the murder of Normans by the local population, a heavy fine was levied on any village where a dead body was discovered on the assumption that it was presumed to be Norman, unless it could be proved to be English. The fine was known as the *murdrum,* from which the word murder is derived, and the coroner's long association with sudden death began as many of the early coroners' inquests dealt with this 'Presumption of Normanry' only rebuttable by the local community, and a large fine thus avoided, by the 'Presentment of Englishry'.

In response to legal, administrative and social changes, the coroner system continued to adapt over the centuries, but in the nineteenth century major changes took place in relation to the investigation of death in the community.

Despite the fact that autopsy had been performed in Italy as early as 1286 and continued to develop there for both public health and forensic purposes, prior to 1836 no attempts had been made in this country to certify any medical cause of death. The method of recording the number of deaths also left much to be desired, and consisted of two women 'searchers' who were appointed in each parish, and who would view the dead bodies and record the numbers of deaths.

Not only was this system very inaccurate, and often caused panic in the population during times of epidemic when higher numbers of deaths were recorded than were actually occurring, but corruption also presented problems as searchers were bribed not to inspect some bodies too closely. Following a Commons Select Committee on Parochial Registration in 1833, registration of births and deaths was introduced in the first Births and Deaths Registration Act in 1836, which also imposed duties on the coroners concerning, among other things, the issue of burial orders.

In addition, concern that uncontrolled access to numerous poisons and inadequate medical investigation of the actual cause of death were leading to

many undetected homicides resulted in further changes: the Coroners Act of 1887 diminished coroners' fiscal responsibility, leaving them to become more concerned with determining the circumstances and the actual medical causes of sudden, violent and unnatural deaths.

Death certification

The statutory basis for this is contained in s22 of the Births and Deaths Registration Act 1953 which provides that 'In the case of the death of any person who has been attended during his last illness by a registered medical practitioner, that practitioner shall sign a certificate in the prescribed form stating to the best of his knowledge and belief the cause of death.'

It is essential that care is taken to ensure that the Medical Certificate of Cause of Death is completed properly and will not be rejected by the Registrar of Births and Deaths. This avoids both unnecessary distress to grieving relatives waiting in a register office trying to register a death, and subsequent anger directed at the individual doctor by those bereaved whose grief has been added to in this manner. This involves a knowledge and recognition of those deaths that must be reported to the coroner (defined below); in such a case the coroner's office should be contacted by telephone at the earliest possible opportunity for further guidance and advice.

The Registrar of Births and Deaths scrutinizes all Medical Certificates of Cause of Death, and has a statutory duty under s41(1) of the Registration of Births and Deaths Regulations 1987 to report the death to the coroner if it is one–

(a) in respect of which the deceased was not attended during his last illness by a registered medical practitioner;

(b) in respect of which the registrar
  (i) has been unable to obtain a duly completed certificate of the cause of death; or
  (ii) has received such a certificate with respect to which it appears to him, from the

particulars contained in the certificate or otherwise, that the deceased was not seen by the certifying medical practitioner either after death or within 14 days before death; or

(c) the cause of which appears to be unknown; or

(d) which the registrar has reason to believe to have been unnatural or to have been caused by violence or neglect or by abortion, or to have been attended by suspicious circumstances; or

(e) which appears to the registrar to have occurred during an operation or before recovery from the effect of an anaesthetic; or

(f) which appears to the registrar from the contents of any medical certificate of cause of death to have been due to industrial disease or industrial poisoning.

Arrangements usually exist at a local level for notifying deaths that occur within 24 hours of admission to hospital. This is not a statutory requirement, but it avoids the registrar otherwise questioning a certificate where it appears that the patient may not have been in hospital long enough to enable the cause of death to be fully established, or where it appears that the patient was not attended during the last illness by a registered medical practitioner other than treatment given in extremis by hospital staff.

Section 41(1) of the Registration of Births and Deaths Regulations defines most, but not all, of the instances when a death must be reported to the coroner. One exception that must be considered by any forensic or prison doctor is a death in custody which, rather than being notified through the registrar, will be reported directly to the coroner by the appropriate prison or police authority. Any medical practitioner must be aware, however, that since judicial review of a coronial decision in just such a case, a prisoner who dies while a patient in hospital is still considered in legal terms to be in custody whether under guard or not. Such deaths must, therefore, be reported to the coroner whether natural or not, rather than being registered in the normal manner.

In respect of deaths in custody, cases in recent years have demonstrated the increasing impact of the Human Rights Act 1998, particularly Schedule 1, Article 2 dealing with the right to life, and have emphasized the importance of a thorough investigation and inquest into any death in prison or police custody, highlighting the role of the coroner's inquest in fulfilling the obligation of the state to ensure that there has been a suitable enquiry into all such deaths. Practice here is evolving as case law in this area develops, but there have already been significant changes to the nature of the narrative verdicts that juries may consider and return in some deaths in custody, and the Middleton judgment in the House of Lords has been followed by the increased use of narrative verdicts here.

Where the death is entirely natural and does not fall into any of the categories mentioned above, however, care must be taken to ensure that the certificate is completed correctly, and the correct format employed, to ensure that the Medical Certificate of Cause of Death is acceptable to the Registrar of Births and Deaths. Advice on this was given in a letter to doctors from the Office of Population Censuses and Surveys in 1990, which reminded doctors that the certificates served both a legal and a statistical purpose, and indicated some of the common certification errors that occur.

The letter pointed out that there is no need to record the mode of dying, as this does not give any assistance in deriving mortality statistics, and stressed that it is even more important not to complete a certificate where the mode of dying, for example shock, uraemia or asphyxia, was the only entry. The need to avoid the use of abbreviations was emphasized, as these may mean different things to different doctors and can lead to inaccuracy and ambiguity, for example 'M I' which might mean mitral incompetence or myocardial infarction, or 'M S' which might mean mitral stenosis or multiple sclerosis.

If the cause of death is one often recognized as employment-related, but is known not to be in the case in question, the addition of the words 'non-industrial' on the certificate after the cause of death can avoid subsequent rejection by the registrar.

An immediately available and useful set of notes and directions is contained in books of blank Medical Certificates of Cause of Death, and compliance with these will avoid many of the common problems that arise. This will assist with the correct inclusion and positioning of any relevant antecedent diseases or conditions, and will help to ensure that part I, and where appropriate part II, are filled in correctly and in a logical sequence.

There are significant and similar numbers of failures to recognize which deaths are reportable in all grades of doctor from junior to senior [3]. Any doctor, regardless of seniority, who is uncertain about an aspect of death certification or referral is best advised to seek the guidance of the local coroner's office at the earliest opportunity to resolve the matter and to avoid consequent problems of distress to relatives (and doctors).

Problems can also arise from a doctor's well-intentioned desire to keep certain sensitive diagnoses off the Medical Certificate of Cause of Death. To withhold such information seems not to be lawful [4] as the doctor's statutory duty is to state 'to the best of his knowledge and belief the cause of death' on the certificate.

The proportion of all registered deaths in England and Wales reported to coroners has now risen to about 46%, the highest ever recorded.

Natural deaths

If further enquiry reveals that the cause was natural, a post-mortem examination is not required, the coroner will issue a Form 100A, notifying the registrar that the death was due to natural causes, and the attending doctor will then be advised to complete a Medical Certificate of the Cause of Death in the usual manner.

In many cases reported to coroners, however, a post-mortem examination is still required to ascertain the cause of death and, if this reveals that the cause of death is natural, the coroner will issue a Form 100B, to notify the registrar of the cause of death, and that the coroner will be taking no further action.

The registrar, having received either the Medical Certificate of the Cause of Death from the attending doctor or Form 100B from the coroner, is able to register the death and issue a disposal certificate to allow arrangements to be made to dispose of the body.

In 2006, post-mortem examinations were conducted on 110 200 of the 229 600 deaths reported to coroners. This proportion has declined steadily and, for the first time, in 2005 post-mortem examinations were conducted on fewer than half of all deaths reported to coroners.

Unnatural deaths and inquests

If the cause of death is found not to be natural, either from the history of the circumstances of the death or from the post-mortem examination, the coroner has a statutory duty to conduct an inquest under s8(1) of the Coroners Act 1988, which provides that:

Where a coroner is informed that a body of a person ('the deceased') is lying within his district and there is reasonable cause to suspect that the deceased–

(a) has died a violent or unnatural death;
(b) has died a sudden death of which the cause is unknown; or
(c) has died in prison, or in such a place or in such circumstances as to require an inquest under any other Act, then, whether the cause of death arose within his district or not, the coroner shall as soon as practicable hold an inquest into the death of the deceased either with or, subject to subsection (3), without a jury.

The issue of what constituted an 'unnatural death' for the purposes of an inquest was explored by the Court of Appeal in *R (Touche)* v. *Inner North London Coroner* [2001] QB 1206, CA. Here a woman had died from severe hypertension and cerebral haemorrhage following the delivery of twins by Caesarean section, and there was medical evidence that the death would probably have been avoided had her blood pressure been monitored post-operatively. The court ruled that, even if a death arose from what was essentially a recognized natural cause, it should be considered as potentially 'unnatural' for the purposes of an inquest if there was evidence that neglect could have contributed to the death.

Prior to the Coroners (Amendment) Act 1926, every inquest had to be held with a jury, but in most inquests now, the coroner sits alone. Section 8(3) of the Coroners Act 1988, however, provides that:

If it appears to a coroner, either before he proceeds to hold an inquest or in the course of an inquest begun without a jury, that there is reason to suspect–

(a) that the death occurred in prison or in such a place or in such circumstances as to require an inquest under any other Act;

(b) that the death occurred while the deceased was in police custody, or resulted from an injury caused by a police officer in the purported execution of his duty;

(c) that the death was caused by an accident, poisoning or disease notice of which is required to be given under any Act to a government department, to any inspector or other officer of a government department or to an inspector appointed under section 19 of the Health and Safety at Work etc. Act 1974; or

(d) that the death occurred in circumstances the continuance or possible recurrence of which is prejudicial to the health or safety of the public or any section of the public, he shall proceed to summon a jury in the manner required by subsection (2).

The conduct of an inquest is governed by The Coroners Rules 1984, and the function and range of an inquest, as well as the controversial subject of what used to be referred to as 'lack of care', but is now more properly considered as 'neglect', was usefully examined and reaffirmed by the Court of Appeal in *R* v. *North Humberside Coroner, ex parte Jamieson* [1994] 3 WLR 82.

Rule 36 of the Coroners Rules 1984 (Matters to be ascertained at inquest) provides that:

(1) The proceedings and evidence at inquest shall be directed solely to ascertaining the following matters, namely–

   (a) who the deceased was;

   (b) how, when and where the deceased came by his death;

   (c) the particulars for the time being required by the Registration Acts to be registered concerning the death.

(2) Neither the coroner nor the jury shall express any opinion on any other matters and Rule 42 (Verdict) provides that:

   No verdict shall be framed in such a way as to appear to determine any question of –

   (a) criminal liability on the part of a named person, or

   (b) civil liability.

An inquest is a fact-finding enquiry rather than a fault-finding trial, and the proceedings are inquisitorial rather than adversarial in nature. The Master of the Rolls, giving the judgment of the Court in *R* v. *North Humberside Coroner*, cited above, stated that it is the duty of the coroner to 'ensure that the relevant facts were fully, fairly and fearlessly investigated'.

The coroner initially examines a witness on oath, after which relevant questions may be put to the witness by any of those with a proper interest in the proceedings, either in person or by counsel or solicitor. Those who have this entitlement to examine witnesses are defined by Rule 20 of the Coroners Rules, although the coroner has discretion to include other people who do not appear to have a 'proper interest'.

Evidence given on oath before a coroner may subsequently be used in proceedings in other courts, and Rule 22 provides that:

(1) no witness at an inquest shall be obliged to answer any question tending to incriminate himself, and

(2) where it appears to the coroner that a witness has been asked such a question, the coroner shall inform the witness that he may refuse to answer.

This protection against self-incrimination applies only to criminal offences, not to possible civil or disciplinary proceedings, and it does not allow a witness to refuse to enter the witness box itself.

Of deaths reported to coroners in 2006, inquests were held on 29 300. The commonest verdicts were death by accident or misadventure, recorded in 34%, natural causes (25%), suicide (12%) and industrial disease (9%), the last representing an increase from 5% in 1984, the long latent period in the development of mesothelioma being a significant factor here.

Disposal arrangements

The Births and Deaths Registration Act 1926 prohibits disposal of a body except where there is a registrar's certificate or on the coroner's order and, as stated above, the registrar, having received either the Medical Certificate of Cause of Death from the attending doctor, or Form 100B from the coroner, is able to register the death and issue a disposal certificate to allow for arrangements to be made to dispose of the body. This disposal certificate is then delivered to the undertaker, who must notify the registrar after the burial takes place. In cases where an inquest is to be conducted, a Burial Order must be issued by the coroner to enable the burial to take place. In Scotland, the registrar's acknowledgement of registration (Form 14) is required by the cemetery or crematorium superintendent before disposal may take place.

Cremation

Strict controls exist where a cremation is requested, to prevent evidence of crime being lost, and the cremation regulations prescribe the use of particular forms, dependent upon the situation:

Form B is signed by the registered medical practitioner who issued the Medical Certificate of Cause

of Death and who must, for this purpose, have viewed the body after death.

Form C is a confirmatory certificate signed by a doctor who has been registered for at least five years, and who was not involved in the care of the patient, and who must have examined the body after death, and seen and questioned the doctor who signed Form B. The doctors should not be professional partners, or related to each other or to the deceased. Form C can now be dispensed with in hospital deaths where a post-mortem has been conducted.

Form D is issued after a post-mortem examination conducted where the medical referee of the crematorium requires further information to confirm the cause of death.

Form E is a cremation certificate issued by a coroner, and replaces Forms B and C. It can be issued whether or not the coroner has decided to hold an inquest. The Scottish equivalent issued by the procurator fiscal (Form E (1)) includes the medical cause of death. Cremation in England and Wales of persons dying abroad requires authority from the Secretary of State (or Scottish Ministers).

Form F is the authority to cremate the body from the medical referee of the crematorium.

Form G is the completion certificate from the cremation superintendent, once the cremation has taken place.

Form H is used where a body has undergone anatomical examination according to the Anatomy Act 1984.

Where a request is made to take a body out of the country for disposal abroad, whether it was originally a coroner's case or not, this can only be done with a coroner's Out of England Order. This is to ensure that a body is not lost from the jurisdiction until it is certain that there has been no foul play. The same also applies to requests for a burial at sea.

Death certification in Northern Ireland

The coroner system in Northern Ireland is similar to that operating in England and Wales, although there are certain differences. Coroners in Northern

Ireland are appointed by the Lord Chancellor, unlike those in England and Wales who are appointed by the local authority, the appointment then being subject to the approval of the Home Secretary before it can take effect. In Northern Ireland, only barristers and solicitors are eligible to become coroners, whereas in England and Wales doctors of no less than five years standing are also eligible. The Medical Certificate of Cause of Death in Northern Ireland, unlike the certificate in England and Wales, does not have a Notice to Informant; the medical practitioner in Northern Ireland is required to issue a Medical Certificate of Cause of Death if he/she has attended and treated the deceased within 28 days, rather than 14 days as in England and Wales, and is satisfied that the cause of death was natural.

The medical practitioner in Northern Ireland has a statutory duty to refer reportable deaths to the coroner, in addition to the registrar, and a statutory obligation not to issue a certificate in those cases, whereas in England and Wales the doctor who has attended the deceased in the final illness has the statutory duty to report deaths to the coroner. It is, of course, a standard and appropriate practice for doctors in England and Wales to report relevant deaths to the coroner themselves at the earliest opportunity, despite the absence of a statutory obligation to do so.

Where a death is reported in England and Wales the coroner shall (that is, must) hold an inquest if the death falls within s8(1) of the Coroners Act 1988 as discussed earlier. In Northern Ireland the relevant statute, the Coroners Act (Northern Ireland) 1959 (as amended) states that the coroner may hold an inquest, thus introducing an element of discretion.

The jurisdiction of the coroner in England and Wales arises from the presence of a body within his/her district, irrespective of where the death occurred, and therefore also covers deaths that occur abroad when the body is returned to the district. In Northern Ireland, however, the coroner only has jurisdiction if the death takes place, or the body is found, within the district.

As in England and Wales, there are rules in operation, the Coroners (Practice and Procedure) Rules (Northern Ireland) 1963 (as amended). In jury cases, coroners in England and Wales can accept a majority verdict as long as no more than two jurors disagree, whereas in Northern Ireland, only a unanimous verdict can be accepted from a jury.

Death certification in Scotland

Section 24 of the Registration of Births, Deaths and Marriages (Scotland) Act 1965 places a duty on a registered medical practitioner who has attended the deceased during the last illness to complete a Medical Certificate of Cause of Death. This certificate, like the Northern Ireland one, has no Notice to Informant. If no doctor has attended the deceased during the final illness, any other doctor who knows the cause may complete the certificate.

There is no coroner system in Scotland, where the law officer responsible for enquiring into all sudden and unexpected or unnatural deaths is the procurator fiscal, who has a statutory duty to investigate the following categories of death:
- deaths where the cause is uncertain;
- deaths from accidents caused by any vehicle, aeroplane or train;
- deaths from employment, whether from accident, industrial disease or industrial poisoning;
- deaths due to poisoning;
- deaths where suicide is a possibility;
- deaths occurring under anaesthetic;
- deaths resulting from an accident;
- deaths following an abortion or attempted abortion;
- deaths appearing to arise from neglect;
- deaths in prison or police custody;
- death of a newborn child whose body is found;
- deaths occurring not in a house, and where the deceased's residence is unknown;
- deaths caused by drowning;
- death of a child from suffocation, including overlaying;
- deaths from food poisoning or infectious disease;

- deaths from burning or scalding, fire or explosion;
- deaths of foster children;
- deaths possibly arising from defects in medicinal products;
- any other violent, suspicious, sudden or unexplained deaths.

The medical practitioner in Scotland has a duty to report deaths in these categories to the procurator fiscal, as does any citizen under a general duty, and the Registrar of Births, Deaths and Marriages has a specific statutory duty to inform the procurator fiscal of these deaths under the 1965 Act.

The jurisdiction of the procurator fiscal is coterminous with that of the civil jurisdiction of the sheriff in whose court he appears, although where the death is criminal and the body has been moved from one jurisdiction to another, the area where the crime was originally committed will determine which fiscal supervises the investigation.

The procurator fiscal's enquiries are made in private, regardless of how the death was caused, although a public enquiry may be held if the relatives persuade the fiscal of the need for this. In practice, much of the investigation will be conducted by the police. Opinion may also be sought from medical practitioners involved in the care of the deceased and from pathologists, and independent experts in technical matters, if relevant. As in criminal investigations, the fiscal prepares a precognition including any witness statements, reports and conclusions.

The fiscal has a common law power to order a post-mortem examination but, if difficulties are anticipated, may apply for a warrant in suspicious cases granting authority to two named pathologists to conduct the examination.

In non-suspicious cases, the procurator fiscal will only instruct a post-mortem examination if the circumstances justify it, and the post-mortem rate for natural deaths is significantly lower than in England and Wales. If a death is thought to be natural and the deceased's primary care physician cannot issue a certificate, a police surgeon may be asked to undertake an external examination and report the results of this to the fiscal, who may then decide to accept a certificate from the police surgeon.

If a death occurred in custody or was caused by an accident in the course of employment, the Fatal Accidents and Sudden Deaths Inquiry (Scotland) Act 1976 obliges the fiscal to hold a Fatal Accident Inquiry (FAI) in public before a sheriff. Such an inquiry may also be held in some discretionary circumstances where it appears to the Lord Advocate to be in the public interest to do so; this will include some sudden, suspicious or unexplained deaths or where there was significant public concern. The procurator fiscal, or occasionally Crown counsel, will lead the evidence, and parties may be legally represented. The purposes and procedures of FAIs are now under government review.

Proposals for reform in England and Wales

Only a brief overview of some of the proposals from the detailed inquiries set up in the wake of Dr Shipman's conviction is possible. Reading the original reports is highly recommended for those with a particular interest.

Both the Fundamental Review into Death Certification and Investigation [5] and the Third Report of The Shipman Inquiry (Death Certification and Investigation of Deaths by Coroners) [6] have recommended an increased level of medical input into the process of death investigation, coupled with organizational and structural reform to the service itself.

The Fundamental Review recommended, among other proposed changes, a statutory medical assessor in each coroner's area, who would appoint a panel of doctors to provide all community second certifications and a regional structure to the coronership.

The Third Report of The Shipman Inquiry proposed an alternative structural change, creating both judicial coroners and medical coroners for each region and a radically reformed coronership which will seek to establish the cause of all deaths, supported by trained investigators.

The Home Office itself, having received both reports, produced a Position Paper in March 2004 entitled 'Reforming the Coroner and Death Certification Service' [7], representing the Government's response to the reviews and expressing its intention to introduce a new system combining an independent check on all deaths with professional oversight of death patterns, based on one national jurisdiction for England and Wales, divided administratively into local coroner areas with one local coroner and deputies, coroner's officers with a more clearly defined and consistent investigative role, and a medical team to support each office.

The draft bill subsequently published in 2006 stated the aims of providing a better service to the bereaved, creating a national framework and leadership, yet ensuring a locally based service, and of providing more effective investigations and inquests.

The Government's proposals included the establishment of a family charter setting out what the bereaved can expect from the service, the creation of one national jurisdiction for England and Wales, divided into local coroner areas to improve consistency of service, the appointment of a Chief Coroner, the creation of a Medical Adviser to the Chief Coroner to ensure a high level of medical oversight and advice to the service, the creation of a Coronial Council, with members drawn from professional stakeholders and lay organizations, increased powers of investigation and evidence gathering, and powers to impose reporting restrictions on certain inquests.

At the time of writing the law is as stated above. No date has yet been set for the introduction of the Coroners Bill, but amendments to the draft take into account pre-legislative scrutiny by the Constitutional Affairs Select Committee, and representations from various interested parties. The same duty to investigate deaths will apply when a death occurs abroad and the body is returned to a coroner's jurisdiction, but the Chief Coroner will have an obligation to assist in obtaining evidence abroad where a coroner requests assistance; when a coroner makes a report to an organization with the power to take action to prevent deaths in the future, that organization will have a duty to respond (both reports and responses will be monitored by the Chief Coroner and summarized in the annual report to the Lord Chancellor who, in turn, lays it before Parliament); it has been confirmed that inquests into workplace deaths will still continue to be heard with a jury, but coroner's juries will now consist of between seven and nine people; the coroner will not be able to impose reporting restrictions, but the Ministry of Justice has published a discussion document (www.justice.gov.uk) intending to strengthen the editors' code of conduct relating to sensitive reporting; the revised Bill will list the decisions by coroners that can be appealed, such as a decision not to request a post-mortem or the determination at the end of an inquest; the Chief Coroner will have responsibility for ensuring appropriate arrangements are in place for providing coroners' officers with training and guidance; registered medial practitioners will have an obligation to report relevant deaths to the coroner (reform of the death certification system is also in prospect); the coroner system – but not the judicial decisions of coroners – will be inspected by HM Inspectors of Court Administration (HMICA).

REFERENCES

1. Knight B (1991) *Simpson's Forensic Medicine*, 10th ed. London: Edward Arnold.
2. Health Departments of Great Britain and Northern Ireland Working Party (1983) *Cadaveric Organs for Transplantation, A Code of Practice Including the Diagnosis of Brain Death*. Department of Health.
3. Start RD, Delargy-Aziz Y, Dorries CP, Silocks PB, Cotton DWK (1993) Clinicians and the coronial system; ability of clinicians to recognize reportable deaths. *BMJ* **306**: 1038–41.
4. Schutte PK (1991) Problems in death certification. *The Police Surgeon* **39**: 31–2.
5. *Death Certification and Investigation in England, Wales and Northern Ireland. The Report of a Fundamental*

Review 2003. Cm 5831. Available at www.archive 2. official-documents.co.uk/document/cm58/5831/ 5831 pdf

6. *The Shipman Inquiry. Third Report. Death Certification and Investigation of Deaths by Coroners.* Cm 5854. Available at www.the-shipman-inquiry.org. uk/thirdreport.asp

7. *Reforming the Coroner and Death Certification Service, a Position Paper.* Cm 6159. Available at www. archive2.official-documents.co.uk/document/cm61/ 6159/6159 pdf

FURTHER READING

Henssge C, Knight B, Krompecher T, Madea B, Nokes L (1991) *The Estimation of the Time of Death in the Early Post Mortem Period.* London: Edward Arnold.

Office of Population Censuses and Surveys (1990) *Completion of Medical Certificates of Cause of Death.* London: OCPS.

Department for Constitutional Affairs (2007) *Statistics of Deaths Reported to Coroners: England and Wales 2006.*

The Coroners Rules 1984. London: HMSO.

The notes and directions accompanying books of Medical Certificates of Cause of Death.

Matthews P (2002 and subsequent supplements) *Jervis on Coroners,* 12th edn. London: Sweet and Maxwell.

Dorries C (2004) *Coroners' Courts. A Guide to Law and Practice'* 2nd edn, Oxford: Oxford University Press.

R v. North Humberside Coroner, ex parte Jamieson [1994] 3 W L R 82, CA.

R v. Inner North London Coroner, ex parte Touche [2001] Q B 1206, CA.

R v. Her Majesty's Coroner for the Western District of Somerset ex parte Middleton, (2004) HL 10.

Births and Deaths Registration Act 1953.

Registration of Births and Deaths Regulations 1987.

The Coroners Act 1988.

The Treasure Act 1996.

Coroner Reform: The Government's Draft Bill Cm 6849 (2006).

19

Dealing with a major disaster

Anthony Busuttil

A major disaster (etymologically, an abnormal star) or an emergency may be defined as: 'any event that occurs with or without warning, and causes or threatens to cause death or injury, damage to property or to the environment and disruption of the community, and whose effects are of such a scale that they cannot be dealt with by the emergency services, the National Health Service (NHS) and the local authorities as part of their everyday activities and therefore requires the mobilization and organization of special and extra services'. This includes natural disasters – flooding, tsunami, earthquakes; terrorist activity; major public transport incidents (air, train, ships, road traffic); public services problems (gas explosion).

Incidents in the USA are classified according to three ascending levels of scale related to the responses required:

- A *Level I disaster* is one in which local emergency response personnel and organizations are able to contain and deal effectively with the disaster and its aftermath.
- A *Level II disaster* requires regional efforts and mutual aid from surrounding communities.
- A *Level III disaster* is of such a magnitude that local and regional assets are overwhelmed, requiring state wide or federal assistance.

Since the 1990s there have been multidisciplinary plans in place in the UK to deal with emergencies. Recent events like the Asian tsunami and the London bombings have necessitated continual restructuring and reorganization of the Disaster Victim Identification (DVI) response team; the Centre for International Forensic Assistance (CIFA) now works closely with the police, supplying a list of appropriately trained and skilled '-ologists'. The plans must also be updated and tested with periodic exercises to ascertain that all runs well, and to discover any problems requiring solutions before the real event. It also helps the team to become familiar with the equipment and with each other.

From the police point of view, a major incident does not require them to carry out activities which they would not deal with in their everyday work, but such tasks appear to be more complicated because of the large scale of events, the heightened interests of the community and the public media, and the necessity to bring the incident to a swift conclusion, so enabling the particular community to return to normality.

Police objectives in the aftermath of a major incident

The forensic medical examiner will be working closely with the police in such emergencies, so there should be a complete understanding of the primary objectives of police activity:

Clinical Forensic Medicine, third edition ed. W.D.S. McLay. Published by Cambridge University Press. © Cambridge University Press 2009.

1. In conjunction with the other emergency services (mainly the ambulance and fire services) the first priority is the saving of life. The task of the police is to facilitate the recovery and removal of casualties from the site of the incident, then to ensure their treatment on site and transport to hospital by those who are appropriately trained and equipped to carry out such duties. In so doing they should not put themselves and others at risk by attempting to carry out some of these tasks themselves.

2. In the disruption and disorder amounting to chaos which may be experienced by those actively involved in or affected by the incident, and inevitably also by those responding to it, the police co-ordinate the responses and activities of all the emergency services and other organizations involved in the salvage and response operations. They will strive to restore order as promptly and effectively as possible.

3. Whatever the nature of a major incident, some form of enquiry, and often more than one enquiry, must look at causation of the incident. In addition to an enquiry, a criminal trial and almost certainly civil litigation might ensue.

   In the light of this, the police regard any major incident site as a scene of crime requiring a thorough investigation (see Chapter 15). It has to be preserved as much as practicable, and to be managed in as structured a manner as other incidents of a smaller scale. Thus, the fewer people at the scene, particularly those who are not essential to the rescue efforts and to the investigation, the better. The police, together with scene of crime officers, forensic scientists and photographers, will proceed with preserving the evidence; they will also keep out those who have no business to be there.

   One of the cardinal aspects of crime scene investigation is to photograph the body in the original position in which it was found. This also holds true in a major incident; bodies should be moved only if they hamper the activities of the rescuers and their access to the living, or if they would be lost or further damaged if they are not moved, or if they are too exposed to the public gaze and the attention of the media where they are. If they must be moved, statements will be obtained in due course from those carrying out this displacement, to ensure full documentation and continuity of evidence gathering.

4. Although the police have to carry out an investigation in all instances, others will have a legitimate, and sometimes a statutory, right to proceed with their own specialized investigations. As appropriate to the incident, these include the Air Accident Investigation Branch, the Maritime Accident Investigation Branch, British Rail Inspectorate, the Board of Trade, the Department of Transport, and the Health and Safety Executive, or a combination of these. The investigation initiated by any of these bodies is independent of that carried out by the police, but the police have a duty to facilitate such additional investigations, and to co-ordinate their efforts and collaborate with these other bodies. Companies and other establishments whose premises, personnel and equipment (for example, an aircraft company) have been involved in a disaster may wish to carry out their own private investigation which would also be assisted by the police.

5. In the British Isles, the police traditionally accept the role of collating and disseminating information about casualties involved in the disaster. The casualties of a major incident are various:

   (a) The injured, who require treatment on site and, when necessary, transport for further treatment in hospital.

   (b) The deceased, who require to be identified accurately and promptly, and their remains returned to their relatives accompanied by the appropriate documentation for disposal according to their wishes. Life may be pronounced extinct on site either immediately or after triage and resuscitation; there will often be other deaths en route to hospital or in hospital after treatment. All the fatalities related to a particular incident should be dealt with by the same mortuary team.

Although it has generally been customary for a doctor to diagnose death, there are no statutory obligations requiring this and, indeed, this duty has now been devolved to paramedics and ambulance personnel. When severe mutilation or burning has taken place, even personnel who are not medically qualified may take on this role. It is prudent to have a medical practitioner subsequently confirm death, preferably with the body still *in situ*. This event must be documented fully with the name of the doctor and the timing. The time that life was formally pronounced extinct is often the time inserted in the death certificate, with the consequent influence on probate and other civil legal matters, not least if members of the same family have succumbed together (commorientes).

(c) The uninjured survivors who do not need treatment, but urgently desire to pass on messages to their relatives.

(d) Evacuees who may be shocked, have no roof over their heads and have lost property; they urgently require shelter and somewhere to rest and recuperate. A survivor reception centre will be set up by the local authority (social work and housing departments) with the co-operation of such voluntary organizations as the Red Cross, Salvation Army and Women's Royal Volunteer Service.

(e) Relatives and friends, urgently seeking accurate and full information about those who may have been involved in the incident. Difficulties of communication with those dealing with the incident will result in people taking to their cars and making a visit to the scene, adding further to the chaos.

It is salutary to remember that all the survivors, injured and uninjured, in an incident are potential witnesses whose personal details must be accurately recorded, and the information that they can supply about the incident carefully documented in statements.

In conjunction with the ambulance services and the NHS, detailed, well-rehearsed and updated plans are in existence to deal with the casualties on site and to transfer them to designated hospitals.

A *casualty bureau* established by the police receives enquiries and collects and collates information about missing persons over the telephone, by fax or as written documents (for example, primary care or hospital or dental notes). However, doctors and dentists are better equipped to interpret and transcribe the medical/dental records, yet another role for some of the police doctors. When information becomes available about those involved in the disaster, the bureau arranges for messages to be passed on through local police forces. This involves a major deployment of resources by the police and the putting into operation of sophisticated telephone call interception and diversion techniques. For disasters with large numbers of fatalities (and international involvement) it is important to standardize documentation for ease of use and understanding; at present the Interpol DVI form is widely used.

6. If there are any deaths in a disaster, the coroner (in Scotland, the procurator fiscal) must be informed at a very early stage, and instructions obtained. All police officers in such an incident have a role to play as coroner's officers or as agents of the procurator fiscal.

There is a requirement to ensure continuity of the chain of evidence and for a full investigation of each death. After being photographed and labelled on site, bodies are transferred, perhaps through an interim collection point established close to the site of the disaster, to a mortuary. The body collection point may be an open-air area, a building such as a gymnasium or swimming pool, or an inflatable tent. The labelled bodies (the label is attached to a limb) are placed into sealable body bags (also labelled) at the scene; these labels have now been largely standardized on a national level and are devised in a manner that is unique and indelible. The body bags should not be opened again for any reason until the body has reached the mortuary and the post-mortem examination commences.

If the incident has involved several deaths there may be an early requirement for a temporary mortuary plan to be set into motion – usually by the police on the instructions of the coroner or procurator fiscal, and in close collaboration with the local authority. This must be equipped, manned and fully commissioned as soon as possible, usually within 24 hours; appropriate secure and reliable communication links are established at an early stage with the casualty bureau and the coroner or procurator fiscal.

An identification commission, chaired by the coroner or procurator fiscal, carries out formal identification of the deceased, with set criteria required for such identification to be held as valid.

7. In any large or unusual incident there is potential for superimposed criminal activity such as looting. Commonly, members of the public with no direct involvement in the incident seek to observe the incident with their own eyes, and travel far and wide to do this; an even stranger phenomenon is the quest to collect souvenirs of such incidents. These activities hamper both the emergency services and the investigators.

The police will set up cordons to attempt to prevent such incidents and will be responsible for the security of the scene. Attempts will also be made at an early stage to ensure that the public are not exposed unduly to scenes of carnage and suffering; screens may have to be erected for this purpose. Roadblocks and diversions will be put in place for similar purposes.

8. There is a legitimate quest by the public media for accurate and up-to-date information about the incident and the evolution of the emergency responses to it. All such communications are channelled through a police press office staffed by trained personnel. This office will be the only source of information, ensuring that it is strictly and carefully controlled. The press have to be given appropriate facilities and kept fully briefed; they should also be able to ask questions at the regular press conferences held for them.

Planning for disasters

The effectiveness of the response to a major incident is greatly enhanced by appropriate planning, by regular training, testing and exercising and by continuous updating and modification of plans. Local authorities are obliged only by their general duty of care to formulate such plans; a failure to do so or to issue public warnings can lead to successful litigation. Following severe flooding in Cardiff in 1979 property owners were awarded substantial damages against Cardiff City Council and South Glamorgan County Council because they had issued no public warnings (www.nscwip.info/publication/interimreport/background.aspx).

Planning of this nature must ensure a carefully co-ordinated team effort, involving all those who have a legitimate and essential role to play when disaster actually strikes. This can be summarized as follows:
- Major incident declared
- Exact location and assessment of the situation
- Type of incident, e.g. explosion and fire in tall building, release of gas in underground system
- Access routes that are safe to use
- Number, type, severity of casualties
- Emergency services now present and required

Ambulance service

The ambulance service carries the principal responsibility for:
(a) Saving lives;
(b) Prompt dispatch of sufficient ambulances, medical, paramedical and other logistical support to the incident site;

(c) Overall management and safety on site of NHS staff and of resources;

(d) Setting up and management of triage and casualty clearing areas;

(e) Alerting receiving hospitals;

(f) Setting up on site effective communications systems with other medical facilities;

(g) A proper interface with the police and other emergency services, especially the fire brigade;

(h) Effective and efficient evacuation in order of priority of all casualties to the appropriate hospitals.

The forensic physician

There is a tendency for doctors to volunteer their professional services or attempt to join in the work of the emergency services, particularly in a well-publicized incident which involves numerous casualties: a doctor who has worked closely with the police will feel that his/her professional services and clinical skills could be required in a major incident to assist with the treatment of casualties on site. This inclination to help should be avoided at all costs, and only those doctors who have been specifically called out and to whom specific duties have been pre-assigned, should attend. When they so do, they should be briefed fully and in detail as to the very specific tasks which are allotted to them and they should stick strictly to these.

There are duties which forensic medical examiners can apply themselves to on site. Where the place of doctors called out specifically by the police is written into disaster plans, and rehearsed during major incident exercises, the police doctors and all other emergency services become totally familiar with these roles.

Once living casualties have been removed, and the incident site made safe, forensic physicians are eminently qualified to carry out several tasks. In liaison with the coroner or procurator fiscal and the pathologist called out to the incident (the supervising pathologist) they may visit the scene, formally pronounce life extinct and assist with placing the bodies in bags after they have been tagged and photographed *in situ*, and their exact location identified accurately on a map or by some other means. Relatives and others who wish to pay their respects are often keen to visit the exact spot where specific bodies were found.

In liaison with police, any human remains have to be identified as such, and collected. If the incident involves several fatalities and extensive mutilation, as in an aircraft crash, an early decision is taken about which body parts are to be specifically labelled, and tagged similarly to the intact bodies. All body parts have to be identified (sometimes difficult in rural areas, because of admixed animal remains) and collected not only from the aesthetic and humanitarian points of view but also because these form an important adjunct to the pathological examination. A portion of skin with a tattoo, prosthesis, a portion of a jaw, a finger or fingers might be enough to be able to state that a particular person has perished in the particular disaster. Furthermore, these fragments may contain vital evidence in terms of embedded foreign bodies that they have been in the vicinity of an explosive device.

Advice on kitting out with protective clothing the personnel concerned in body retrieval, and briefing them about health and safety matters, may often require an input from police doctors. This must be co-ordinated and integrated with the informed advice from the local environmental health department and consultants in communicable diseases.

A watchful eye is kept on all personnel for the development of features suggesting the onset of an acute post-traumatic stress reaction. All participants in the disaster need to feel cared for by those to whom they answer, and this caring attitude has to be maintained throughout the incident. This topic is explored further in Chapter 20.

Amenities for the bereaved who visit the scene or who wish to view the bodies of the deceased should be carefully attended to. As part of the mortuary plans for major incidents, appropriate facilities for the bereaved to view the body in dignified surroundings, then to recuperate and collect their thoughts should be provided. Formal visual identification is not usually resorted to, and thus the viewing of bodies can be delayed until they are in a more presentable state, and perhaps even until they have been embalmed, if the investigations are prolonged and bodies have to be repatriated. Adequate medical support to deal with acute bereavement reactions and with the stress on relatives' physical and psychological health is no less important.

As part of the response by the police and by the local authority in providing full support and care for evacuees and for the wider local community, the professional skills of police doctors may also be called upon in dealing with emergency medical problems in this displaced community.

Mortuary phase

The establishment of a temporary mortuary is likely with a significant number of fatalities. This will be in a building (for example, hanger, ice rink, warehouse) or temporary transportable units separated from the local hospital or public mortuary to ensure that their activities can proceed normally during the disaster investigation. The temporary site may require to have attached to it facilities for radiological examination of the cadavers, odontological identification, fingerprinting, the storage of specimens (toxicological, histological, DNA) removed from the deceased, and the refrigerated interim storage of the cadavers and other retrieved human remains. Space must also be provided for storing securely the personal effects of the deceased. Facilities such as washrooms and canteens for personnel working in and around the temporary mortuary are also needed.

When the body bags are eventually opened in the mortuary, standard forms (such as those produced by Interpol) are used to log all relevant information derived from the external, and if indicated, the internal examination of the bodies.

In carrying out their examinations, the pathologists value the assistance of medically qualified persons in transcribing the autopsy findings during the post-mortem examinations: it does expedite the documentation of this information and it also shields inexperienced personnel from the sights necessarily associated with the mortuary.

All the information gathered has to be written down contemporaneously; doctors are better able to cope with the swift and accurate transcription of this. It may perhaps be worth noting that tape-recording of this information is a recipe for a further disaster, given the multitude of tapes erased, lost or reused.

Identification

Definitive identification of an individual who has perished in a major disaster is ultimately the responsibility of the coroner or the procurator fiscal, who must be convinced that there is an adequate match on a number of predetermined criteria. In practice, such decisions are often taken on a committee basis by the Identification Commission, chaired by the coroner or the fiscal, on which the police and other relevant agencies involved in the investigation are represented. For example, it may be decided that identification would only be accepted if two of the following three items match: personal features, fingerprints and odontological details.

Identification is often a lengthy process of gradual elimination and exclusion. Computer programs such as CRISIS (Zeebrugge incident), HOLMES (Lockerbie air disaster) or Plassdata (Asian tsunami) may be used to assist with such investigations and are continually being developed and updated.

The main identification methods used are:

Visual: this method is rarely favoured in major incidents, and is obviously useless in the presence of mutilation, burning or fairly advanced decomposition; this method is not only inhumane, but often one fraught with potential for error. In their state of emotion and shock, bereaved relatives may find themselves coming to the wrong conclusion.

Photographs: The use of photographs from family albums, from passport and visa applications for matching purposes is to be treated with great caution, but may be helpful for screening and supplementary identification.

Personal and somatic details:

(a) General information: approximate age, ethnic features, height, weight, build, colour of hair and eyes, length of hair, balding, facial characteristics, pierced ear lobes, body hirsutism, and so on.

(b) Specific information: for example scars, tattoos, birthmarks, amputations, circumcision, old injuries.

(c) Occupational data: carbon pigmentation of the facial skin in miners, callosities on hands and feet in manual workers.

(d) Medical complaints: psoriasis, eczema.

Clothing: this is described in layers, photographed and subsequently (particularly if intact) laundered or dry-cleaned to enable its demonstration to the relatives. Patterns of suits and dresses, labels and sites of previous repair may all be useful.

Personal effects:

(a) Contents of pockets: all items in the pockets are removed, catalogued and described. Note that any documents carried by the deceased may be useful, particularly if a series of them are present bearing the same name and address.

(b) Jewellery: if firmly attached to the body (rings, earrings) may be particularly useful. These items may have to be cleaned before they are shown to the bereaved. If the body is mutilated, these items may be displaced internally into other parts of the body e.g. necklaces into the thorax.

All items retrieved are eventually returned to the bereaved.

Fingerprints (and palm prints): in the UK they can only be matched with prints retained on criminal records and perhaps on the files of the armed forces. If these become of major importance in identification, prints may be taken from personal items in the office, workplace or home for comparison purposes (this had to be done in the Piper Alpha disaster).

Fingers dehydrated after death or partially decomposed may still yield good prints if they are appropriately treated; it is often necessary to have fingerprint experts working in the temporary mortuary to prevent the necessity for removal of the fingers or the hands.

Details of the feet: footprints are kept on record by some armed forces. Chiropodists retain a vast amount of detail about feet, and their records may assist in identification.

Teeth: the work of the forensic dentist is detailed in Chapter 17.

Radiological: features may assist in ageing the individual, particularly in children. In addition, anatomical abnormalities such as a cervical rib, metallic foreign bodies (prostheses, metal sutures) may be demonstrated. The three-dimensional configuration of the frontal sinuses are unique to individuals.

If the disaster involves the possibility of an explosive device or gunshot injuries, extensive radiography is used in the attempt to identify such a device from shrapnel and other foreign material embedded in the bodies of the deceased. Personnel in the mortuary require proper protection during radiological examinations.

DNA: serological tests have been totally superseded by DNA profiling. The reader is referred to Chapter 16.

Facial reconstruction: computerized or soft tissue building-up techniques may have to be resorted to.

Table 19.1 shows the success of various methods of identification in the Lockerbie air disaster.

Table 19.1. Identification methods used in the Lockerbie investigation

Numbers of deceased identified	Method used
18	Odontology alone
78	Odontology and fingerprints
118	Odontology and methods other than fingerprinting, mainly personal effects
13	Fingerprints alone
17	Fingerprints with methods other than odontology
14	Methods other than odontology and fingerprinting

Table 19.2. The duties of responders described in the Civil Contingencies Act. Further detail of what these duties mean and how they should be performed are set out in associated regulations and guidance

	Duties
Category 1	
Emergency services – Police (including British Transport Police), Fire and Ambulance Service	Assess local risks and use this to inform emergency planning
Local authorities	Put in place emergency plans
NHS and health bodies (primary care trusts, acute trusts, foundation trusts)	Put in place business continuity management arrangements
Health Protection Agency	Put in place arrangements to make information available to the public about civil protection matters, and maintain arrangements to warn, inform and advise the public in the event of an emergency
Environment Agency	Share information with other local responders to enhance co-ordination
	Co-operate with other local responders to enhance co-ordination and efficiency
	A specific duty placed on local authorities is to provide advice and assistance to business and voluntary organizations about business continuity management
Category 2	
Utility companies – gas, electricity, water and sewerage, public communications providers (Internet, landlines and mobiles)	Share information with Category 1 responders to enhance co-ordination
Transport companies – bus and train operators	Co-operate with Category 1 responders to enhance co-ordination and efficiency
Highways Agency	
Health and Safety Executive	
Strategic Health Authorities	
Voluntary organizations	

Special instances

Some disasters will involve the spillage of chemical agents and corrosives, or irrespirable gases, or even the leakage of radioactivity. Before the retrieval of any fatalities commences, expert advice must be obtained to ensure that none of the personnel involved in their recovery is exposed to dangerous situations which can be catered for and avoided. Chapter 9 of *Emergency Planning in the NHS* deals specifically with chemical contamination incidents [1].

Operational debriefing

After the investigation of the incident has been completed, it is essential that all the relevant documents are made available for any eventual court or inquiry purposes.

Similarly the lessons learnt from each individual incident are unique and it is essential that in any final debrief after the incident, the doctors called by the police should be fully involved.

Statutory operational duties

The Civil Contingencies Act 2004 (a full copy of the Act, or a short guide, can be downloaded from www.UKresilience.gov.uk) describes the civil protection duties to be undertaken by different categories of responders, and divides responders into two categories (see Table 19.2).

REFERENCE

1. Welsh Office, Health and Social Work Department (1993) *Arrangements to Deal With Health Aspects of Chemical Contamination Incidents.* Health Services Guidelines – HSG (93)38 – Chapter 9 – Emergency Planning in the NHS. London: HMSO, pp. 32–7.

FURTHER READING

Interpol DVI Guide (1997) Available at www.interpol.int/ Public/DisasterVictim/guide.pdf

ACPO Emergency Procedures Manual (1995) London: HMSO.

Adshead G, Canterbury R, Rose S (1994) Current provision and recommendations for the management of psycho-social morbidity following disaster in England. *Criminal Behaviour & Mental Health* **4**: 181–208.

Alexander D, Wells A (1991) Reactions of police officers to body-handling after a major disaster. A before and after comparison. *British Journal of Psychiatry* **159**: 547–55.

Allen AJ (1991) *The Disasters Working Party – Planning for a Caring Response.* Department of Health, London: HMSO.

Auf der Heide E (1995) *Community Medical Disaster Planning and Evaluation Guide.* Dallas: American College of Emergency Physicians.

Auf der Heide E (1996) Disaster planning, part II: disaster problems, issues, and challenges identified in the research literature. *Emergency Medical Clinics of North America* **14**: 453–80.

Busuttil A, Green M, Jones JSP (2000) *Deaths in Major Disasters – the Pathologist's Role.* London: Royal College of Pathologists.

Clark DH (1991) Dental identification in the Piper Alpha oil rig disaster. *Journal of Forensic Odonto-Stomatology* **9**(2): 37–46.

Drabek TE, Hoetmer GJ (1991) *Emergency Management: Principles and Practice for Local Government.* Washington, DC: International City Management Association.

Home Office (1994) *Dealing with Fatalities During Disasters – Report of the National Working Party.* London: HMSO on behalf of Emergency Planning College.

Gersons B, Carlier L (1992) Post-traumatic stress disorder: the history of a recent concept. *British Journal of Psychiatry* **161**: 742–9.

Moody GH, Busuttil A (1994) Identification in the Lockerbie air disaster. *American Journal of Forensic Medicine and Pathology* **15**(1): 63–9.

Scanlon TJ (1992) *Disaster Preparedness – Some Myths and Misconceptions.* Easingwold: Home Office Emergency Planning College.

Hogan D, Burstein JL (eds.) (2002) *Disaster Medicine* Philadelphia: Lippincott Williams & Wilkins.

O'Leary M (ed.) (2004) *The First 72 Hours: A Community Approach to Disaster Preparedness* Lincoln: iUniverse Publishing. Available at www.iuniverse.com/bookstore/book_detail.asp?&isbn=0-595-31084-2.

Tierney KJ, Lindell MK, Perry RW (2001) *Facing the Unexpected: Disaster Preparedness and Response in the United States.* Washington: Joseph Henry Press. Available at www.nas.edu

20

Occupational health of police officers

W. D. S. McLay

Although, in constitutional terms, constables are independent holders of an office under the Crown, the Police (Health and Safety) Regulations 1999 conferred on them the status of employees for the purposes of health and safety legislation. The terms of the European Framework Directive for Health and Safety require police forces to compile risk assessments covering officers and civilian employees, many of whom undertake essentially operational tasks formerly done by police officers. Employers must take all reasonable steps to protect the workforce, but an onus remains on employees to take proper care of themselves and their colleagues.

Forces have introduced occupational health units with a varying remit. Despite the availability of specialist occupational health advice, forensic physicians are, in practice, often on hand to take immediate action or to provide clinical reassurance.

Fitness for the tasks set by society entails a basic level of physical health and stamina in recruits; injury and ill-health will reduce the effectiveness of serving officers, and there may come a time when capacity for continued service must be assessed. The occupational health physician's concern is to look far beyond management concepts of reducing the number and duration of sickness absences.

The operational hazards of police work [1] are diverse and unpredictable, but much has been done to improve techniques of self-protection, accompanied by the introduction of safety equipment including stab-proof vests, side-handled batons, CS spray and rigid handcuffs. Despite all of these, officers continue to be injured. The stress occasioned by involvement in violent incidents – whether as a direct victim of assault, or in policing public disorder or as a rescuer in a major incident – is not difficult to appreciate. What is often viewed less sympathetically is the distress caused by minor tragedies such as attendance at a cot death or the delivery of news about an unexpected bereavement. Procedural and organizational factors, too, arouse much unexpressed anger among the lower ranks. It is not enough to have in place a mechanism to treat post-traumatic stress in the individual officer: it is necessary to mitigate needless anxiety by paying careful attention to relationships between senior officers and their subordinates, by ensuring that operational demands are well thought out and reasonable and by improving communication between the ranks.

Conditions of service of police officers

On appointment as police officers, candidates expect to serve an ordinary working life of 30 years. They may also opt to retire after 25 years, but with entitlement to a reduced pension, on reaching the

Clinical Forensic Medicine, third edition ed. W. D. S. McLay. Published by Cambridge University Press. © Cambridge University Press 2009.

age of 50. The recruitment of older men and women, an outcome encouraged by a lengthy, controversial and only partly implemented report [2] will result in still shorter service.

Constables and sergeants reach their age limit at 55 but, subject to the chief constable's approval and the applicant's medical fitness, late entrants may continue to serve beyond this age to qualify for a full pension. Chief officers (chief constables, deputy and assistant chief constables and Metropolitan commanders) may also retire at age 55, although they are entitled to serve for another 10 years.

In response to the positive encouragement of female recruitment, the proportion of policewomen in Great Britain is about 20%, but they remain under-represented in the higher ranks. A recruit may be as young as 18½, the age at which cadets transfer to the regular force. Selection is based on standardized examinations, interviews and medical fitness.

During the first two years, service is probationary and may be terminated if the chief constable considers the individual unlikely to become an efficient officer. Such a decision is properly taken in the light of inefficiency in a professional sense, concerns about integrity and attitude or because, within that time, some medical condition debarring further service has come to light.

Conditions of work

The conventional picture of the British 'bobby' is of an officer pounding the beat, but (despite strenuous and much publicized efforts to get officers back on the streets) today's police officers spend much of their time in a car or behind a desk, where little expenditure of energy is required. When activity is called for, it is usually in sudden bursts as, for example, in a chase. It is important to encourage police officers to play games or be involved in sports from an early stage in service, and to reinforce this when they marry, a time when other interests seem more pressing: stamina and agility are assets to the operational officer.

Lifestyle can be influenced for the better. Local health education units will provide posters and other printed material for display and distribution. Commercial organizations in the food industry will help to mount exhibitions, and advise on improved canteen catering. 'Sponsored slims' for a good cause are surprisingly popular (the British Heart Foundation is a suitable source of publicity material (see www.bhf.org.uk/publications.aspx)). The statutory prohibition of smoking in workplaces has not lessened the need to discourage the habit.

Unpleasant conditions cannot be separated from police work! Officers are deployed to cover both sociable and unsociable hours, so must work shifts, in all weathers, learning from their first hours on the beat to cope with the wicked, the pathetic, the dying and the bereaved, the frightened victim of rape and the indignant householder who knows his/her stolen property is unlikely to be recovered. Accidents occur when roads are wet and busy; crime is not confined to daylight hours. The police officer is at the beck and call of society, yet his/her work is ever more minutely scrutinized. Each is personally answerable for the decisions taken in trying circumstances; this responsibility adds a great deal of stress to the officer's working day.

Shifts by themselves disrupt the normal pattern of anyone's life, and the need to ensure proper coverage by rotating the shifts exacerbates the disruption. No system has been devised which does not to some extent impair effective working, but different forces use different patterns and methods; any rotation not based on a forward change from early to late to night is working against the physiological clock. Impaired judgement [3] and driving performance [4] are well documented.

Recruits

Equal opportunities policies present problems in measuring physical fitness, for any standards adopted cannot apply equally to males and females. The policy to be adopted under the Disability Discrimination Act 1995 (DDA) is laid out in Home Office circulars of 2004 to be found on the knowledgenetwork.gov.uk/HO site. Recruits will not have to complete a pre-employment medical questionnaire (PEMQ) until they have shown their skills and abilities successfully at an assessment centre. Recruits assessed as at risk of premature ill-health retirement (whether or not the disability is covered by the DDA) are excluded from ill-health benefits under the Police Pension Scheme, but pay reduced contributions.

Although it is difficult to define the necessary physical attributes for police work, you should take care to become acquainted with work-related activities and the skills necessary to perform these. Guidance available on the website cited above is mainly negative in outlook, suggesting that some medical conditions are, or may be, incompatible with service as a police officer. You must bear in mind an individual whose service will stretch for the following 30 years; much of the officer's career may be spent on the beat, or on a variety of tasks requiring a reasonable degree of physical fitness. Only a small proportion of officers are essentially administrators, and the number of protected posts to which unfit officers can be assigned has diminished. Some recruits have the unrealistic expectation that it is feasible to opt for a particular type of police work (popular ones are the mounted or traffic branches) in which they will spend their whole service. As noted above, the recruiting net is now cast more widely to encourage older applicants.

Accidents cannot be foreseen, nor can illnesses be predicted, but these may well reduce the candidate's potential. Be reluctant to accept the overweight candidate (especially someone with an adverse family history), the even mildly hypertensive or the young person with a tachycardia who assures you he/she is normally very calm. Rejected candidates often appeal to consultant physicians; these practitioners are not good at taking stress or any other occupational factor into account, so tend to give an opinion that such an individual is fit for appointment. If a medical examination induces overreaction, what will a confrontation on the street do? It is unwise to take too prescriptive an attitude to these matters: approval for fitness for appointment is the force medical officer's prerogative, so err on the side of safety; subsequent invaliding from the force is expensive. In all of these cases, it is important not to be pushed into hasty decisions if correspondence with the applicant's primary care physician, or even referral for further investigation, will help you reach a proper conclusion.

Even less easy to quantify than physical illness are attitudinal problems or other psychological difficulties. These are more likely to be spotted by recruiting staff during extended interviews than by a doctor. Nevertheless, the line of questioning you choose may well reveal concerns which you want to discuss with police staff. In this respect, the candidate is not a patient, and must be clearly told that the history he/she gives will have a bearing on the outcome of the selection process. If it is your decision to reject, the details driving you to this conclusion are no concern of lay staff, but you may have a duty to urge the examinee to consult his/her primary care physician, and then to communicate with the doctor yourself.

Cadets, special constables and civilian employees

Standards for the first of these should be very high, because it is wrong to allow them to waste time as cadets, and wrong for the resources of the service to be wasted on training if they are doubtful candidates for the force.

Special constables have a mainly auxiliary role, but they may be faced with the same hazards as their regular colleagues. You must remember that physical or psychological incapacity on their part could easily put the regular partner at risk. The Police Federation is made responsible by the Police Act 1919 for the welfare of special constables, but the police authority is responsible for insuring them against injury. Community support officers have been introduced with the aim of providing a uniformed presence on the street, tackling in particular 'the social menace of antisocial behaviour'. These functions are performed without the powers held by police officers.

Most civilian employees (often now called support staff) are office bound, and no unusual features are of importance in considering their fitness. Nevertheless, police forces are large, complex organizations employing, for example, spray painters and garage mechanics whose sensitivity to allergenic materials could cause problems; risk assessments for these posts are also required. Scenes of crime officers and photographers, too, must be able to work in circumstances trying from both physical and psychological points of view. As a deliberate policy, very many civilians (among these are community support officers) have been recruited to perform work formerly done by police officers; some of this work must be considered operational, carrying with it the stresses implicit in such tasks.

Traffic wardens or other employees undertaking similar duties form a group of civilians who must be capable of both patrol and points duty in inclement weather as well as having the stability to cope with discourtesy and worse from the outraged motorist. They must be able to read road vehicle registration numbers at a distance, identify the colour of a car and read the small print on driving licences and insurance certificates.

Specialists

Members of an underwater search unit are subject to the Diving at Work Regulations 1997, and must be examined at intervals by doctors approved under these regulations or by an Employment Medical Adviser (Health and Safety Executive). *The Medical Examination and Assessment of Divers (MA1)* includes advice on return to diving after serious injury or illness, whether or not work related. You may access this on the Executive's website: www.hse.gov.uk/diving/ma1.pdf.

For Large Goods or Passenger Carrying Vehicle drivers, complete the official form, D4, supplied by the Driver and Vehicle Licensing Agency. Insulin-dependent diabetic police drivers must advise the Agency of their condition, and should test their blood glucose level before driving. Perhaps we should also arrange to test [5] the night vision of all our drivers, whose impairment is not revealed by standard Snellen charts. The regulations are available on the Agency website, where the *At a Glance* guide for medical practitioners, last updated in September 2007, is also to be found (www.dvla.gov.uk/medical/ataglance). The most recent edition of *Fitness to Drive* [6] was published in 2006. Both are invaluable sources for all questions you are likely to face in this area.

Some forces now use helicopters with civilian pilots (the Civil Aviation Authority is responsible for air-crew standards in the UK; the website is www.caa.co.uk). Police officer crew do not operate at heights posing great barometric hazards, but they must have good Eustachian function and hearing (again, regular screening is mandatory).

Authorized firearms officers (AFO) are required to work long and uncomfortable hours in difficult environments, but they also carry a heavy psychological burden. These officers undergo intensive physical training as well as shooting practice. In an occupational health context, it is as well to remember the need to ensure that firing ranges are adequately ventilated; permanent staff should have a periodic check on blood lead and porphyrin levels. Although instructors and trainees wear ear protectors in the range, their freedom from noise-induced hearing loss should be checked regularly by audiometry.

All these specialists are regularly exposed to incidents and unpleasant sights from which psychological distress may arise. Further reference is made to stress below.

Physical and chemical hazards

Police officers encounter many physical and chemical substances, including toxins spilled as a result of traffic or industrial accidents, carbon monoxide and other fumes produced in fires and asbestos fibres released during vandalism or demolition.

During patrol in derelict premises, or in poor lighting conditions, they meet unguarded electric cables, unsafe stairways, unexpected obstacles. They are at risk of assault in all its forms, of injury in road accidents on duty or while assisting at the scene of one. Even before any official issue, many officers equipped themselves with body armour; it has proved difficult to manufacture any material proof against both bullets and knives. There is intermittent pressure for the arming of police officers carrying out normal duties, but they do now routinely carry incapacitating sprays (CS aerosol). They may find themselves affected by the cloud of irritant material.

Motorcyclists are at risk from both road noise and the necessarily loud communication equipment in their helmets.

All operational personnel have the benefit of officer safety training designed to give officers a greater understanding of the techniques of maintaining a safe space around them by demeanour and dominance, rather than simply by threats and the use of a baton. This is backed up by improved equipment in the form of extending batons and rigid handcuffs (and expertise in their use). Such equipment has brought problems in its train, for the increased weight is uncomfortable and may exacerbate back pain; it is a serious hindrance to those in ordinary motor vehicles. From the point of view of the forensic medical examiner, the equipment has introduced new patterns of injury. Another piece of equipment, the Taser (Thomas A Swift's electronic rifle), has been introduced; it is designed to disable by sending a pulse of high voltage current along wires connected to barbed darts fired into the upper body (see also Chapter 6).

Biological hazards

Blood-borne virus diseases are discussed in Chapter 14. Occupational health staff have an important role in educating officers to treat all body fluids as hazardous, yet at the same time affirming that simple precautions are adequate, if conscientiously followed. Biting and spitting (commonly practised by drug abusers in the course of arrest, or as a means of intimidating officers and others) are, at most, an unlikely prelude to the transfer of human immunodeficiency virus (HIV). On the other hand, inoculation of a very much smaller quantity of infected material through the skin or mucous membranes could cause hepatitis.

Stress and alcohol

Pursuit of the efficient use of expensive police manpower has led to the replacement of many officers by civilians, when the duties of the post do not require the holder to exercise police powers. As a consequence few such posts are available for the unfit officer, unless on a very short-term basis. Changes in the style of policing, in public attitudes and in the investigation of complaints against the police all contribute to a rise in stress. So, too, do unexpected changes in duty hours. Careful management in this, as in other supervisory aspects, will ameliorate working conditions, reducing the resentment officers feel when they consider themselves to be treated in a cavalier manner.

Attendance at mass disasters and the use of firearms are examples already mentioned of events causing great stress to those involved. A better account of an incident by the participants is likely after an interval during which they have had time to collect their thoughts: there are sound reasons, therefore, to keep over-officious investigators at bay. The actions taken by police officers will be of interest to journalists. There is a need to protect them, and their relatives, from intrusive questioning; relatives certainly must be kept well informed about the wellbeing of the officers. Where an officer is involved in the death of a civilian, some form of public inquest will surely follow; adequate support must be provided by those not required to judge the wisdom of the officer's conduct.

Few are unscathed by major or life-threatening incidents; emotions become engaged. Immediate supervisors need training in recognition of signs of exhaustion, physical or emotional, in those on duty; they must take active steps, as far as practicable, to protect their staff. The very normality of a measure of distress is difficult for many police officers to accept, or to admit to. The concept of post-incident debriefing is now scorned [7], perhaps because it was expected to lessen the incidence of post-traumatic stress disorder (PTSD) in emergency personnel [8], and has not been shown to do so [9]. In addition, 'psychological' or 'counselling' were words often attached to the process, implying illegitimately a form of psychotherapy. In 2005 the National Institute for Health and Clinical Excellence (NICE) issued guidance on PTSD [10], emphasizing the need for practical support in the immediate aftermath of major incidents by, for instance, handing leaflets to participants! The guidance note does carry classic anecdotal accounts of the development of PTSD and describes currently favoured treatments. Post-traumatic stress disorder is accepted as a basis for both litigation and criminal injuries compensation.

Stress at work, in turn, leads to conflict at home. Domestic pressures are themselves a prime source of stress, although it is more usual to lay emphasis on that arising at work. Quite apart from the more dramatic incidents referred to above, maladroit supervision, frustration, lengthy investigation of sexual abuse cases and the delivery of death messages are all part of the relentless pressure felt by many officers. The expense to employers in ensuring that stressed workers are adequately catered for [11] is dwarfed by the claims of successful litigants.

Alcohol abuse is a widespread problem in the working population, and it seems unlikely that police officers are differently affected than others. The consequences to their own careers and to the standing of the police when drunken officers become involved with members of the public are dire. It is to be hoped that most chief officers treat alcohol abuse in their force as demanding appropriate counselling rather than as a purely disciplinary matter. Good management includes the acceptance of an alcohol policy supported also by the representative organizations. Few officers with an established, severe alcohol problem return to productive work. So often initial improvement (perhaps under the threat of disciplinary action) is not maintained.

Sick leave

Police officers are subject to the Statutory Sick Pay Scheme, as if they were normal employees. The Police Regulations 2003 provide that police officers have six months fully paid sick leave, then six months on half pay; after twelve months, no payment is made. The chief constable has personal discretion to modify the strict application of the rules, discretion likely to be exercised if the absence results from injury on duty. By the Police (Scotland) Regulations 2004, greater power over leave is retained by Scottish Ministers.

Forces should have routines for monitoring sickness absence, both to minimize it and for welfare purposes. Officers on sick leave, or with a pattern causing concern, may be referred for an opinion. To assist you in reaching a fair conclusion you should be ready to seek advice from the officer's own doctor (the response from primary care physicians to requests of this kind is patchy) or from a consultant if he attends hospital. You must comply with the provisions of the Data Protection Act 1998 and have valid registration with the Information Commissioner's Office when information is sought or provided for employment purposes. Duties under the Act are reinforced by the General Medical Council's publications *Consent: Patients and Doctors Making Decisions Together* (2008), *Confidentiality* (2004) and *Good Medical Practice* (2006) [12], all of which are circulated to registered medical practitioners in the UK.

Very occasionally, a difference of opinion arises between an officer's own doctor who considers that sick leave is justified, and the force medical officer who takes a contrary view. The police authority, within 28 days of becoming aware of such a dispute, must appoint (preferably with the agreement of the first two) a third medical practitioner to arbitrate; this opinion is binding on the authority. Your own opinion will have much greater value if you make yourself familiar with the officer's circumstances at home and at work. The www.dwp.gov.uk/medical site carries up-to-date online learning for doctors on matters related to disability and benefits.

Residential convalescent homes in the UK provide police officers with a wide range of rehabilitation to aid recovery from illness and injury. Physiotherapy is the most widely applied treatment, but the benefits of occupational therapy [13] should be better recognized.

Maternity leave

Running in parallel with the statutory maternity provisions, policewomen are entitled to a year on maternity leave (three months being paid at the ordinary rate, but nine months without pay or housing allowance where this remains applicable). Proper arrangements must be made to protect pregnant officers when they have notified their condition. A European directive lays a duty on employers to protect new and nursing mothers (in effect, they may not work in an operational role, even if they wish to).

Pensions

The 1987 Police Pension Scheme closed to new members in 2007, when the New Police Pension Scheme came into being. Officers had three months to opt whether or not to transfer on favourable terms. The new scheme altered the basis for calculation from sixtieths to seventieths of salary per year and increased the 'normal' length of service from 30 to 35 years. Guides to the scheme may be found (for England, Wales and Northern Ireland) on the police.homeoffice.gov.uk/human-resources/police-pensions site and at sppa.gov.uk/pensions_reform.police.htm (for Scotland).

Officers may themselves request pensioning because of ill-health, or this may be proposed to the police authority by the chief constable on the force medical adviser's recommendation. In terms of the regulations, you must judge the officer to be permanently disabled for the ordinary duties of a member of the force. It has already been emphasized that the scope for 'tucking away' an unfit officer has been much reduced and there may be little option but the unpalatable one of premature discharge. Each case must be looked at individually, but the factors suggested include ability to run and walk reasonable distances, and stand for reasonable periods; to exercise reasonable physical force in restraint and retention in custody; to sit for reasonable periods, to write, read, use the telephone and use (or learn to use) IT; to make decisions and report situations to others; to evaluate information and to record details; and to understand, retain and explain facts and procedures. An enhanced pension and lump sum are payable if the officer is permanently disabled for any regular employment. Entitlement to both levels of payment is reviewable by the police authority at five-year intervals. An officer receives an injury award where he/she has ceased to be a member of a police force and is permanently disabled as a result of an injury received without his/her own default in the execution of his/her duty. The award consists of a gratuity and a pension, both of which are related to the loss of earning capacity of the officer. The police authority must review the level of these awards at intervals. An appeal mechanism is in place, so you must ensure that full notes are kept and that you can justify your decision.

REFERENCES

1. Mitchell M, Cowan M, Hamilton R, Jackson J, Speed E (1998) *Facing Violence: Assessing the Training and Support Requirements of Police Constables in Scotland.* Crime and Criminal Justice Research Findings no.26. Edinburgh: the Stationery Office for the Scottish Office.

2. Sheehy P (1993) *Inquiry into Policing Responsibilities and Rewards.* CM 2280. London: HMSO.

3. Ahmed-Little Y (2007) Implications of shift work for junior doctors. *BMJ* **334**: 777–8.

4. Nabi H, Guéguen A, Chiron M, *et al.* (2006) Awareness of driving while sleepy and road traffic accidents. *BMJ* **333**: 75–7.

5. Jory W (2001) Testing night vision for driving (letter). *BMJ* **322**: 672.

6. Carter T (2006) *Fitness to Drive: A Guide for Health Professionals.* London: RSM Press for Department of Transport. ISBN 1-85315-651-5.

7. Gersons BPR, Olff M (2005) Coping with the aftermath of trauma. *BMJ* **330**: 1038–9.

8. Everly GS Jr, Boyle SH, Lating JM (1999) The effectiveness of psychological debriefing with vicarious trauma: a meta-analysis. *Stress Medicine* **15**: 229–33.

9. Raphael B, Meldrum L, McFarlane AC (1995) Does debriefing after psychological trauma work? *BMJ* 1995 **310**: 1479.

10. NICE (2005) *Clinical Guideline 26. Post-traumatic Stress Disorder (PTSD): The Management of PTSD in Adults and Children in Primary and Secondary Care.* London: Gaskell and The British Psychological Society. ISBN 1-904671-25-X.

11. McLay D, Shuttleworth C (2005) Occupational health. In: Payne-James J, Byard RW, Corey T, Henderson C, eds. *Encyclopedia of Forensic and Legal Medicine.* London: Elsevier, pp. 377–8.

12. General Medical Council booklets. *Confidentiality* (2004), *Consent: Patients and Doctors Making Decisions Together* (2008), *Good Medical Practice* (2006). London: GMC. Available at www.gmc-uk.org/publications/index.asp

13. Pratt J, McFadyen A, Hall G, Campbell M, McLay D (1997) A review of the initial outcomes of a return-to-work programme for police officers following injury or illness. *British Journal of Occupational Therapy* **60**(6): 253–8.

Index